Gynecologic Oncology Handbook

Gynecologic Oncology Handbook

An Evidence-Based Clinical Guide

Second Edition

Michelle F. Benoit, MD
Gynecologic Oncology
Seattle, Washington

M. Yvette Williams-Brown, MD, MMS
Assistant Professor of Obstetrics and Gynecology
Gynecologic Oncology
Dell Medical School
The University of Texas at Austin
Austin, Texas

Creighton L. Edwards, MD
Professor of Obstetrics and Gynecology
Division of Gynecologic Oncology
Baylor College of Medicine
Houston, Texas

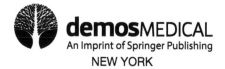

demosMEDICAL
An Imprint of Springer Publishing
NEW YORK

Visit our website at www.demosmedical.com

ISBN: 9781620701195
ebook ISBN: 9781617052965

Acquisitions Editor: David D'Addona
Compositor: diacriTech

Medicine is an ever-changing science. Research and clinical experience are continually expanding our knowledge, in particular our understanding of proper treatment and drug therapy. The authors, editors, and publisher have made every effort to ensure that all information in this book is in accordance with the state of knowledge at the time of production of the book. Nevertheless, the authors, editors, and publisher are not responsible for errors or omissions or for any consequences from application of the information in this book and make no warranty, expressed or implied, with respect to the contents of the publication. Every reader should examine carefully the package inserts accompanying each drug and should carefully check whether the dosage schedules mentioned therein or the contraindications stated by the manufacturer differ from the statements made in this book. Such examination is particularly important with drugs that are either rarely used or have been newly released on the market.

Library of Congress Cataloging-in-Publication Data

Names: Benoit, Michelle F., author. | Williams-Brown, M. Yvette (Marian Yvette), author. | Edwards, Creighton L., author.
Title: Gynecologic oncology handbook : an evidence-based clinical guide / Michelle F. Benoit, M. Yvette Williams-Brown, Creighton L. Edwards.
Description: 2nd edition. | New York : Demos Medical Publishing, [2017] | Includes bibliographical references and index.
Identifiers: LCCN 2017013585| ISBN 9781620701195 | ISBN 9781617052965 (e-book)
Subjects: | MESH: Genital Neoplasms, Female—therapy | Genital Neoplasms, Female—diagnosis | Postoperative Complications | Intraoperative Complications | Pregnancy Complications, Neoplastic | Handbooks
Classification: LCC RC280.G5 | NLM WP 39 | DDC 616.99/465—dc23 LC record available at https://lccn.loc.gov/2017013585

Printed in the United States of America by McNaughton & Gunn.
17 18 19 20 21 / 5 4 3 2 1

The second edition is dedicated to our mentor and friend,
Dr. Creighton Edwards, an outstanding clinician, educator, and role
model. He taught us to treat the whole patient, to stand up for what
is right, and gave us the resolve to always keep trying. He is our John
Wayne of medicine: he showed us that "courage is being scared to
death but saddling up anyway."
—Michelle and Yvette

Contents

List of Tables

List of Figures

Preface

This handbook is structured to provide comprehensive care for the gynecologic cancer patient. It is directed toward clinicians at all levels of training and the chapters are tiered in this fashion. Basic diagnosis, workup, staging, and treatment are outlined first. Specific surgical and adjuvant therapies are then recommended reflecting the most current standards of care. Finally, the evidence-based medicine is summarized in support of recommended treatments. Thus, the medical student can have a dedicated overview, the resident can refer to directed patient care protocols, and the fellow and practicing physician can support their clinical decisions with easily accessible literature.

The updated second edition furthers the content to include: the latest cancer-screening information, new surgical technology and platforms, novel cytotoxic chemotherapy in addition to targeted and immunotherapy treatments, vaccination information, and the most current clinical trial outcomes. The 8th Edition AJCC staging guidelines have also been incorporated, providing accurate instructions for staging to keep the reader at the forefront of medicine. With this additional information, we provide a comprehensive and contemporary reference for clinical practice.

It continues to be our honor to assemble this handbook for our friends and colleagues. We again acknowledge the dedication it has taken from the physicians, support staff, and especially our patients, to design and participate in the trials that have advanced our knowledge of these difficult gynecologic cancers. In particular, we would like to acknowledge Hong Xiu Ji, MD, PhD, and Mr. James Romnes, PA, for providing the histology images. We hope the information provided herein can continue to guide high-quality care and reflect our commitment to the subspecialty.

Michelle F. Benoit, MD
M. Yvette Williams-Brown, MD, MMS
Creighton L. Edwards, MD

CANCER SCREENING, PREVENTION, AND PREINVASIVE GYNECOLOGIC DISEASE

1

Cervical Cancer Screening

The Lower Anogenital Squamous Terminology (LAST) project has developed terminology for lower anogenital tract preinvasive disease to create a unified histopathological nomenclature with a single set of diagnostic terms. It is recommended for all human papilloma virus (HPV) associated preinvasive squamous lesions regardless of anatomic site or sex/gender and has been adopted by the World Health Organization (WHO) (1).

In March 2012, the American Society of Colposcopy and Cervical Pathology (ASCCP) and College of American Pathologists definitively changed intraepithelial neoplasia from a three tier diagnosis to a two tier diagnosis. Therefore, preinvasive pathology from the cervix, anus, vulva, and vagina is classified as cervical-squamous intraepithelial lesion (SIL), anal-SIL, vulvar-SIL, and vaginal-SIL, respectively. Intraepithelial neoplasia is further categorized as Low-Grade LSIL (-IN 1) or High-Grade HSIL (-IN 2/-IN 3).

THE HUMAN PAPILLOMA VIRUS (HPV)

HPV has been found to cause over 90% of cervical cancers. It is a double stranded, circular DNA virus. The virus is organized into three regions: the upstream regulatory regions, the early region containing genes E1–E7, and the late region containing genes L1–L2.

- The early, or E, region proteins are related to viral gene regulation and cell transformation:

    E1: ATP-dependent helicase for replication.

    E2: transcriptional regulatory activities, regulates E6/7.

    E3: ubiquitin ligases.

    E4: structural proteins, expressed in late stages. These proteins disrupt the intermediate filaments and cornified cell envelopes. They facilitate the release of assembled virions. Produces koilocytosis.

    E5: stimulates cell growth, complexes with EGFR. It is lost during cancer development.

    E6: binds to and degrades p53, preventing cell death and promoting viral replication.

    E7: binds to and inactivates tumor suppressor protein, Rb, cooperates with activated Ras; it activates cyclins E and A.

    E6 and E7: the two primary oncoproteins of HPV.

- The late, or L, proteins are necessary for the virion capsid production:

    L1: major capsid

    L2: minor capsid

- HPV infection is limited to the basal epithelial cells in the lower reproductive tract. HPV binds to alpha 6 integrin on the host cell, stimulating mitosis when normally it would go dormant. The basal cells then divide with the potential for malignant transformation.
- HPV can be detected by either viral DNA, viral RNA, or by using cellular markers. Detection of HPV DNA is either by polymerase chain reaction (PCR) or hybridization. HPV RNA detection methods look for expression of E6/E7 by detecting mRNA. Finally, viral proteins or cellular proteins such as p16 or Ki-67 can be detected by immunohistochemistry (IHC) to determine HPV infection.
- Transmission is via direct contact. The majority of sexually active persons will acquire HPV at least once in their lives. HPV has also been detected in 3% of sexually naïve persons. The use of condoms reduces the rate of HPV infection by 50%. Fomite transmission has not been definitively documented.
- Most exposures produce a transient productive viral infection. One third of women develop low-grade cytological changes. Most changes clear spontaneously within 2 years. Less than 20% of women are still HPV+ at 2 years. Long-term or persistent infections occur in fewer than 10% of women at 2 years. Rates of HPV infection differ by age: if older than 29 years, there is a 31% infection rate; if younger than 29, there is a 65% rate of infection.
- The Addressing THE Need for Advanced HPV diagnostics (ATHENA) study documented the prevalence of cervical cytologic abnormalities. The prevalence of cytologic abnormalities in 42,209 women 21 years old or older undergoing screening was 7.1%. Liquid-based cytology (LBC) and HPV testing were performed. Atypical squamous cells of undetermined significance (ASC-US) and HPV positive patients were referred for colposcopy. The prevalence of high risk (HR) HPV, HPV 16, and HPV 18 was 12.6%, 2.8%, and 1.0%, respectively. HR HPV was detected in 31% of women aged 21 to 24 years, 7.5% of women aged 40 to 44 years, and 5% of women older than 70 years (2). Currently, virus typing in cervical HSIL (-IN 2/3) patients has revealed that HPV 16 is present in 45.3%, HPV 18 is present in 6.9%, and HPV 31 is present in 8.6%.

PAP SMEARS

Papanicolaou (Pap) smears (cytology), introduced in the 1950s, have promoted a significant decrease in the rates of cervical cancer. Between 1955 and 1992, the incidence and death rates of cervical cancer in the United States decreased by more than 60% (3).

- The false-negative rate of Pap smears is between 6% and 25%. The conventional Pap smear has a sensitivity of 51% and a specificity of 98% (4). The rate of cervical cancer following a negative normal Pap test is 7.5/100,000 women/year; for all women with HPV-negative testing there are 3.8 cervical cancers/100,000 women/year. For women who are both HPV negative and Pap cytology negative the rate is 3.2 cervical cancers/100,000 women/year. Liquid based cytology (LBC) screening has been widely adopted. LBC has the same sensitivity and specificity as conventional Pap smears. The Thin Prep and Mono Prep Pap tests both use a filter for cell separation. SurePath uses density centrifugation for cell separation. LBC is neither more sensitive nor more specific than conventional cytology for detecting high-grade cervical dysplasia (5). However, there are advantages to LBC: reflex HPV testing can be performed as well as testing for other pathogens and STDs.

- The Bethesda system of **Pap smear reporting** has three basic components: descriptive interpretation, statement of adequacy, and categorization of the interpretation (optional). The adequacy communicates the quality of the specimen. There are three optional interpretive categories: within normal limits, benign cellular changes, and epithelial cell abnormality. Cytology management algorithms can be found at www.asccp.org.
  - Epithelial cell abnormalities can be divided into either squamous or glandular cell changes:
    - Squamous cell cytology abnormalities are reported as LSIL, HSIL, squamous cell carcinoma, or atypical squamous cells (ASC). ASC is divided into ASC-US (the risk of cervical HSIL (-IN 2/3) is 7%–17%) or ASC-H (the risk of cervical HSIL (-IN 2/3) is 40% and the risk of invasive cancer is 1 in 1000).
    - Glandular cell cytology abnormalities include atypical glandular cells (AGC), adenocarcinoma in situ (AIS), and adenocarcinoma. AGC is divided into AGC–not further classified, or AGC–favor neoplasia.
  - Per the ALTS trial: reviewing ASC Pap patients alone (with a median rate of ASC being 5% per lab), the rate of cervical LSIL (-IN 1) was 26.1% and the rate of cervical HSIL (-IN 2/3) was 9.2%. In the LSIL Pap arm of the ALTS trial, the rate of cervical HSIL (-IN 2/3) was 15%. HPV DNA testing identified more cases of cervical HSIL (-IN 2/3) than a single repeat Pap and referred equivalent numbers of women for colposcopy. Cost-effective modeling revealed that HPV DNA testing was cheaper than colposcopy. Thus, all three methods (immediate colposcopy, re-Pap, and HPV testing) were found to be safe and effective, but HPV testing was the preferred approach for triage (6,7).

    Based on a study using data collected from nearly 1 million women undergoing cotesting and approximately 400,000 women undergoing cytology screening alone, women with ASC-US, HPV+ have a 5-year cervical HSIL (-IN3) risk of 6.8%. Women with LSIL (without HPV results) have a 5-year cervical HSIL (-IN3) risk of 5.2%; thus, equal management was recommended for women at equal risk (8).
  - Atypical squamous cells, cannot exclude high grade squamous intra-epithelial lesion (ASC-H) is relatively proportional to HSIL. Immediate colposcopy and endocervical curettage (ECC) are recommended. If no cervical SIL (-IN 1/2/3) is found, a repeat Pap smear at 6 and 12 months, or HPV testing at 12 months, is recommended.
  - LSIL is found at a median rate of 2.6%. In the ALTS study, 83% of LSIL Pap tests were found to harbor HR HPV. Cervical HSIL (-IN 2/3) was identified in 15% to 30% of these patients. LSIL Pap smear tests should be dispositioned to colposcopy and ECC if HR HPV+ or unknown HPV status. The caveats to this are: if the patient is postmenopausal or HR HPV–. Repeat cotesting in 12 months or reflex HPV testing on recent cytology can be done for this subgroup of women.
  - HSIL is found at a median rate of 0.7%. Cervical HSIL (-IN 2/3) is found in 53% to 66% of women with HSIL. Therefore, all patients with HSIL

should receive colposcopy with ECC and directed, random, or random four quadrant biopsy, or be dispositioned to an immediate ablation or excisional procedures. If no cervical HSIL (-IN 2/3) is found on biopsy, and the exam was satisfactory with a negative ECC, ablation or excisional procedures should be considered. Colposcopy and cytology every 6 months for 1 year should be done if loop electrocautery excision procedure (LEEP) is declined or the patient is nulliparous. If repeat HSIL is found at Pap smear, LEEP should definitively be performed.

○ Abnormal glandular cells of unknown significance (AGUS) Pap smears should be managed with a colposcopy, directed or random biopsy, ECC, HPV testing, and endometrial biopsy (EMB) based on risk factors (such as age over 35 years, unopposed estrogen exposure, and/or abnormal uterine bleeding).

○ A meta-analysis of Pap smear results was performed to review progression and regression rates at 24 months after the first abnormal Pap. Progression to HSIL from ASC-US was 7.1%, and LSIL 20.8%. Progression to invasive cancer was 0.2% for ASC-US, 0.15% for LSIL, and 1.44% for HSIL. Regression to normal was 68.2% for ASC-US, 47.4% for LSIL, and 35% for HSIL (9).

HPV TESTING

HPV testing can be used as a cotest or stand-alone test in cervical cancer screening; HPV testing increases the sensitivity of detecting cervical histopathology, including adenocarcinoma (Table 1.1).

- **ATHENA study using HPV as first-line screening test**: the 3-year cumulative incidence rates (CIRs) of cervical HSIL (-IN 3+) in cytology-negative women was 0.8% (95% CI: 0.5%–1.1%), 0.3% (95% CI: 0.1%–0.7%) in HPV-negative women, and 0.3% (95% CI: 0.1%–0.6%) in cytology- and HPV-negative women. The sensitivity for cervical HSIL (-IN 3+) of cytology was 47.8% compared to 61.7% for the hybrid strategy (cytology if 25–29 years old and cotesting with cytology and HPV if >30 years old) and 76.1% for HPV as a primary test. Specificity for cervical HSIL (-IN 3+) was 97.1%, 94.6%, and 93.5%, respectively. HPV as the sole and primary screen test detects significantly more cases of cervical HSIL (-IN 3+) in women older than 25 years than either cytology or the hybrid strategy, although it requires more colposcopies (11).

- **Guidance for use of primary HR HPV testing for cervical cancer screening:** primary HR HPV screening is at least as effective as cytology. A negative HR HPV test provides greater reassurance of no histologic cervical HSIL (-IN 2/3), than negative cytology. Because of equivalent or superior effectiveness, primary HR HPV screening can be considered as an alternative to current cytology-based cervical cancer screening methods. Cytology alone and cotesting remain the screening options specifically recommended in major guidelines. Based on limited data, triage of HR HPV-positive women using a combination of genotyping for HPV 16 and 18 and reflex cytology for women positive for the other 12 HR HPV genotypes is a reasonable approach for managing HR HPV-positive women. Rescreening after a negative primary HR HPV screen should occur no sooner than every 3 years. Primary HR HPV screening should not be initiated prior to age 25 (12).

Table 1.1 HPV-Based Cervical Cancer Screening Tests*

Marker	Test name	Manufacturer	Target molecule	Target HPV genotypes	HPV genotyping	Technology
HPV DNA	Amplicor	Roche	L1	13 carcinogenic	No	PCR
	careHPV	QIAGEN	Full genome	13 carcinogenic and HPV66	No	Hybridization
	Cervista	Hologic	L1	13 carcinogenic and HPV66	Partial (HPV16 and HPV18)	Hybridization
	CLART	Genomica	L1	13 carcinogenic and 22 noncarcinogenic	Yes	PCR
	COBAS 4800	Roche	L1	13 carcinogenic and HPV66	Partial (HPV16 and HPV18)	Real-time PCR
	eHC	QIAGEN	Full genome	13 carcinogenic, HPV66, and HPV82	Partial (HPV types 16, 18, and 45)	Hybridization
	GP5+/6+ EIA	Not commercialized	L1	13 carcinogenic and HPV66	No	PCR
	HC2	QIAGEN	Full genome	13 carcinogenic	No	Hybridization
	HPV QUAD	Autogenomics	E1	13 carcinogenic and HPV66	Partial (HPV types 16, 18, 31, 33, and 45)	PCR
	HR-HPV Dx PCR	BioRad	n/a	13 carcinogenic and HPV66	No	PCR

(continued)

Table 1.1 HPV-Based Cervical Cancer Screening Tests* (*continued*)

Marker	Test name	Manufacturer	Target molecule	Target HPV genotypes	HPV genotyping	Technology
	Infinity HPV	Autogenomics	E1	13 carcinogenic and 13 noncarcinogenic	Yes	PCR
	InnoLiPA	Innogenetics	L1	13 carcinogenic and 15 noncarcinogenic	Yes	PCR
	Linear array	Roche	L1	13 carcinogenic and 24 noncarcinogenic	Yes	PCR
	Multiplex HPV genotyping kit	Multimetrix	L1	13 carcinogenic and 11 noncarcinogenic	Yes	PCR
	Papillocheck	Greiner	E1	13 carcinogenic and 11 noncarcinogenic	Yes	PCR
	RT HPV	Abbott	L1	13 carcinogenic and HPV66	Partial (HPV16 and HPV18)	Real-time PCR
	n/a	Becton Dickinson	n/a	13 carcinogenic and HPV66	Partial (HPV types 16, 18, 31, 45, 51, 52, and 59)	Real-time PCR

(*continued*)

Table 1.1 HPV-Based Cervical Cancer Screening Tests* *(continued)*

Marker	Test name	Manufacturer	Target molecule	Target HPV genotypes	HPV genotyping	Technology
HPV RNA	Aptima	GenProbe	E6/E7 mRNA	13 carcinogenic and HPV66	No	TMA
	NucliSENS EasyQ HPV	BioMerieux	E6/E7 mRNA	HPV types 16, 18, 31, 33, and 45	Yes	NASBA
	OncoTect	Invirion/InCellDx	E6/E7 mRNA	13 carcinogenic	n/a	In situ hybridization
	PreTect Proofer	Norchip	E6/E7 mRNA	HPV types 16, 18, 31, 33, and 45	Yes	NASBA
HPV protein	E6 protein	Arbor Vitae	E6	HPV types 16, 18, and 45	n/a	Immunoassay
	Cytoactiv	Cytoimmun	L1	Carcinogenic types, not specified	n/a	Immunostain
Cellular protein	CINtec plus	mtm Laboratories	p16[INK4a]/Ki-67	n/a	n/a	Immunostain
	ProExC	Becton Dickinson	MCM2/Top2A	n/a	n/a	Immunostain
FISH	oncoFISH	ikonisys	3q/TERC	n/a	n/a	FISH

FISH, fluorescence in situ hybridization; NASBA, nucleic acid sequence–based amplification; PCR, polymerase chain reaction; TMA, transcription-mediated amplification.

*Cross-hybridization with noncarcinogenic HPV types described.

Source: Ref. (10). Schiffman M, Wentzensen N, Wacholder S et al. Human papillomavirus testing in the prevention of cervical cancer. *J Natl Cancer Inst.* March 2, 2011;103(5):368–383.

CYTOLOGIC GUIDELINES

Cytologic guidelines can be found at: www.asccp.org (Current Cytology Algorithms)

- Screening:
  - Initiation: begin screening at age 21 regardless of sexual history with the exception of those who are infected with HIV or otherwise immunocompromised.
  - Screening method and intervals—ages 21 to 65: cytology every 3 years, or ages 21 to 29: cytology every 3 years then at age 30 to 65 cytology plus HR HPV cotesting every 5 years. HR HPV testing alone is also a consideration between ages 25 and 65.
  - For those in low resource settings, visual inspection with acetic acid (VIA) as triage is recommended, which can proceed to immediate treatment based on risk assessment.
  - End screening: discontinuation of screening is recommended for women with an intact cervix who are aged 65 years and older and who have had three or more consecutive normal Pap tests (cytology) or two consecutive negative cotests, or two consecutive negative HPV tests within a 10-year period. Screening should not be restarted for any reason even including a new partner. For women with a hysterectomy performed for benign indications, screening can be discontinued. Women with a supracervical hysterectomy should continue screening until age 65 years and can discontinue screening when three or more consecutive normal Pap tests (cytology) or two consecutive negative cotests, or two consecutive negative HPV tests within a 10-year period with the most recent performed within the past 5 years.
- Annual screening indefinitely is recommended for women with a history of intrauterine DES exposure.
- For HIV positive women: screening should begin within 1 year of sexual activity or within the first year of HIV diagnosis if already sexually active, but no later than 21 years of age. Annual cytologic testing should continue up to age 29. HPV testing should not occur. If three consecutive annual negative cytology-alone tests are normal, follow-up cytology testing should occur at 3-year intervals. For those over the age of 30, annual screening should continue with cytology alone or cotesting. After three negative annual cytology-alone tests results that are normal, follow-up screening can be every 3 years. Women who have one negative cotest result can have their next cervical cancer screening in 3 years: cervical cancer screening should continue throughout her lifetime and not be discontinued.
- Women with a history of an abnormal Pap over 65 years old should continue screening until there are three or more consecutive normal Pap tests (cytology) or two consecutive negative cotests, or two consecutive negative HPV tests within in a 10-year period. Women with a history of cervical HSIL (-IN 2/3) should continue screening for 20 years after diagnosis and/or treatment—screening interval guidelines may be followed if normal Pap smears are obtained. Women with a history of hysterectomy due to cervical HSIL (-IN 2/3) should continue vaginal Pap smear screening for 20 years after surgery—screening interval guidelines can be followed if a normal Pap smear is obtained. Women with a history of cervical cancer should continue annual screening indefinitely with cytology alone. If screening is inadequate, screening until age 75 can be considered (USPTF).

- Based on the relative risk of underlying cervical HSIL (-IN 2/3) or cervical cancer, women can be categorized into three groups based on Pap and HR HPV results with management protocols to follow risk categorization. Approximately 20% will be categorized low risk and fall into routine 3-year screening protocols, 50% will be in the moderate risk category and need repeat testing in 1 year, and 30% will fall into the high-risk category with recommended colposcopy.
- ASC-US HPV negative women have a low risk of cervical HSIL (-IN 2/3) and it is recommended they have cotesting in 3 years. ASC-US HPV+ women over the age of 30 should be managed:
  - Repeat cotesting in 12 months. If the repeat cytology test is ASC-US or higher or the HPV test is still positive, these women should be referred to colposcopy. Otherwise contesting should occur in 3 years.
  - Immediate HPV genotype specific testing for HPV 16/18. If HPV 16/18 results are positive, then direct colposcopy referral should occur. If negative for both 16/18 genotypes, then cotesting in 12 months should follow. If follow-up testing remains abnormal, then these women should be referred to colposcopy.
- Prevalence of anal HPV with known cervical dysplasia: prevalence of anal HPV was 32.5%. The prevalence of abnormal anal cytology was 17.6%. Women with cervical HR HPV were more likely to have concurrent anal HR HPV (OR 3.6, 95% CI: 1.19–10.77) (13).

  See **Cervical SIL (-IN 1/2/3) Management Protocols in the Preinvasive Disease** section.

NOTABLE TRIALS

- HPV typing for management of HPV positive ASC-US cervical cytology results: ASC-US linked to HPV 16, 18, 31, 33, 58 warrants immediate colposcopy. Management of HPV 45, 52 is uncertain. HPV 51, 39, 68, 35, 59, 56, 66 are probably low enough to recommend 1 year retesting to permit viral clearance, deferring colposcopy for up to 40% of HPV positive ASC-US women, half of whom would be cotest negative at 1-year follow-up (14).

HPV VACCINATION

- The HPV **prophylactic** vaccination is encouraged in both females and males between the ages of 9 and 26 years old.
  - There is hope that this vaccine will decrease the global incidence rates of head and neck and anogenital cancers.
  - Initial vaccines consisted of the L1 capsids either with the quadrivalent vaccine for HPV 6, 11, 16, and 18; or the bivalent vaccine for HPV 16 and 18.
  - The nonavalent HPV vaccine is now available. It includes HPV types 6, 11, 16, 18, 31, 33, 45, 52, and 58. In a randomized phase III trial, vaccine or placebo were given at day 1, month 2, and month 6. Tissue was obtained by biopsy or definitive therapy (conization). Efficacy against high-grade disease, related to all vaccine HPV types, was 97%. Efficacy against cervical HSIL (-IN 2/3) was 96%. Efficacy against vulvar HSIL (-IN 2/3) or vaginal HSIL (-IN 2/3) was 100%. It was approved December 10, 2014.
  - The CDC recommends a two dose abbreviated HPV vaccine 6 to 12 months apart for persons aged 11 to 12 years. Adolescents who receive their two

shots less than 5 months apart or those who receive the vaccine series after the age of 15 are required a 3rd dose of the HPV vaccine. This is based on data demonstrating that two doses of HPV vaccine in young adolescents aged 9 to 14 years produces an immune response similar or higher than the response in young adults aged 16 to 26 years who receive the standard 3-dose series over a 6-month time period.

o VIVIANE study: this was a randomized controlled trial of 5,747 women over the age of 25 years vaccinated with the 3-shot bi-valent HPV series; 15% had prior HPV infection documented. At month 84, in women seronegative for the corresponding HPV type in the according-to-protocol cohort for efficacy, vaccine efficacy against 6-month persistent infection or cervical HSIL (-IN 1+) associated with HPV 16/18 was significant in all age groups combined (90.5%, 96.2% CI: 78.6–96.5). Vaccine efficacy against HPV 16/18-related cytological abnormalities (ASC of undetermined significance and low-grade squamous intraepithelial lesion) and cervical HSIL (-IN 1+) was also significant. There was noted to be significant cross-protective efficacy against 6-month persistent infection with HPV 31 (65.8%, 96.2% CI: 24.9–85.8) and HPV 45 (70.7%, 96.2% CI: 34.2–88.4). In the total vaccinated cohort, vaccine efficacy against cervical HSIL (-IN 1+) irrespective of HPV was significant (22.9%, 96.2% CI: 4.8–37.7). Thus, in women older than 25 years, the HPV 16/18 vaccine continues to protect against infections, cytological abnormalities, and lesions associated with HPV 16/18 and cervical HSIL (-IN 1+) irrespective of HPV type, and infection with nonvaccine types HPV 31 and HPV 45 over a 7-year follow-up period (15).

o There are data to support that the nonavalent vaccine will prevent up to 90% of cervical cancers instead of the prior 70% protection provided by the quadrivalent vaccine.

o Insurance tends to cover the above age ranges, but anyone can receive this vaccine if they pay out of pocket for it.

- There is possible **therapeutic** effect:
  o From the FUTURE I and FUTURE II trials, a retrospective analysis of these two randomized trials in patients ages 20 to 45 who were treated for cervical HSIL (-IN 2/3) by LEEP: 360 were vaccinated 377 were not. There was a 2.5% recurrence rate in the vaccination group, 7.2% in the control group. This demonstrated a 64.9% reduction in high-grade disease of the cervix in women who underwent a surgical procedure for cervical HSIL (-IN 2/3) and were vaccinated. The vaccine was given prior to their excisional procedure. The HR for recurrence was 2.84 (95% CI: 1.3–6.0; $p < 0.01$) even after evaluating for positive endocervical cytology and positive margin status. This post hoc analysis was not specifically designed to address the question of a therapeutic benefit (16).

REFERENCES

1. Darragh TM, Colgan TJ, Cox JT, et al. The Lower Anogenital Squamous Terminology Standardization Project for HPV-Associated Lesions: background and consensus recommendations from the College of American Pathologists and the American Society for Colposcopy and Cervical Pathology. *Arch Pathol Lab Med.* 2012;136(10):1266-1297.

2. Wright TC Jr, Stoler MH, Behrens CM, et al. The ATHENA human papillomavirus study: design, methods, and baseline results. *Am J Obstet Gynecol.* 2012;206: 46.e1-46.e11.

3. https://report.nih.gov/nihfactsheets/viewfactsheet.aspx?csid=76

4. Nanda K, McCrory DC, Myers ER, et al. Accuracy of the Papanicolaou test in screening for and follow-up of cervical cytologic abnormalities: a systematic review. *Ann Intern Med.* May 16, 2000;132(10):810-819.

5. Siebers AG, Klinkhamer PJ, Arbyn M, et al. Cytologic detection of cervical abnormalities using liquid-based copared with conventional cytology: a randomized controlled trial. *Obstet Gynecol.* December 2008;112(6):1327-1334.

6. ASCUS-LSIL Traige Study (ALTS) Group. Results of a randomized trial on the management of cytology interpretations of atypical squamous cells of undertermined significance. *Am J Obstet Gynecol.* 2003;188:1383-1392.

7. ASCUS-LSIL Traige Study (ALTS) Group. A randomized trial on the management of low-grade squamous intraepithelial lesion cytology interpretations. *Am J Obstet Gynecol.* 2003;188:1393-1400.

8. Katki HA, Schiffman M, Castle PE, et al. Benchmarking CIN 3+ risk as the basis for incorporating HPV and Pap cotesting into cervical screening and management guidelines. *J Low Genit Tract Dis.* April 2013;17(5 Suppl 1):S28-S35.

9. Melnikow J, Nuovo J, Willan AR, et al. Natural history of cervical squamous intraepithelial lesions: a meta-analysis. *Obstet Gynecol.* 1998;92(4, Pt. 2):727-735.

10. Schiffman M, Wentzensen N, Wacholder S, et al. Human papillomavirus testing in the prevention of cervical cancer. *J Natl Cancer Inst.* March 2, 2011;103(5):368-383.

11. Wright TC, Stoler MH, Behrens CM, et al. Primary cervical cancer screening with human papillomavirus: end of study results from the ATHENA study using HPV as the first-line screening test. *Gynecol Oncol.* 2015;136:189-197.

12. Huh WK, Ault KA, Chelmow D, et al. Interim guidance for use of primary HR HPV testing for cervical cancer screening. *Gynecol Oncol.* 2015;136:178-182.

13. Lamme J, Pattaratornkosohn, Mercado-Abadie J, et al. Concurrent anal HPV and abnormal anal cytology in women with known cervical dysplasia. *Obstet Gynecol.* August 2014;124(2):242.

14. Schiffman M, Vaughan LM, Raine-Bennett TR, et al. HPV typing for management of HPV positive ASC-US cervical cytology results. *Gynecol Oncol.* 2015;138:573-578.

15. Wheeler CM, Skinner SR, Del Rosario-Raymundo MR, et al. Efficacy, safety, and immunogenicity of the human papillomavirus 16/18 AS04-adjuvanted vaccine in women older than 25 years: 7-year follow-up of the phase 3, double-blind, randomised controlled VIVIANE study. *Lancet Infect Dis.* October 2016;16(10):1154-1168.

16. Kang WD, Choi HS, Kim SM, et al. Is vaccination with quadrivalent HPV vaccine after loop electrosurgical excision procedure effective in preventing recurrence in patients with high-grade cervical intraepithelial neoplasia (CIN2-3)? *Gynecol Oncol.* August 2013;130(2):264-268.

Preinvasive Disease

The Lower Anogenital Squamous Terminology (LAST) Project developed terminology for lower anogenital tract preinvasive disease to create a unified histopathological nomenclature with a single set of diagnostic terms. It is recommended for all human papillomavirus (HPV)-associated preinvasive squamous lesions regardless of anatomic site or sex/gender and has been adopted by the World Health Organization (WHO) (1).

In March 2012, the ASCCP and College of American Pathologists definitively changed intraepithelial neoplasia from a three-tier diagnosis to a two-tier diagnosis. Therefore, biopsy pathology from the cervix, anus, vulva, and vagina is classified as cervical-squamous intraepithelial lesion (SIL), anal-SIL, vulvar-SIL, and vaginal-SIL, respectively. Intraepithelial neoplasia is further categorized as low-grade LSIL (-IN 1) or high-grade HSIL (-IN 2/3). Histologic management guidelines can be found at: www.asccp.org.

CERVICAL-SILs

- Characteristics: cervical SILs are asymptomatic; Pap smear screening (cytology) or positive high risk (HR) HPV testing are the main means of detection. The median age at diagnosis has ranged from 23 years old in the ASCUS/LSIL Triage Study (ALTS) trial (2) to 34 years old in a Norwegian population. Risk factors for cervical SIL are HPV infection, immunosuppression, smoking, a history of sexually transmitted diseases (STDs), and multiple sexual partners. The use of oral contraceptives is also linked to an increased risk of HPV infection. The use of oral contraceptives was previously thought to be only a marker for exposure more than a cause; however, studies suggest that the hormones in oral contraceptive pills may cause changes in cervical cells that make them more susceptible to infection (33).
- Immunosuppression can significantly contribute to increased rates of dysplasia and cancer: for those infected with HIV, the relative risk for invasive cervical cancer (ICC) is five times higher (3). The risk of invasive cancer varies by CD4 count: HIV-infected women with baseline CD4$^+$ T-cells of $\geq$ 350, 200 to 349, and less than 200 cells per microliter had a 2.3, 3.0, and 7.7 times increase in the incidence of invasion, respectively, compared with HIV-uninfected women (p(trend) = 0.001) (4). The standardized incidence ratio for ICC is 9.2 for HIV-infected patients (5).
- For immunosuppressed solid organ transplant patients, the relative risk for cervical SIL is 13.6 (6). The relative risk of a transplant patient having ICC is 5 (7).
- Cervical intraepithelial lesion terminology is two-tiered: LSIL (-IN 1) is categorized as a low-grade lesion and HSIL (-IN 2/3) are combined into the category of high-grade lesions. Classification is according to the amount of epithelium

involved: cervical LSIL (old CIN 1) demonstrates atypia in the lower third of epithelium; cervical HSIL (old CIN 2/3) demonstrates atypia from the middle third to throughout the entire epithelium. The microscopic appearance is nuclear atypia, disorganization/depolarization, parakeratosis, and abnormal mitotic figures. Most lesions occur in the transformation zone. There is no distinction between cervical HSIL (-IN 3) and carcinoma in situ (CIS); thus, it is recommended that CIS terminology not be used.

- Biomarker interpretation: p16 immunohistochemistry (IHC) is recommended when the differential diagnosis is between -IN 2/-IN 3 and a precancer mimic or if the pathologist is entertaining a hematoxylin and eosin (H&E) stain morphologic interpretation of -IN 2. p16 IHC may also be used as an adjunct to biopsy specimen assessment when interpreted as -IN 1 that are high risk for missed high-grade disease due to a prior cytologic interpretation of HSIL, atypical squamous cells cannot exclude high grade (ASC-H), or atypical glandular cells not otherwise specified (AGC[NOS]). If there is difficulty in stratifying LSIL from HSIL, p16 IHC can be performed on the specimen and if positive then the lesion is categorized as HSIL. Those results with a prior -IN2 diagnosis can have p16 IHC staining: if that staining is negative it would then fall to the lower LSIL category and if p16 positive, upgrade into the HSIL category (Table 1.2).

Table 1.2 Management of Abnormal Pap and/or HR HPV Tests

Abnormal screening result	Management	Risk of cervical HSIL (-IN 2/3)
ASC-US, HR HPV–	Routine screening in 3 y	Low
ASC-US, HR HPV unknown	Cytology in 12 m, colposcopy for any abnormality, if normal routine screening	Moderate
Normal cytology, HR HPV+, HPV genotyping unknown or negative LSIL, HR HPV–	Cytology plus HPV testing in 12 m; colposcopy for any abnormality; if both normal, repeat cytology plus HPV testing in 3 y	Moderate
ASC-US, HR HPV+, Normal cytology, HR HPV+ on two consecutive tests Normal cytology, HR HPV+, HPV genotyping+ LSIL, HR HPV+ or unknown	Age 25 or above: colposcopy Age 21–24: cytology in 12 m but colposcopy for ASC-H or HSIL or worse, and at 24 m with colposcopy for any abnormality; if all normal routine screening	High Moderate
HSIL ASC-H	Colposcopy	High

(continued)

Table 1.2 Management of Abnormal Pap and/or HR HPV Tests (*continued*)		
Abnormal screening result	**Management**	**Risk of cervical HSIL (-IN 2/3)**
AGC AIS	Colposcopy with ECC, EMB if abnormal bleeding, chronic anovulation, or age 35 or above	High

AGC, atypical glandular cells; AIS, adenocarcinoma in situ; ASC-US, atypical squamous cells of undetermined significance; ECC, endocervical curettage; EMB, endometrial biopsy; HPV, human papillomavirus; HR, high risk; HSIL, high-grade squamous intraepithelial lesion: LSIL, low-grade squamous intraepithelial lesion.

- **Colposcopy:** microscopic evaluation of the cervix at 8× to 25× can visualize tissue abnormalities. Application of 3% to 5% topical acetic acid (vinegar) for 3 to 5 minutes can dehydrate the surface cells and unmask tissue changes such as acetowhite epithelium and atypical vessels. Directed biopsy can sample these areas for cervical SIL (-IN 1,2,3). If no abnormalities are seen, then an endocervical curettage (ECC) and random or four-quadrant biopsies can be performed, with highest yield from the transformation zone. An adequate colposcopy is visualization of the entire cervix, its transformation zone, and the vaginal fornices. An ECC should usually be done if the patient is not pregnant. Histologic confirmation with biopsy should occur before ablative therapy is performed (i.e., cryotherapy) (Table 1.3).
- Treatment of cervical LSIL (-IN 1) can vary. In the ALTS for cervical cancer study, 41% of cervical LSIL (-IN 1) diagnoses were downgraded to normal and 13% were upgraded to cervical HSIL (-IN 2/3). In one study, 90% of women with LSIL (-IN 1) spontaneously regressed in 24 months (8). If cervical LSIL (-IN 1) is diagnosed after a Pap test that showed HSIL or ASC-H, more aggressive management should be considered. If cervical SIL (-IN 1) is diagnosed after an atypical squamous cells of undetermined significance (ASC-US) or LSIL Pap, HPV testing every 12 months or repeating a Pap smear in 6 months can be considered. If cervical LSIL (-IN 1) persists for 2 years, a loop electrosurgical excision procedure (LEEP) can be considered. Before using any ablative (cryo or laser) therapy, a negative ECC should be obtained (Table 1.4).
- Management of cervical HSIL (-IN 2/3) diagnosed at colposcopic biopsy:
  - Surveillance: surveillance can be offered for women of reproductive age with cervical HSIL (-IN 2, 2/3), given that the patient is reliable, and had an adequate colposcopy. Cure rates with treatment are about 90%, whereas spontaneous regression rates are about 40%. Thus, treatment is recommended as primarily ablative techniques in women ages 21–24. Surveillance is colposcopy and cytology every 6 months up to 24 months if adequate colposcopy. Routine screening may resume after two normal cytology tests and colposcopy examinations followed by a normal cytology test and negative HR HPV test a year later.

Table 1.3 Management of Colposcopic Findings

Indication for colposcopy	Findings at colposcopy: no lesion, normal biopsy, or cervical LSIL (-IN1)	Findings at colposcopy: cervical HSIL (-IN 2/3)	Risk of cervical HSIL (-IN 2/3)
Normal cytology, HR HPV+ on two consecutive tests Normal cytology, HR HPV+, HPV genotyping+ ASC-US on two consecutive tests ASC-US, HR HPV+ LSIL	Age 25 or above: cytology plus HR HPV testing in 12 m; colposcopy for any abnormality; if both normal, cytology alone if younger than 30 or cytology plus HR HPV testing if older than 30 in 3 years; if testing at 3 years is normal, routine screening is done Ages 21–24: cytology alone in 12 months; colposcopy for ASC-H or HSIL or higher and at 24 months with colposcopy for any abnormality; if all normal, routine screening	Diagnostic excisional procedure	Low Low
AGC, NOS	Cytology plus HR HPV testing in 12 and 24 months; colposcopy for any abnormality; if all normal, repeat cytology plus HR HPV testing in 3 years; if cytology and HR HPV testing at 3 years is normal, routine screening	Diagnostic excisional procedure	Low
HSIL; ASC-H	Age 25 or above: cytology plus HR HPV testing in 12 and 24 months if colposcopy adequate and ECC negative; if both normal, routine screening; treatment is also an option Age 21–24: colposcopy and cytology in 6 and 12 months, if colposcopy adequate and ECC negative; if all normal, routine screening Treatment if colposcopy is inadequate	Diagnostic excisional procedure	Low Moderate High
AGC, favor neoplasia, AIS	Diagnostic excisional procedure		High

AGC, atypical glandular cells; AIS, adenocarcinoma in situ; ASC-US, atypical squamous cells of undetermined significance; ECC, endocervical curettage; HPV, human papillomavirus; HR, high risk; HSIL, high-grade squamous intraepithelial lesion; LSIL, low-grade squamous intraepithelial lesion.

Table 1.4 Risk of Progression to Cervical -IN 3

Lesion	% Regression	% Persistent	% Progress to cervical -IN 3
LSIL (-IN1)	57	32	11
HSIL (-IN 2)	43	35	22
HSIL (-IN 3)	32	35	NA

NA, not applicable.

- ○ Ablation therapy: some authors caution excisional therapy in reproductive-aged women due to risk of adverse reproductive outcomes (preterm labor, cervical stenosis, and infertility).
    - ■ Cryotherapy: criteria for application are adequate colposcopy, the lesion is completely visible, it does not cover more than 75% of the ectocervix, and the lesions can be covered with the cryoprobe. Due to risk of cryotherapy failure, this procedure is not recommended in women over 40 years old.
    - ■ Laser: the same criteria should be met as for cryotherapy but laser can be used for lesions larger than 2 cm, for multifocal lesions, or both, with or without vaginal involvement
    - ■ Excisional therapy: may be used for primary treatment or if criteria for ablation are not met. For the conization procedure, it is necessary to remove 5 to 7 mm of cervical stroma and perform an ECC. There is evidence of skip lesions and multifocality, especially in glandular lesions, so one should, therefore, not solely remove the acetowhite lesion.
        - □ LEEP: office-based procedure
        - □ Cold knife conization (CKC): if there is suspicion for malignancy and margin status is important, if there has been prior cervical treatment, or if cervical atrophy is present, a CKC is recommended. This is a general anesthesia-based procedure.
- • Follow-up after treatment for cervical HSIL (-IN 2/3) is based on categorization into low- or high-risk groups.
    - ○ Low risk is LEEP or CKC with negative margins or those who had ablative therapies. Follow-up consists of cytology plus HR HPV testing in 12 and 24 months; colposcopy for any abnormality; if all are normal, cytology plus HR HPV testing in 3 years; if cytology and HPV testing at 3 years are normal, routine screening for 20 years. Annual cotesting or annual cytology until two negative annual tests is another option.
    - ○ High risk is those with LEEP- or CKC-positive margins or those with positive post-procedure ECC. Follow up is cytology and ECC at 4 to 6 months (preferred), but repeat excision is acceptable. If re-excision is not possible, then hysterectomy is acceptable; then cytology plus HR HPV testing in 12 and 24 months; colposcopy for any abnormality; if all are normal, repeat cytology plus HR HPV testing in 3 years; if cytology and HPV testing are normal at 3 years, then routine screening for 20 years. Annual cotesting or annual cytology until two negative annual tests is another option. There are data to support the spontaneous resolution of positive margins in 56% of women (9).

- Additional indications for conization beyond treatment of cervical-HSIL (-IN 2/3), and a positive ECC are: evaluation of microscopic invasive cancer, treatment of Stage IA1 cervical cancer, evaluation of significant cytologic/histologic discrepancy, and evaluation of an unsatisfactory colposcopic exam. CKC may be a more favorable procedure for glandular lesions.
- The addition of a postconization ECC to cone biopsy for adenocarcinoma in situ (AIS) of the cervix provides prognostic information. Women who have both a negative ECC and negative cone margin have a 14% risk of residual AIS and if they desire fertility can be managed conservatively. A positive ECC post-cone or internal positive margin has significant risk of residual disease and 12% to 17% will have cancer (10).
- Glandular precancerous changes include AIS. This is histologically represented as: crowding of cells, atypia, pseudostratification, and increased mitotic activity. To distinguish atypia versus AIS, the degree of mitotic activity and pseudostratification should be taken into account. To diagnose an invasive lesion, atypical glands extend beyond the depth normally involved by endocervical glands, which is approximately 5 to 6 mm from the surface.
- Notable Trials:
  - Relevance of random biopsy at the transformation zone when colposcopy is negative. The ATHENA study (addressing the need for advanced HPV diagnostics) trial screened 47,000 plus women with cytology and HR HPV DNA genotyping. Colposcopy was performed in all women with abnormal cytology or positive HPV results. A single random biopsy was taken at the squamnocolumnar junction (SCJ) if colposcopy was adequate and no lesions were seen. This single random biopsy increased the detection of high-grade disease, diagnosing cervical HSIL in 20.9% (-IN 2) and 18.9% of (-IN 3) (11).
  - Alternative treatment to LEEP/CKC: 59 patients with cervical HSIL (-IN 2/3) were randomized to a 16-week treatment of self-applied vaginal suppositories of imiquimod or placebo. Imiquimod is a topical immune response modulator, is a toll-like seven receptor agonist affecting the upregulation of interferon alpha and activation of the dendritic cells. The suppository dose was 6.25 mg, one suppository per week for weeks 1 and 2, in weeks 3 and 4 two suppositories per week, then until 16 weeks three suppositories per week. At night, avoid intercourse those nights, and suspend application during the first 3 days of menses. Dose modification was to 3.125 mg. The main outcome was regression to cervical LSIL (-IN 1) or less. Secondary outcomes were complete histologic remission, HPV clearance, and tolerability. Histologic regression was observed in 73% versus 39% $p = 0.009$. Complete remission was 47% in the imiquimod group compared to placebo 14%, $p = 0.008$. All patients at baseline tested HPV positive and HPV clearance rates increased in the imiquimod group 60% versus placebo group 14% $p < 0.001$. No high-grade side effects were observed (12).
  - HPV typing for management of HPV-positive ASC-US cervical cytology results: ASC-US linked to HPV 16, 18, 31, 33, 58 warrants immediate colposcopy. Management of HPV 45, 52 is uncertain. HPV 51, 39, 68, 35, 59, 56, 66 are probably low enough to recommend 1-year retesting to permit viral

clearance deferring colposcopy for up to 40% of HPV + ASC-US women, half of whom would be cotest negative at 1 year follow-up (13).

○ Trichloroacetic acid has been investigated in the treatment of 241 women with cervical HSIL (-IN 2/3) and 179 with cervical LSIL (-IN 1). The regression rate was 87.7% for cervical HSIL (-IN 2/3) and 82.3% for cervical LSIL (-IN 1). Clearance of HPV 16/18 was found in 73.5% of cervical HSIL (-IN 2/3) and 75% of cervical LSIL (-IN 1). Topical 85% TCA was applied to the ectocervix and a saturated cotton swab was inserted into the distal cervical canal one time (14).

VULVAR-SIL

- **Characteristics**: vulvar squamous intraepithelial lesions (prior vulvar intraepithelial neoplasia [VIN]) can present with pruritus, a mass lesion, or hyperpigmentation. They can also be asymptomatic. The median age at diagnosis is 46 years old. Vulvar SILs are classified according to the amount of epithelium involved: vulvar LSIL (-IN 1) demonstrates atypia in the lower third of epithelium, vulvar HSIL (-IN 2/3) demonstrates atypia from the middle third of epithelium, to throughout the entire epithelium. 3-4.8% of vulvar HSIL patients who receive treatment can still progress to cancer. 88% of untreated patients have been found to develop invasive disease (15,31); 12% to 23% of women with vulvar HSIL (-IN 3) are found to have invasive disease at the time of -IN 3 excision (16); however, most of these diagnoses have less than 1-mm depth of invasion. One third of invasive cancers have coexisting vulvar HSIL (-IN 3). Solitary lesions have the highest risk of progression. Spontaneous regression has occurred with a range of 10% to 56%. But, because this is a precancerous lesion, treatment is the standard of care. Recurrence is higher when associated with positive margins, ranging from 17% to 46%. It is important to remember that L/H-SIL is a histologic biopsy diagnosis, not a screening diagnosis.
- Risk factors for vulvar-SIL are a history of other genital tract dysplasia (25% have another lower reproductive tract dysplasia), smoking, immunosuppression, HPV infection, and a history of other STDs.
- The Vulvar Oncology Subcommittee of the International Society for the Study of Vulvar Diseases (ISSVD) classifies VIN into three categories congruent with the LAST Project. Terminology for vulvar SIL is: vulvar-LSIL and vulvar HSIL and differentiated-type VIN (DVIN) (17).
  ○ LSIL of the vulva: vulvar LSIL (prior VIN1) flat condyloma, or HPV effect.
  ○ HSIL of the vulva
    ▪ VIN usual type: this encompasses the former VIN 2/3 subtypes of: warty, basaloid, and mixed types. The microscopic appearance of the basaloid type is thickened epithelium with a flat, smooth surface, numerous mitotic figures, and enlarged hyperchromatic nuclei.
    ▪ VIN warty type: the warty type is condylomatous in appearance, and microscopically cells contain numerous mitotic figures with abnormal maturation. The usual type is the most common, typically occurring in younger, premenopausal women. Risk factors include HPV, smoking, and immunosuppression. Lesions are often multifocal.
  ○ DVIN differentiated type: this encompasses the former category of simplex type. These lesions comprise less than 5% of VIN. They typically occur in

postmenopausal women and are associated with lichen sclerosis, but not HPV. Lesions are usually unifocal and p53 positive. This lesion is probably a precursor to HPV-negative vulvar cancer (18).

- Most often vulvar SILs are found between 3 and 9 o'clock on the vulva, in non–hair-bearing areas. The lesions are often multifocal and can be macular, papular, warty, white, red, gray, or brown. Diagnosis is with colposcopy and biopsy using 3%–5% acetic acid applied to the perineum for 5 minutes.
- Treatment is varied. Wide local excision with 5-mm margins (skinning vulvectomy) is appropriate, as is CO_2 laser ablation, or cavitron ultrasonic surgical aspiration (CUSA). Topical treatment for vulvar-HSIL can be with: 5-fluorouracil (5-FU) (5% 5-FU cream once daily per week; may increase to two or three times weekly as tolerated by the patient as this medication can cause a significant chemical burn) or imiquimod 5% cream (three times a week, i.e., Monday, Wednesday, Friday, but may decrease frequency to once per week if significant vulvar swelling reaction occurs). Imiquimod should not be used in immunocompromised patients.
- Recurrent disease is common, approaching 50% if margins are positive, versus 15% if negative margins are obtained.
- Benign lesions: can mimic vulvar dysplasia. It is imperative to biopsy these lesions to confirm the histologic diagnosis prior to any treatment.
  - Warty lesions are of three main types: condyloma acuminatum, sessile plaques, and keratotic verruca vulgaris. Of patients with vulvar warts, 22% to 32% have concomitant cervical SIL (-IN 1/2/3); therefore, screening colposcopy of the entire lower genital tract is recommended. Treatment can be with topical solutions, such as imiquimod or trichloroacetic acid; laser ablation; CUSA; or surgical resection.
  - Micropapillomatosis labialis is asymptomatic and can appear as small areas of mucosal papillomas. No HPV DNA has been isolated in these lesions. Treatment is not necessary.
  - Lichen sclerosis can present with pruritus. The vulvar skin is paper thin and biopsy shows blunted rete pegs. Treatment is with clobetasol steroid cream to the perineum twice daily for 6 weeks. To promote thickening of the vulvar skin, applying a 2% compounded testosterone cream twice weekly may also be useful. There is an increased risk for malignant transformation to a well-differentiated squamous cell cancer with this lesion.
  - Hyperplastic dystrophy can also present with pruritus. Biopsy shows thickened and widened rete pegs and hyperkeratosis. Treatment is with 1% hydrocortisone cream to the perineum twice daily.

VAGINAL SQUAMOUS INTRAEPITHELIAL NEOPLASIA (VAGINAL-SIL)

- Most patients are asymptomatic. Occasionally, patients complain of vaginal discharge or postcoital or postmenopausal bleeding. Most lesions are found because of an abnormal Pap smear.
- Risk factors are HPV infection, other genital tract dysplasia, and immunosuppression.
- Vaginal SIL is classified into two tiers: vaginal LSIL (-IN 1) demonstrates atypia in the lower third of the epithelium, and vaginal HSIL (-IN 2/3) demonstrates atypia into the middle third of the epithelium up to the entire epithelium.

Microscopic abnormalities include nuclear atypia, cellular depolarization, para-keratosis, and abnormal mitotic figures.

- The most common location of vaginal dysplasia is the posterior vaginal fornix. Vaginal SIL is often multifocal. Diagnosis is made with colposcopic directed biopsy after application of 3-5% acetic acid for 5 minutes.

- There are data to suggest an association of vaginal SIL in posthysterectomy women in whom surgery was done for cervical dysplasia: 5%- developed vaginal SIL within 10 years.

- Treatment can be with laser ablation, surgical excision, or topical suppository creams: 5% 5-FU cream can be used. There are many regimens, but our recommended dosing for 5-FU is once weekly for 10 weeks. This may be decreased to once every 2 to 3 weeks if the patient becomes symptomatic due to development of a vaginal chemical burn. Monthly maintenance dosing can be considered. Recurrence rates range from 0% to 38%. Compounded 2.5% imiquimod cream can also be applied via an intravaginal applicator every other night for 16 weeks. It may be necessary to decrease the dosing frequency to once per week if significant vaginal swelling reaction occurs.

- No large long-term follow-up studies have been done to evaluate the risk of vaginal SIL and progression to vaginal cancer. One study from Finland evaluated 23 patients and showed a 78% rate of regression, 13% persistence, and 8% progression to cancer. Another study evaluated vaginectomy specimens and showed a 28% incidence of cancer (19). An 18% incidence of recurrence was demonstrated after vaginectomy.

SILs and HIV

- One third of people with HIV are infected heterosexually. Cervical dysplasia in women with HIV has a more negative outcome. Screening for cervical cancer in HIV-positive women is recommended annually for 3 years beginning within 1 year of onset of sexual activity or within the first year after HIV diagnosis (if already sexually active), but no later than 21 years old. If three consecutive normal Pap smears are obtained, every 3-year cytology can follow. If over 30 years old, cotesting can occur. Cervical cancer screening should continue throughout her lifetime and should not be discontinued. In HIV-positive women, cervical-SIL was found in 14% of women with a normal Pap versus 3% if HIV negative. Of posthysterectomy, HIV-positive women with no prior abnormal Paps, 30% had abnormal vaginal cuff cytology, 29% confirmed vaginal-SIL 2/3 lending consideration to Pap testing in this population (20).

- Current guidelines suggest measuring a baseline (pretreatment) viral load. A drug is considered efficacious if it lowers the viral load by at least 90% within 8 weeks. The viral load should continue to drop to less than 50 copies within 6 months. The viral load should be measured within 2 to 8 weeks after treatment is started or changed, and every 3 to 4 months thereafter. Anyone with a viral load over 100,000 should be offered treatment, as should anyone with an AIDS-defining illness or a CD4 count less than 200.

- Highly active antiretroviral therapy (HAART) includes at least three active antiretroviral medications. Typically two drugs are a nucleoside or nucleotide reverse transcriptase inhibitor (NRTI) plus a third medication. This third medication can be a nonnucleoside reverse transcriptase inhibitor (NNRTI), a protease inhibitor (PI), or another NRTI such as abacavir (Ziagen).

- If cervical LSIL (-IN 1) is diagnosed, some clinicians treat immediately. Others may delay treatment if the Pap was a non-HSIL Pap prior to biopsy confirmation of cervical-LSIL (-IN 1). It is important to check the viral load and CD4 counts. If there is a high viral load and a low Group 1 CD4 count, delay in treatment can be detrimental. For a diagnosis of cervical HSIL (-IN 2/3), conization should be performed.
- Analysis of two large studies (HIV Epidemiology Research Study [HERS] Group, and Women's Interagency HIV Study [WIHS]) showed that there was a 45% immediate failure rate/disease persistence at 6 months for HIV-positive women treated for cervical HSIL (-IN 2/3) by LEEP. For those who had a normal Pap smear at 6 months, there was a 56% recurrence rate. The median recurrence-free period was 30 months. 60% of persistent or recurrent disease was low grade. 73% of patients in this study were not on HAART (32).
- Conization margins are very important in HIV-positive patients. Those patients with positive margins had 100% recurrence versus a 30% to 50% recurrence with negative margins. This is compared to an 8% to 15% recurrence rate in HIV-negative women with negative margins. There is an association with a decreased recurrence rate with the use of HAART and higher CD4 counts in two studies (one for each factor). If the CD4 is greater than 500, 30% were found to regress.
- 7% of HIV-positive women with condyloma in the perineal or pararectal area can develop vulvar-SIL (-IN 2/3) within a 3-year period. HIV-positive women are seven times more likely to develop vulvar SIL than HIV-negative women.
- HPV vaccination is recommended for HIV-infected persons per routine guidelines.

Uterine Precancer

- Symptoms are usually postmenopausal bleeding (PMPB).
- Imaging can assist in determining risk of cancer. Endometrial stripe thickness on pelvic ultrasound is the best imaging test (Figure 1.1).
  - EMS thickness is set at an upper limit of 4 mm for postmenopausal women. All women with PMPB should be considered for sampling, but the risk of cancer is less with a smaller EMS (21).
  - EMS thickness is not a 100% reliable screening method for patients with PMPB, however, as 27.6% of patients with type II cancers had an EMS $\leq$ 5 mm. Patients with continued PMPB and an endometrial biopsy (EMB) that was negative or nondiagnostic should undergo further evaluation with a method not previously used (saline infusion sonography [SIS], hysteroscopy with directed sampling, or dilation and curettage [D&C]) (22).
- Diagnosis is by tissue sampling. Sampling methods can include endometrial biopsy, cytology retrieved at time of sonohysterography, hysteroscopy and directed biopsy, or D&C. If complex atypical hyperplasia (CAH) or EIN (endometrial intraepithelial neoplasia) is found on EMB, D&C can be used to reliably rule in or out G1 cancer (23).
- There are two means of categorizing uterine precancer

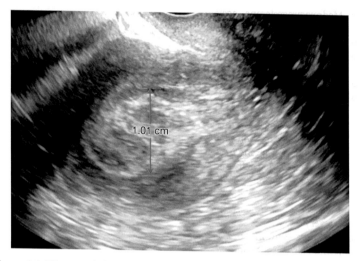

Figure 1.1 Ultrasound demonstrating thickened endometrial stripe.

- ○ WHO-94 schema: with risk of progressing to cancer if left untreated (%)

Simple hyperplasia	1%
Complex hyperplasia	3%
Simple hyperplasia with atypia	9%
Complex hyperplasia with atypia	27% more than 2.1 mm in size

- ○ **Endometrial** intraepithelial neoplasia (**EIN**) schema: this is the preferred terminology per ACOG/SGO.
  - ▪ Benign: benign endometrial hyperplasia (prior WHO-94 simple hyperplasia and complex hyperplasia)
  - ▪ **EIN** (premalignant): atypical endometrial hyperplasia of more than 1 mm in size (this includes the prior WHO-94 categories of simple and complex hyperplasias with atypia)
  - ▪ Malignant endometrial adenocarcinoma endometrioid type well differentiated (Grade 1 cancer).
- As per GOG 167, the risk of concurrent uterine cancer found at the time of hysterectomy done for CAH is 42.6% (24):
- **Surgical treatment** for EIN: Total hysterectomy with removal of the uterus intact provides effective treatment for premalignant lesions. Hysterectomy can be performed with a bilateral salpingo-oophorectomy in patients with confirmed premalignant disease.
- **Medical treatment** for EIN: Medical treatment may be acceptable for patients who desire future fertility or for those with medical comorbidities prohibiting surgical management. Progesterone counterbalances the mitogenic effects of estrogens and induces secretory differentiation. Options include:

- ○ Medroxyprogesterone acetate 10 to 20 PO mg/day, or cyclic 12 to 14 days/month
- ○ Depot medroxyprogesterone 150 mg IM every 3 months
- ○ Micronized vaginal progesterone 100 to 200 mg/day or cyclic 12 to 14 days/month
- ○ Megestrol acetate 40 to 600 PO mg/day
- ○ Levonorgestrel IUD:
  - Mirena IUD: 52 mg in steroid reservoir to be replaced ever every 6 years; releases 20 mg daily: this declines to a rate of 14 mg daily after 5 years, still in the range of clinical effectiveness.
  - Skyla IUD: 13.5 mg in a steroid reservoir to be replaced every 3 years. It releases 15 mcg daily and declines to 5 mcg daily after 3 years.
  - Liletta IUD: 52 mg levonorgestrel in steroid reservoir, replaced every 3 years.
  - Kyleena IUD: 19.5 mg levonorgestrel in a steroid reservoir, to be replaced every 5 years.
- Regression rates for EIN or G1 cancer with medical treatment:
  - ○ With medroxyprogesterone acetate:
    - 10 PO mg daily 12 to 14 days/month, for 3 months 80% to 90% (25).
    - 10 PO mg daily for 6 months: EIN and G1 endometrioid adenocarcinoma:
      - □ 65.8% complete response (CR) for EIN
      - □ 48.2% CR for G1 cancer
      - □ 28% persistent or progressive disease
      - □ 23% had a CR followed by recurrence
  - ○ Mirena IUD—varying degrees of response have been found:
    - Up to 90% if simple or complex hyperplasia but only 67% if EIN.
    - 90% in EIN, 54% in G1 endometrioid cancer (26).
    - Mirena IUD for 12 months of use overall response rate (ORR) 58%: ORR 85% in those with EIN, and 33% RR in those with G1 cancer (27).
  - ○ Notable Trials:
    - Meta-analysis: 344 women (77.7%) demonstrated a response to hormonal therapy. Median follow up was 39 months, and a durable CR was seen in 53.2%. The CR rate was significantly higher for those with hyperplasia than for those with cancer (65.8% vs. 48.2%, $p = 0.002$). The median time to CR was 6 months (range, 1–18 months). Recurrence after an initial response was noted in 23.2% with hyperplasia and 35.4% with cancer ($p = 0.03$). Persistent disease was observed in 14.4% of women with hyperplasia and 25.4% of women with cancer ($p = 0.02$). During the respective study periods, 41.2% of those with hyperplasia and 34.8% with a history of cancer obtained pregnancy ($p = 0.39$), with 117 live births reported (28).
    - Medical management was given to 153 women (PO or IUD) for endometrial hyperplasia or cancer due to inappropriate surgical candidacy or desire for fertility preservation. The average age at diagnosis was 49.6 years. Patients with hyperplasia were compared to patients with cancer. The patients who had hyperplasia responded at a higher rate than those with cancer, showing a CR of 66–70% compared to a rate of 6–13% for those with cancer. 11 to 23% of patients with hyperplasia had an initial response but subsequently recurred, compared to 19–30% of those with

cancer. For those patients with hyperplasia, 11–19% did not respond to medical management at all, compared to 57–75% of those with cancer, ($p < 0.001$). In those patients with cancer, the levonorgestrel-IUD, when compared to oral progesterone regimens, did demonstrate a difference in response. In those patients with hyperplasia, outcomes were significantly different only during the 9- 12-month post-treatment follow-up period, where systemic hormone therapy demonstrated a better response with less disease persistence or progression compared to the levonorgestrel-IUD. Three women were able to conceive (29).

- Treatment was given to 344 women with complex hyperplasia (CH) or CAH who were treated either with IUD or oral progestins over a 12-year period with a median follow-up of 58.8 months. Those with CH treated with an IUD had a 12.7% relapse, those treated with oral progestins had a 30.3% relapse. A body mass index (BMI) ≥ 35 yielded an HR of 18.93 for failure to regress. Oral progestins used were: norethisterone 5 mg TID, medroxyprogesterone 10 mg daily for 10 months, or Megace 180 mg daily or BID. Relapse was associated with diabetes mellitus, EMS greater than 9 mm, or BMI greater than 35, but was not associated with CAH versus CH (30).

REFERENCES

1. Darragh TM, Colgan TJ, Cox JT. The Lower Anogenital Squamous Terminology Standardization Project for HPV-Associated Lesions: background and consensus recommendations from the College of American Pathologists and the American Society for Colposcopy and Cervical Pathology. *Arch Pathol Lab Med.* 2012; 136(10):1266-1297.
2. Castle PE. A descriptive analysis of prevalent vs. incident cervical intraepithelial neoplasia grade 3 following minor cytologic abnormalities. *Am J Clin Pathol.* 2012;138(2): 241-246.
3. Grulich AE, van Leeuwen MT, Falster MO, et al. Incidence of cancers in people with HIV/AIDS compared with immunosuppressed transplant recipients: a meta-analysis. *Lancet.* 2007;370:59-67.
4. Abraham AG, D'Souza G, Jing Y. Invasive cervical cancer risk among HIV-infected women: a North American multicohort collaboration prospective study. *J Acquir Immune Defic Syndr.* April 1, 2013;62(4):405-413.
5. Fordyce EJ, Wang Z, Kahn AR, et al. Risk of cancer among women with AIDS in New York City. *AIDS Public Policy J.* 2000;15:95.
6. Porreco R, Penn I, Droegemueller W, et al. Gynecologic malignancies in immunosuppressed organ homograft recipients. *Obstet Gynecol.* 1975;45:359.
7. Chin-Hong PV, Kwak EJ, AST Infectious Diseases Community of Practice. Human papillomavirus in solid organ transplantation. *Am J Transplant.* 2013;13:189-200.
8. Schlect NF. Human papillomavirus infection and time to progression and regression of cervical intraepithelial neoplasia. *J Natl Cancer Inst.* 2003;95(17):1336-1343.
9. Sawaya GF, Smith-McCune K. Cervical cancer screening. *Obstet Gynecol.* 2016;127(3): 459-467.
10. Tierney KE, Lin PS, Amezcua C, et al. Cervical conization of adenocarcinoma in situ: a predicting model of residual disease. *Am J Obstet Gynecol.* April 2014;210:366e.
11. Huh WK, Sideri M, Stoler, et al. Relevance of random biopsy at the transformation zone when colposcopy is negative. *Obstet Gynecol.* October 2014;124(4):670.
12. Grimm C, Polterauer S, Natter C, et al. Treatment of cervical intraepithelial neoplasia with topical imiquimod. A randomized controlled trial. *Obstet Gynecol.* July 2012;120:1.
13. Schiffman M, Vaughan LM, Raine-Bennett TR, et al. HPV typing for management of HPV positive ASC-US cervical cytology results. *Gynecol Oncol.* 2015;138:573-578.

14. Geisler S, Speiser S, Speiser L, et al. Short-term efficacy of trichloroacetic acid in the treatment of cervical intraepithelial neoplasia. *Obstet Gynecol.* February 2016;127:2.
15. Jones RW. Vulvar intraepithelial neoplasia III: a clinical study of the outcome in 113 cases with relation to the later development of invasive vulvar carcinoma. *Obstet Gynecol.* 1994;84(4):741-745.
16. Modesitt SC. Vulvar intraepithelial neoplasia III: occult cancer and the impact of margin status on recurrence. *Obstet Gynecol.* 1998;92(6):962-966.
17. Darragh TM, Colgan TJ, Cox T, et al. The Lower Anogenital Squamous Terminology Standardization project for HPV associated lesion: background and consensus recommendations from the College of American Pathologists and the American Society for Colposcopy and Cervical Pathology. *Int J Gynecol Pathol.* 2013;32:76-115.
18. Bornstein J, Bogliatto F, Kaefner HK, et al. The 2015 International Society for the Study of Vulvovaginal Disease (ISSVD) terminology of vulvar squamous intraepithelial lesions. *Obstet Gynecol.* February 2016;127(2):264-268.
19. Ireland D. The management of the patient with abnormal vaginal cytology following vaginal hysterectomy. *BJOG.* 1988;95(10):973-975.
20. Smeltzer S, Ua X, Schmeler K, et al. Abnormal vaginal Pap test results after hysterectomy in human immunodeficiency virus-infected women. *Obstet Gynecol.* July 2016;128(1):52.
21. American College of Obstetricians and Gynecologists. ACOG Committee Opinion No. 440: the role of transvaginal ultrasonography in the evaluation of postmenopausal bleeding. *Obstet Gynecol.* 2009;114:409-411.
22. Billingsley CC, Kenne KA, Casino CD, et al. The use of transvaginal ultrasound in type II endometrial cancer. *Int J Gynecol Cancer.* 2015;25:858-862.
23. Suh-Burgmann E, Hung YY, Armstrong MA. Complex atypical endometrial hyperplasia: the risk of unrecognized adenocarcinoma and value of preoperative dilation and curettage. *Obstet Gynecol.* September 2009;114(3):523-529.
24. Trimble CL, Kauderer J, Zaino R, et al. Concurrent endometrial carcinoma in women with a biopsy diagnosis of atypical endometrial hyperplasia: a Gynecologic Oncology Group study. *Cancer.* February 15, 2006;106(4):812-819.
25. Committee on Gynecologic Practice, Society of Gynecologic Oncology. The American College of Obstetricians and Gynecologists Committee Opinion No. 631. Endometrial intraepithelial neoplasia. *Obstet Gynecol.* May 2015;125(5):1272-1278.
26. Westin S. et al. SGO Annual Meeting Abstract 41, March 2016. Gynecol Oncol Vol 141, Supplement 1, June 2016. Challenging the paradigm of progesterone-only therapy for early endometrial cancer: results of a prospective trial of the levonorgesterel intrauterine system pages 18-19 Westin SN, Sun CCL, Broadus N et al.
27. Broaddus R, et al. Prospective phase II trial of the levonorgesterol intrauterine system (Mirena) to treat complex atypical hyperplasia and grade 1 endometrioid endometrial cancer. *Gynecol Oncol.* 2012;125:s9.
28. Gunderson CC, Fader AN, Carson KA, Bristow RE. Oncologic and reproductive outcomes with progestin therapy in women with endometrial hyperplasia and grade 1 adenocarcinoma: a systematic review. *Gynecol Oncol.* May 2012;125(2):477-482.
29. Hubbs JL, Saig RM, Abaid LN, et al. Systemic and local hormone therapy for endometrial hyperplasia and early adenocarcinoma. *Obstet Gynecol.* June 2013;121(6):1172-1180.
30. Gallos ID, Ganesan R, Gupta JK, et al. Prediction of regression and relapse of endometrial hyperplasia with conservative therapy. *Obstet Gynecol.* June 2013;121(6):1165.
31. Sideri M. Squamous vulvar intraepithelial neoplasia: 2004 modified terminology ISSVD Vulvar Oncology Subcommittee. *J Reprod Med.* 2005;50(11):807-810.
32. Massad L, Stewart MD, Fazzari J. Outcomes after treatment of cervical intraepithelial neoplasia among women with HIV. *J Low Genit Tract Dis.* 2007;11(2):90-97.
33. Moreno V, Bosch FX, Munoz N, et al. Effect of oral contraceptives on risk of cervical cancer in women with human papillomavirus infection: the IARC multicentric case-control study. *Lancet* 2002; 359(9312):1085-1092.

Tubo-Ovarian Cancer Screening

SCREENING TEST

A good **screening test** is both sensitive (high probability of detecting disease) as well as specific (high probability that those with disease will be identified). An ideal screening test has a sensitivity of 100% and a specificity of 95%. Screening tests are typically not designed to diagnose disease; rather, they identify subjects who need further diagnostic tests or procedures. A positive predictive value (PPV) of 10% or greater is the goal of any screening test. This means that 1 diagnosis per 10 interventions is needed for the test to be considered worthwhile.

CA-125

CA-125 alone has a sensitivity of 83%; specificity of 59%; PPV of 16%; and NPV of 97%.

HE4

HE4 alone has a sensitivity of 78%; specificity of 95%; PPV of 80%; and NPV of 99%. It has no sensitivity for borderline tumors.

RISK OF MALIGNANCY INDEX

- The risk of malignancy index (RMI) incorporates ultrasound findings with menopausal status (M) and the CA-125 level. It is written as: RMI = $U \times M \times$ CA-125. A score of either 0, 1 or 3 is given to the U. U=0 for an ultrasound with no features of malignancy. $U = 1$ for an ultrasound score of 1. $U = 3$ for an ultrasound score of 2 to 5. A score of either 1 or 3 is given for menopausal status. $M = 1$ for premenopausal women or $M = 3$ for postmenopausal women (19).
- On ultrasound, 1 point is given for each of the following morphologies: multiloculation, solid components, bilaterality, ascites, or intra-abdominal metastasis. The stated sensitivity is 81%, specificity is 85%, PPV is 48%, and NPV is 96%. If the calculated level of RMI is greater than 200, referral to a gynecologic oncologist is recommended.

MORPHOLOGY INDEX

- The Ueland morphology index (MI) assesses ovarian tumors based on tumor volume and wall structure. When the MI is less than 5, most adnexal masses are found to be benign with a NPV of 99%. If the MI is greater than 5, the PPV has been stated at 40% (1).
- The Kentucky University Algorithm has identified women at higher risk for ovarian cancer. A baseline ultrasound is obtained. If it is abnormal, it is repeated within 6 weeks. If the repeat ultrasound is found to still be abnormal, a CA-125

is drawn and the MI is calculated. The stated sensitivity is 85%, the specificity is 98%, the PPV is 14%, and the NPV is 99%. Disease was found at an earlier stage (i.e., stage migration) if there was strict adherence to these guidelines. 64% of cancers were found at Stage I (2).

RISK OF OVARIAN MALIGNANCY ALGORITHM

- The combination test of HE4 and CA-125 is called the **predictive probability algorithm** or **risk of ovarian malignancy algorithm (ROMA)**. This predictive algorithm is calculated for premenopausal and postmenopausal women separately, using the following equations. To calculate the algorithm the assay values obtained from the HE4 EIA and CA-125 II assays are inserted into the applicable equation.
  - Premenopausal woman:
    Predictive index (PI) = −12.0 + 2.38 × LN (HE4) + 0.0626 × LN (CA-125)
  - Postmenopausal woman:
    PI = −8.09 + 1.04 × LN (HE4) + 0.732 × LN (CA-125)
- To calculate the ROMA value (the predictive probability), insert the calculated value for the PI into the following equation: ROMA value % = exp(PI)/(1 + exp(PI)) × 100

The following cut-off points were used in order to provide a specificity level of 75%:
- Premenopausal women:
  - ROMA value ≥13.1% = High risk of finding epithelial ovarian cancer
  - ROMA value <13.1% = Low risk of finding epithelial ovarian cancer
- Postmenopausal women:
  - ROMA value ≥27.7% = High risk of finding epithelial ovarian cancer
  - ROMA value <27.7% = Low risk of finding epithelial ovarian cancer

This test is stated to have a sensitivity of 94%; specificity of 75%; PPV of 58%; and NPV of 97%.

RISK OF OVARIAN CANCER ALGORITHM (ROCA)

This test represents the slope of serial CA-125 levels drawn over a period of time and correlated with patient age. If there is greater than 1% change in the slope of the line, a transvaginal ultrasound (TVUS) is recommended. The UK ROCA study showed a PPV of 19% and a specificity of 99.8%.

COPENHAGEN INDEX

Copenhagen Index (CPH-I) uses the following variables: serum HE4, serum CA-125 and patient age instead of menopausal status, omitting ultrasound characteristics. Comparison of CPH-I, ROMA, and RMI demonstrated an AUC of 0.951, 0.953, and 0.935, respectively. Using a sensitivity at 95%, the specificities for CPH-I, ROMA, and RMI in the validation cohort were 67.3%, 70.7%, and 69.5%, respectively, in the validation study. The coefficients are CPH-I = −14.0647 + 1.0649 × log2(HE4) + 0.6050 × log2(CA-125) + 0.2672 × age/10. The predicted probability is = $e^{(CPH-I)}/(1 + e^{(CPH-I)})$ (3).

OVA-1 TEST

The OVA-1 test utilizes five well-established biomarkers: prealbumin, apolipoprotein A-1, beta$_2$-microglobulin, transferrin, and CA-125. A proprietary algorithm is used to determine the likelihood of malignancy in women with a pelvic mass for whom surgery is planned. The sensitivity is stated to be 92.5%, with a specificity of 42.8%, PPV of 42.3%, and NPV of 92.7%. It is important to remember not to perform this test if the patient has a rheumatoid factor ≥ 250 IU/L or has a triglyceride level >450 mg/dL.

OVARIAN CANCER SYMPTOM INDEX

The ovarian cancer symptom index (SI) associates specific symptoms with ovarian cancer. These symptoms are pelvic/abdominal pain, urinary urgency/frequency, increased abdominal size/bloating, and difficulty eating/feeling full. These symptoms become significant when present for less than 1 year and when they occur greater than 12 days/month. The overall sensitivity was 64% and specificity 88%. For women who are found to have early-stage disease, the sensitivity is stated to be 56.7%, and for women with advanced-stage disease it is 79.5%. When age stratified, the specificity is stated at 90% for women greater than 50 years old and 86.7% for women less than 50 years old (4).

- The SI in combination with a CA-125 has also been used to risk stratify adnexal masses. The combination of CA-125 and the SI has been shown to identify 89.3% of women with cancer, 80.6% of early-stage cancers, and 95.1% of late-stage cancers. The false-positive rate was 11.8% (5).
- The SI in combination with both CA-125 and HE4 has been found to have a sensitivity of 95% and specificity of 80%. If any two of the three tests were positive, a sensitivity of 84% and specificity of 98.5% were found. When all three tests were used, the specificity was 98.5% and the sensitivity was 58% (6).

THE UK COLLABORATIVE TRIAL OF OVARIAN CANCER SCREENING

The UK Collaborative Trial of Ovarian Cancer Screening (UKCTOCS) evaluated 202,638 women aged 50 to 74 years. They were randomized in a 2:1:1 ratio to: no treatment (101,299), annual screening with TVUS (50,623), and annual CA-125 (interpreted as a ROCA) with TVUS as a second-line test (50,624) (designated multimodal screening, MMS). MMS screening was performed using the ROCA algorithm including serial CA-125 level and ultrasound risk factors to include size, volume, and complexity of ovarian cyst. If ultrasound was abnormal, a repeat ultrasound was scheduled either at 3 months or 6 weeks depending on complexity assessment. The sensitivity, specificity, and positive predictive values for all primary ovarian type cancers in 2009 were 89.4%, 99.8%, and 43.3% for MMS, and 84.9%, 98.2%, and 5.3% for TVUS screening. In the MMS arm, 2.9 surgeries were needed per cancer detected, compared to 35.2 in the TVUS group. In the follow-up study published in 2015, the primary outcome was death due to tubo-ovarian cancer. The median follow-up was 11.1 years, and ovarian cancers were diagnosed in 630 (no screening), in 338 (MMS), and 314 (TVUS) women. The mortality reduction over years 0 to 14 using the Cox model was 15% with MMS, and 11% with TVUS, which were **not significant compared to no screening**. This mortality reduction was made up of an 8% relative reduction in mortality during years 0 to 7 (**NS**), and 23% relative reduction in mortality during years 7 to 14 in the MMS versus no screening, and of 2% (**NS**) and 21%, respectively, in the TVUS group versus the no screening group. The total number of surgeries was not reported but 488 benign surgical outcomes (false positives) were documented in the MMS group, 1,634 false positive surgeries in the TVUS group, with surgical complications of 3.1% in the MMS group and 3.5% in the TVUS group. **Prevalent cases of cancer were also removed** from the analysis. Additionally, 792 women in the no screening group, 466 in the MMS group, and 441 in the ultrasound group had a BSO outside of the trial, again confounding the results. The overall ratio of women who had surgery resulting in benign pathology to cancer was 1:2 (792/645) in the no screening group, 2:7 (954:354) in the MMS group, and 6:4 (2075:324) in the TVUS group. There was no total number of women reported who screened positive so we don't know how many surgeries were needed for false-positive screens (7,8).

THE PROSTATE, LUNG, COLON, AND OVARIAN (PLCO) CANCER TRIAL

This study compared CA-125 levels and ultrasound imaging versus observation in 78,216 women aged 55 to 74 with annual TVUS for 4 years and CA-125 for 6 years. 42 of 61 ovarian cancers were found, but 28 (67%) of these were advanced stage. The PPV was 1.1%; the number needed to treat was 20:1. 15% of patients had serious complications related to surgery. There was no evidence of stage migration. Additional data discovered in this trial revealed that 14% of postmenopausal women had simple ovarian cysts, at an 8% incidence; and 32% of these cysts spontaneously regressed. A 15-year follow-up reviewed mortality benefit between arms. Again, 39,105 women were randomized to the intervention arm and 39,111 were in the usual care arm. Median follow-up was 14.7 years in each arm and maximum follow-up 19.2 years in each arm. A total of 187 (intervention) and 176 (usual care) deaths from ovarian cancer were observed, for a risk ratio of 1.06 (95% CI: 0.87–1.30). Risk ratios were similar for study years 0 to 7 (RR = 1.04), 7 to 14 (RR = 1.06) and over 14 years (RR = 1.09). The risk ratio for all-cause mortality was 1.01 (95% CI: 0.97–1.05). Ovarian cancer specific survival was not significantly different across trial arms ($p = 0.16$). Conclusion: extended follow-up of women in the PLCO study indicated no mortality benefit from screening (9,10).

JAPAN SCREENING STUDY

Shizuoka Cohort Study of Ovarian Cancer Screening: this was a prospective randomized controlled trial of ovarian cancer screening. Asymptomatic postmenopausal women were randomly assigned between 1985 and 1999 to an intervention group ($n = 41,688$) or a control group ($n = 40,799$) in a 1:1 ratio. The mean follow-up was 9.2 years. Women in the intervention group had annual pelvic ultrasound and serum CA-125. Women with abnormal ultrasound findings and/or raised CA-125 values were referred for surgical investigation by a gynecological oncologist. 27 cancers were detected in the 41,688 screened women. Eight more cancers were diagnosed outside the screening program. Detection rates of ovarian cancer were 0.31 per 1,000 at the prevalent screen and 0.38 to 0.74 per 1,000 at subsequent screens; they increased with successive screening rounds. Among the 40,779 control women, 32 women developed ovarian cancer. The proportion of stage I ovarian cancer was higher in the screened group (63%) than in the control group (38%), which did not reach statistical significance ($p = 0.2285$) (11).

SERIAL ULTRASOUND OF OVARIAN ABNORMALITIES

In a prospective TVUS study, 39,337 women were included. Ovarian masses were categorized into: (a) normal, (b) simple unilocular cysts, (c) cysts with septations uni- and multicloculated, (d) cysts with solid areas, and (e) solid masses. Septated complex masses without solid areas or papillary projections had a 40% spontaneous resolution rate with a mean time to resolution of 12 months. Indications for surgical evaluation in this screened population were complexity of abnormality increased to cystic with solid area or mostly solid; an increase in volume greater than 50 cm^3 associated with constant or increasing complexity; or if new reported regional pain occurred after a second abnormal ultrasound. Resolution of ovarian masses did occur when followed serially. Resolution by category: unilocular cyst(s) 32.8% resolved at a mean of 55.6 weeks; cyst(s) with septation(s) 43.9% resolved at a mean of 53.0 weeks; cyst(s) with solid area(s) 76.5% resolved at a mean of 7.8 weeks; solid mass 80.6 resolved at a mean of 8.7 weeks. Low risk = unilocular and cysts with septations. High risk = cysts with solid area or solid mass. Thus it is helpful to not just have one ultrasound. Surgery was performed on 557 patients of 39,337 participants with 85 malignancies identified. The PPV for cancer rose from 8% to 25% by reducing false-positive results (12).

GOG 199

GOG 199 was a prospective study of women with confirmed genetic risk of ovarian cancer. At enrollment, women could choose to have ovarian cancer screening or undergo risk reducing surgery to include bilateral salpingoophorectomy. 2,605 women enrolled: there were 1,030 (40%) women in the surgical group and 1,575 (60%) elected to be in the screening group. The primary study outcomes was review of ovarian and breast cancer incidence, also including use of the Risk of Ovarian Cancer Algorithm. Nine neoplastic tubal lesions from 966 RRSO were identified, 8 of which occurred in *BRCA* mutation carriers (13,14).

OPPORTUNISTIC SALPINGECTOMY IN LOW-RISK WOMEN

No difference was found in ovarian function in premenopausal women undergoing hysterectomy versus hysterectomy and bilateral salpingectomy for benign disease. This was determined by assessment of anti-Müllerian hormone (AHM), follicle-stimulating hormone (FSH), antral follicle count, mean ovarian diameter, and peak systolic velocity on postoperative laboratories and imaging. There was no difference in operative time, postoperative stay, time to return to normal activity, and postoperative hemoglobin. Up to 700,000 women have a tubal ligation each year. This procedure can provide significant risk reduction opportunity (15).

OVARIAN CANCER RISK

Ovarian cancer risk after salpingectomy was evaluated in a population-based cohort study on women with prior surgery for benign indications compared to the unexposed population analyzed. The risk reductions for prior hysterectomy was hazard ratio (HR) = 0.79, sterilization HR = 0.72, hysterectomy with BSO HR = 0.06, unilateral salpingo-oophorectomy (USO) compared to

BSO 0.35; all CI did not cross 1. BSO had a 50% lower chance of ovarian cancer than USO (16).

Women who have any abdominal surgery and have completed childbearing could have opportunistic bilateral salpingectomy/salpingo-oophorectomy as an adjunct to surgery (i.e., appendectomy, cholecystectomy, hysterectomy). 15% of ovarian cancers could be prevented annually by BSO at time of hysterectomy. A staged surgery to preserve ovarian function can be performed by bilateral salpingectomy: a Denmark study reduced the risk of ovarian type cancer by 42%, and a Swedish study by 65% with bilateral salpingectomy (20,21).

CHANGING CA-125 "NORMALS"

Future "screening" could focus on detection of advanced stage ovarian cancer when the disease burden is low enough that surgical debulking can primarily achieve no residual disease followed by intraperitoneal (IP) chemotherapy. By making low volume advanced stage ovarian cancer (stage IIIA/IIIB) the target, rather than stage I, the threshold for CA-125 could be raised to 70 U/mL. This would reduce the sensitivity for detecting all ovarian cancers from 75% to 70% but increase the specificity from 95% to 99%. The PPV of a CA-125 at 70 U/mL is then 5%. If the cut-off were raised to 100 U/mL, the sensitivity would be reduced to 60% but specificity increased to 99.9% and the PPV would increase to 31% (17).

SCREENING PELVIC EXAMINATION IN ADULT WOMEN

The American College of Physicians (ACP) recommends against performing screening pelvic examinations in asymptomatic nonpregnant adult women. They cite three cohort studies of 5,633 women including the negative results of PLCO assessing the diagnostic accuracy of a pelvic exam in asymptomatic women mean ages 51 to 58. Only four cases of ovarian cancer were identified in 1 year with a PPV 0% to 3.5%. Examination related "harms" were pain or discomfort ranging from 11% to 60%; and 10% to 80% for fear, embarrassment, or anxiety. Care should be taken with interpretation, of this study (18).

REFERENCES

1. Ueland FR, DePriest PD, Pavlik EJ, et al. Preoperative differentiation of malignant from benign ovarian tumors: the efficacy of morphology indexing and Doppler flow sonography. *Gynecol Oncol.* 2003;91(1):46-50.
2. van Nagell JR Jr, Miller RW, DeSimone CP, et al. Long-term survival of women with epithelial ovarian cancer detected by ultrasonographic screening. *Obstet Gynecol.* 2011;118(6):1212-1221.
3. Karlsen MA, Høgdall EV, Christensen IJ et al. A novel diagnostic index combining HE4, CA125 and age may improve triage of women with suspected ovarian cancer - an international multicenter study in women with an ovarian mass. *Gynecol Oncol.* 2015 Sep;138(3):640-646.
4. Goff BA, Mandel LS, Drescher CW, et al. Development of an ovarian cancer symptom index: possibilities for earlier detection. *Cancer.* 2007;109(2):221-227.
5. Andersen MR, Goff BA, Lowe KA, et al. Combining a symptoms index with CA125 to improve detection of ovarian cancer. *Cancer.* 2008;113(3):484-489.
6. Andersen MR, Goff BA, Lowe KA, et al. Use of a symptom index, CA125, and HE4 to predict ovarian cancer. *Gynecol Oncol.* 2010;116(3):378-383.

7. Menon U, Gentry-Maharaj A, Hallett R, et al. Sensitivity and specificity of multimodal and ultrasound screening for ovarian cancer, and stage distribution of detected cancers: results of the prevalence screen of the UK Collaborative Trial of Ovarian Cancer Screening (UKCTOCS). *Lancet Oncol.* 2009;10(4):327-340.

8. Jacobs IJ, Menon U, Ryan A, et al. Ovarian cancer screening and mortality in the UK Collaborative Trial of Ovarian Cancer Screening (UKCTOCS): a randomised controlled trial. *Lancet.* 2016 Mar 5; 387(10022):945-956.

9. Buys SS, Partridge E, Black A, et al. Effect of screening on ovarian cancer mortality: the Prostate, Lung, Colorectal and Ovarian (PLCO) Cancer Screening Randomized Controlled Trial. *JAMA.* 2011;305(22):2295-2303.

10. Paul F. Pinsky PF, Yu K, Kramer BS, et al. Extended mortality results for ovarian cancer screening in the PLCO trial with median 15 years follow-up. *Gynecol Oncol.* November 2016;143(2):270-275.

11. Kobayashi H, Yamada Y, Sado T, et al. A randomized study of screening for ovarian cancer: a multicenter study in Japan. *Int J Gynecol Cancer.* May–June 2008;18(3):414-420.

12. Pavlik EJ, Ueland FR, Miller RW, et al. Frequency and disposition of ovarian abnormalities followed with serial transvaginal ultrasonography. *Obstet Gynecol.* August 2013; 122(2 Pt 1):210-217.

13. Greene MH, Piedmonte M, Alberts D, et al. A prospective study of risk-reducing salpingo-oophorectomy and longitudinal CA-125 screening among women at increased genetic risk of ovarian cancer: design and baseline characteristics: a Gynecologic Oncology Group study. *Cancer Epidemiol Biomarkers Prev.* March 2008;17(3):594-604.

14. Mai PL, Sherman ME, Piedmonte M, et al. Pathological findings at risk reducing salpingo-ophorectomy among women at increased ovarian cancer risk: results from GOG-199. *J Clin Oncol.* 2012;30(suppl; abstract 1519).

15. Morelli M, Venturella R, Mocciaro R, et al. Prophylactic salpingectomy in premenopausal low-risk women for ovarian cancer: primum non nocere. *Gynecol Oncol.* June 2013;129(3):448-451.

16. Falconer H, Yin L, Grönberg H, et al. Ovarian cancer risk after salpingectomy: a nationwide population-based study. *J Natl Cancer Inst.* January 27, 2015;107(2):dju410. doi:10.1093/jnci/dju410

17. Sopik V, Rosen B, Giannakeas V, et al. Why have ovarian cancer mortality rates declined? Part III. Prospects for the future. *Gynecol Oncol.* September 2015;138(3):757-761.

18. Qaseem A, Humphrey LL, Harris R, et al. Screening pelvic examination in adult women: a clinical practice guideline from the American College of Physicians. *Ann Intern Med.* July 1, 2014;161(1):67-72.

19. Jacobs I, Oram D, Fairbanks J, Turner J, Frost C, Grudzinskas JG. A risk of malignancy index incorporating CA125, ultrasound and menopausal status for the accurate preoperative diagnosis of ovarian cancer. *Br J Obstet Gynaecol* 1990; 97: 922-929.

20. Madsen C, Baandrup L, Dehlendorff C, Kjaer SK. Tubal ligation and salpingectomy and the risk of epithelial ovarian cancer and borderline ovarian tumors: a nationwide case-control study. *Acta Obstet Gynecol Scand.* 2015 Jan;94(1):86-94. Epub 2014 Oct 17.

21. Falconer H, Yin L, Grönberg H, Altman D. Ovarian cancer risk after salpingectomy: a nationwide population-based study. *J Natl Cancer Inst.* 2015 Feb;107.

GYNECOLOGIC CANCERS

2

CHARACTERISTICS

There are approximately 400,000 new cases of cervical cancer worldwide annually. In 2017 there were 12,820 anticipated new cases identified with approximately 4,210 deaths in the United States.

- The most common symptom of cervical cancer is abnormal vaginal bleeding—specifically, postcoital and intermenstrual bleeding, menorrhagia, and postmenopausal bleeding. Other symptoms include pelvic fullness/pain, unilateral leg swelling, bladder irritability, and tenesmus. Cervical cancer is also commonly asymptomatic, found only following an abnormal Pap smear, colposcopic exam, or cervical biopsy.
- Common signs of advanced cervical cancer are a fungating cervical mass, unilateral leg edema, and obstructive renal failure.
- Cervical cancer often results from persistent infection with high-risk HPV types (most commonly 16 and 18). Risk factors associated with cervical cancer are: prior history of sexually transmitted diseases (STDs), early age of first coitus, multiple sexual partners, multiparity, nonbarrier methods of birth control, and smoking.
- Cervical cancer primarily spreads by direct extension from the cervix to the parametria, vagina, uterine corpus, and the pelvis. Other routes of spread include lymphatic and hematogenous dissemination, as well as direct peritoneal seeding.
- Lymph node (LN) metastasis usually occurs in a sequential fashion, traveling first to the parametrial LNs, then to pelvic (obturator, internal, and external iliac), common iliac, para-aortic, then scalene LN.

PRE-TREATMENT WORKUP

The pre-treatment workup of cervical cancer begins with a history and physical exam. Laboratory studies to assess hematologic, renal, and liver functions should be performed. Imaging studies should also be performed to include pelvic imaging and a CXR (Figure 2.1).

- FIGO-approved imaging studies include barium enema, intravenous pyelogram, and chest x-ray. Other modalities such as CT (to assess LNs and evaluate for hydronephrosis), MRI (to assess integrity of tissue planes and extent of cervical disease), or PET/CT (to evaluate for distant metastasis) are non-FIGO-approved staging tests due to the poor availability of these imaging modalities in medically underserved countries. However, advanced imaging is important in depicting important prognostic factors and, when available, is recommended in addition to the clinical examination.
- Cervical conization should be used to evaluate microscopic disease. Conization can differentiate between microinvasive versus invasive early-stage disease.

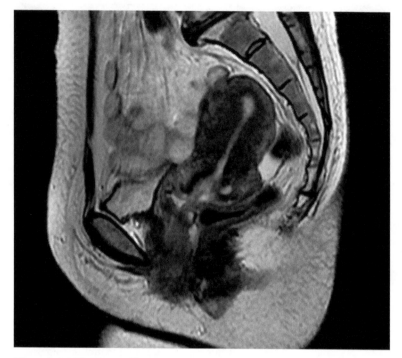

Figure 2.1 MRI of stage IIB squamous cell cervical cancer.

- For lesions that are macroscopic, an office examination or an examination under anesthesia (EUA) with cystoscopy and proctoscopy is indicated.
- If patients cannot tolerate an office exam, or if there is ambiguity about the staging in an office setting, an EUA should be performed. There are data to suggest that EUA can significantly change clinical staging: 23% were upstaged, most to IIA or IIB disease. Patients were down staged less often (9%) to IB2 and IIB. Proctoscopy was not found to be helpful, but cystoscopy identified 8% of patients with stage IVA disease, and a CXR was abnormal in 4% of patients (1).
- Multiple studies have supported the use of PET scans. An analysis of 15 published (FDG)-PET studies on cervical cancer showed that the pooled sensitivity and specificity of FDG-PET for detecting pelvic LN metastasis were 79% (95% CI: 65%–90%) and 99% (95% CI: 96%–99%), compared with 72% (95% CI: 53%–87%) and 96% (95% CI: 92%–98%) for MRI, and 47% (95% CI: 21%–73%) for CT (specificity not available). The pooled sensitivity and specificity of FDG-PET for detecting PA-LNs were 84% (95% CI: 68%–94%) and 95% (95% CI: 89%–98%) (2). A study from Israel (3) revealed a sensitivity of 60%, a specificity of 94%, a PPV of 90%, and an NPV of 74%. PET–CT may not pick up lesions smaller than 1.5 cm. There are data to suggest that treatment modification can occur in 25% of patients based on PET–CT results.

HISTOLOGY

There are several different histologic types of cervical cancer, the most common being squamous (85%). Other types include adenocarcinoma (15%–20%), verrucous carcinoma, adenosquamous carcinoma, clear cell carcinoma, neuroendocrine carcinomas, and undifferentiated types.

- Adenocarcinoma: about 15% have no visible lesion because the lesion arises from the endocervical canal, forming a "barrel-shaped" lesion. Cells frequently stain CEA+. Variants are the more common mucinous endocervical, mucinous intestinal type, signet ring type, and colloid variants. Adenoma Malignum/Minimal Deviation Variant has an infiltrative pattern distinct from those listed elsewhere with cytologically benign appearing cells on low power but moderate nuclear atypia seen on higher power and are seen in patients with Peutz–Jeghers syndrome. There is a three-tiered system developed to classify risk of LN metastasis developed by Silva et al. (4).
  - Pattern A: well-demarcated glands frequently forming clusters or groups with lobular architecture and lacking destructive stromal invasion or LVI. LN metastasis risk: 0%.
  - Pattern B: localized destructive invasion with small clusters or individual tumor cells within desmoplastic stroma often arising from pattern A glands. Often well to moderately differentiated. LVI ±. LN metastasis risk: 4.4%.
  - Pattern C: diffusely infiltrative glands and associated desmoplastic response. Confluent growth filling a 4× field (5 mm) or mucin lakes present, solid poorly differentiated component with LVI. LN metastasis risk: 23.8% (5).
- Verrucous carcinoma: this is a well-differentiated squamous cell carcinoma. It is known to recur locally, but does not metastasize. Historically, these tumors should not be treated with radiation therapy (XRT) because radiation can cause anaplastic transformation; however, recent evidence does not support this. It is associated with HPV6.
- Adenosquamous carcinoma: this is a mixed glandular and squamous carcinoma. It behaves similar to adenocarcinoma.
- Glassy cell carcinoma: this is a poorly differentiated type of adenosquamous carcinoma.
- Clear cell carcinoma: this is a poorly differentiated carcinoma. It is nodular and reddish in gross appearance. It has a hobnail cell shape microscopically. It can be associated with intrauterine DES exposure.
- Neuroendocrine carcinoma: this includes the small cell, large cell, and carcinoid (typical and atypical) carcinomas. Small cell is the most common neuroendocrine tumor in the cervix. It contains adenoid basal cells with scarce myoepithelial differentiation.
- Papillary squamous cell: this is a variant of squamous cell carcinoma. It appears as transitional or cuboidal cells on microscopy.
- Mesonephric adenocarcinoma: remnants of the mesonephric ducts are occasionally seen in the lateral aspects of the cervix, are PAS+, and do not contain intracytoplasmic mucin (Tables 2.1A–D and 2.2).

STAGING

T	FIGO	T criteria
Table 2.1A AJCC 8th Edition and FIGO 2009: T Category		
TX		Primary tumor cannot be assessed
T0		No evidence of primary tumor
T1	I	Cervical carcinoma confined to the uterus (extension to the corpus should be disregarded)
T1a	IA	Invasive carcinoma diagnosed only by microscopy. Stromal invasion with a maximum depth of 5.0 mm measured from the base of the epithelium and a horizontal spread of 7.0 mm or less. Vascular space involvement, venous or lymphatic, does not affect classification
T1a1	IA2	Measured stromal invasion of 3.0 mm or less in depth and 7.0 mm or less in horizontal spread
T1a2	IA2	Measured stromal invasion of more than 3.0 mm and not more than 5.0 mm, with a horizontal spread of 7.0 mm or less
T1b	IB	Clinically visible lesion confined to the cervix or microscopic lesion greater than T1a/IA2. Includes all macroscopically visible lesions, even with superficial invasion
T1b1	IB1	Clinically visible lesion 4.0 cm or less in greatest dimension
T1b2	IB2	Clinically visible lesion more than 4.0 cm in greatest dimension
T2	II	Cervical carcinoma invading beyond the uterus such as the vagina, but not the pelvic wall or to the lower third of the vagina
T2a	IIA	Tumor without parametrial invasion
T2a1	IIA1	Clinically visible lesion 4.0 cm or less in greatest dimension
T2a2	IIA2	Clinically visible lesion more than 4.0 cm in greatest dimension
T2b	IIB	Tumor has spread to the parametrial area.
T3	III	Tumor extending to the pelvic sidewall and/or involving the lower third of the vagina and/or causing hydronephrosis or nonfunctioning kidney
T3a	IIIA	Tumor involving the lower third of the vagina but not extending to the pelvic sidewall
T3b	IIIB	Tumor extending to the pelvic sidewall and/or causing hydronephrosis or nonfunctioning kidney
T4	IVA	Tumor invading the mucosa of the bladder or rectum and/or extending beyond the true pelvis (bullous edema is not sufficient to classify a tumor as T4)

Table 2.1B AJCC 8th Edition and FIGO 2009: N Category

N	FIGO	N criteria
NX		Regional LNs cannot be assessed
N0		No regional LN metastasis
N0(i+)		Isolated tumor cells in regional LN(s) not greater than 0.2 mm
N1		Regional LN metastasis

LN, lymph node.

Table 2.1C AJCC 8th Edition and FIGO 2009: M Category

M	FIGO	M criteria
M0		No distant metastasis
M1	IVB	Distant metastasis (including peritoneal spread or involvement of the supraclavicular, mediastinal, or distant LNs; lung; liver; or bone)

LN, lymph node.

Table 2.1D AJCC 8th Edition and FIGO 2009: Stage Grouping

When T is	And N is	And M is	Then the stage group is
T1	Any N	M0	I
T1a	Any N	M0	IA
T1a1	Any N	M0	IA1
T1a2	Any N	M0	IA2
T1b	Any N	M0	IB
T1b1	Any N	M0	IB1
T1b2	Any N	M0	IB2
T2	Any N	M0	II
T2a	Any N	M0	IIA
T2a1	Any N	M0	IIA1
T2a2	Any N	M0	IIA2
T2b	Any N	M0	IIB
T3	Any N	M0	III
T3a	Any N	M0	IIIA
T3b	Any N	M0	IIIB
T4	Any N	M0	IVA
Any T	Any N	M1	IVB

Source: From Amin MB, Edge SB. *AJCC Cancer Staging Manual* 8th Edition. Chicago, IL: American Joint Committee on Cancer. With permission.

Table 2.2 Cervical Cancer Overall Survival by Stage	
Stage	**5Y survival (%)**
IA	93
IB	80
IIA	63
IIB	58
IIIA	35
IIIB	32
IVA	16
IVB	15

TREATMENT

The treatment of cervical cancer may involve the use of surgery, chemotherapy, radiation therapy (XRT) or a combination of therapies. About 70% of newly diagnosed patients with invasive carcinoma of the cervix have disease limited to the uterine cervix and are, therefore, potential operative candidates. 54 to 84% of these patients will need adjuvant therapies for intermediate or high-risk factors; so thorough investigation of the full extent of disease should be performed. NCI statements support treatment with the fewest number of interventions; thus, if high-risk factors are found on conization, which predict a high probability for the need of adjuvant therapies, it may be prudent to not perform surgery.

- Treatment options by stage:
  - Stage IA1:
    - No LVSI: a simple (type I/extrafascial) hysterectomy or cold knife cone with 3 mm negative margins (if fertility-sparing treatment is desired) are adequate therapies. Intracavitary XRT can be used alone if the patient is not a surgical candidate. If margins on the CKC are positive, repeat CKC should be performed. Consideration of simple trachelectomy if fertility is desired is another option. If margins continue to be positive for carcinoma, a type II radical hysterectomy with pelvic LND can be considered.
    - LVSI: a type II (modified) radical hysterectomy with pelvic LND (P-LND) with/without para-aortic LND should be considered. Whole pelvic (WP) external beam XRT (EBXRT) with brachytherapy can also be considered. If fertility is desired, a cone biopsy with negative 3 mm margins with a pelvic LND, and consideration of para-aortic LND (PA-LND) should be performed. A radical trachelectomy with pelvic LND can also be considered.
  - Stage IA2:
    - A type II or type III radical hysterectomy with P-LND with/without PA-LND can be offered. Similar outcomes have been seen with both types of radical hysterectomy (6) or
    - Pelvic EBXRT with brachytherapy

○ Stages IB1 and IIA1:
  - A type III radical hysterectomy and pelvic LND with/without PA-LND can be offered with consideration of SLN mapping. Surgical candidates are those with lesions that are not bulky or barrel shaped.
  - Definitive treatment can also be primary external beam radiation therapy (EBXRT) and brachytherapy with concurrent cisplatin chemotherapy. Total dosing for XRT should be 80–85 Gy. Similar cure rates are seen with either radical surgery or XRT (7).
○ Stages IB2 and IIA2:
  - A combination of EBXRT and brachytherapy with chemotherapy is the standard of care. Patients with large cervical lesions staged IB2 have a high rate of needing adjuvant therapies after surgical approach and primum non nocere states the least injurious approach be the standard of care. Total dosing with XRT should be ≥85 Gy.
  - A type III radical hysterectomy with P-LND with/without PA-LND can be considered.
  - Surgical LN staging can be considered via extraperitoneal or transperitoneal laparoscopic LND. If negative, tailored field EBXRT and brachytherapy with concurrent cisplatin chemotherapy can be administered. If positive, then the need arises for EBXRT to cover the para-aortic and involved LN basins.
  - Surgery can be considered as adjuvant therapy in certain situations; for example, if there is residual tumor after definitive chemotherapy–XRT or uterine anatomy precludes adequate brachytherapy. Total dose with this approach is 75–80 Gy.
○ Stage IB2, IIA2, IIB, IIIA, IIIB, IVA: CT of chest, abdomen, and pelvis should be obtained:
  - If imaging shows adenopathy:
    □ Positive pelvic adenopathy but negative PA adenopathy: consider laparoscopic LND of pelvic and PA basins or fine needle aspiration (FNA) of suspicious LN:
      – If positive PALN: WP EBXRT and brachytherapy with extended field XRT concurrent with cisplatin chemotherapy.
      – If negative PALN: then WP EBXRT with brachytherapy concurrent with cisplatin chemotherapy (tailored fields).
    □ If no surgical LN evaluation is performed: WP EBXRT with brachytherapy concurrent with cisplatin chemotherapy with/without extended field para-aortic (PA-XRT) can also be considered.
    □ Positive pelvic and PA adenopathy on imaging: consider laparoscopic LND followed by WP and PA EBXRT to affected LN basins with brachytherapy, concurrent with cisplatin chemotherapy.
    □ If distant metastases are seen: systemic chemotherapy with individualized palliative XRT.
○ Stage IVB: chemotherapy should be used for disseminated disease and XRT can be considered for pelvic tumor control or palliation of symptoms including bleeding.

○ If cancer is incidentally found on a postoperative hysterectomy specimen:
  ■ Stage IA1 with LVSI or >stage IA2: imaging should be obtained with pathologic review:
    □ Negative margins and negative imaging:
      – WP EBXRT and brachytherapy with concurrent cisplatin chemotherapy should be offered or
      – A parametrectomy with upper vaginectomy and P-LND with/without PA-LND can be performed
    □ Positive margins or gross residual disease:
      – If imaging is negative for adenopathy: WP EBXRT with concurrent cisplatin chemotherapy with/without brachytherapy based on vaginal margins
      – If imaging is positive for adenopathy: consider debulking of grossly enlarged LN followed by WP and PA EBXRT with concurrent cisplatin chemotherapy with/without brachytherapy based on vaginal margins

- Most randomized trials included 5% to 8% of patients with adenocarcinoma, so they are applicable to cite in treating adenocarcinoma of the cervix.
- Margin status is important in conization. In one study evaluating adenocarcinoma in situ (8), 33% of patients with negative margins had residual disease at the time of hysterectomy and 14% had invasive cancer; 53% of those with positive margins had residual disease and 26% were found to have invasive cancers. In another study, which reviewed patients with invasive squamous cell cancer on conization (9), 24% of patients had residual disease if they had negative margins and 60% were found to have residual disease if they had positive margins.
- The incidence of positive LNs with squamous cell and adenocarcinomas is 5% for stage IA2, 15% for stage IB1, 30% for stage IB2, 45% for stage IIB, and 60% for stage IIIB.
- The incidence of adnexal metastasis with adenocarcinoma is 1.7% compared to 0.5% for squamous cell lesions. According to GOG 49 (10), this is a nonsignificant difference, and all patients with ovarian metastasis had evidence of other extra-cervical disease.
- The rate of an aborted radical hysterectomy for grossly positive LNs is approximately 7% to 8% (11). Per GOG 49, the rate of abandoned radical hysterectomy was 8.3%.
- If a positive LN is found at the time of radical hysterectomy, there are two management options: completion of, or abortion of, radical hysterectomy.
  ○ Some proceed and complete the radical hysterectomy. The rationale is that removal of bulky LNs leaves less residual tumor for XRT to sterilize.
  ○ Another study showed that the local recurrence and distant recurrence rates were not significantly different for LN positive aborted versus completed radical hysterectomy patients. The progression-free survival (PFS) was 74.9 months versus 46.8 months ($p = 0.106$) and the overall survival (OS) was 91.8 months versus 69.4 months ($p = 0.886$) (12). Potter (13) found similar outcomes and the trend favored definitive XRT. Leaving the uterus in situ can help with treatment planning and can move the small bowel out of the treatment field. Debulking of LN greater than 2 cm prior to abortion of hysterectomy may be beneficial additionally.

○ The number of positive LN affects OS. The 5-year survival (YS) decreases for each additional positive LN: 1 node (79%), 2 to 3 nodes (63%), 4+ nodes (40%) (14).

- Surgical staging in locally advanced cervical cancer may be beneficial. In one study, surgical staging of women with locally advanced cervical cancer was suggested to improve overall clinical outcome, as those with positive LNs had a modification in standard XRT fields in up to 43% of patients (15).

- LN debulking can potentially improve the 5 YS in patients with locally advanced cervical cancer (16). One study showed that if grossly metastatic LNs were resected, the survival of women in that group approached the level of those women who had microscopic LN involvement only (50%, 5 YS), which was significantly higher than the women with unresectable LNs (0%) (16). There was a 10.5% incidence of severe XRT-related morbidity and a 1% incidence of treatment-related deaths due to combined therapies.

- A cut through hysterectomy refers to a cancer either found incidentally on final pathology or resected without radical surgery. Treatment of a "cut through" can include adjuvant XRT or a radical parametrectomy. There are data to suggest that the 5 YS is better with adjuvant XRT versus radical parametrectomy with a 68.7% versus a 49% 5 YS. This is stage and margin dependent. The 5 YS for women staged IA2 and IIA was 96% (17), but was much lower for women stage IIB or higher who had a 5 YS of 28%.

- Hydronephrosis found on imaging predicts a worse OS and PFS. Relief of ureteral obstruction has been associated with improved survival. Management with stenting via cystoscopy from below, or antegrade from above, is beneficial for preservation of renal function and enabling full dosing of radiosensitizing chemotherapy (18).

SURGICAL TREATMENT

- Hysterectomy types: Piver classification I–V is based on the degree of resection of vagina, parametria, cardinal ligaments, and uterosacral ligaments (19).
  ○ Class I radical hysterectomy is the same as a simple hysterectomy. It is indicated for stage IA1 cervical cancers without lymphovascular space involvement.
  ○ Class II radical hysterectomy is a modified radical hysterectomy. It involves resection of the medial half of the cardinal and uterosacral ligaments. The uterine artery is taken at its junction with the ureter. The upper one fourth (or 1–2 cm) of the vagina is also removed. This results in a wider local treatment margin than a simple hysterectomy.
  ○ Class III radical hysterectomy is also called a Wertheim/Meigs–Okabayashi hysterectomy. Originally, Wertheim did not include lymphadenectomy, whereas Meigs and Okabayashi did. In this procedure, the cardinal and uterosacral ligaments are completely transected and one third to one half of the vagina is removed. The uterine artery is taken at its origin. The autonomic nerves for bladder and rectal function are also resected, which can result in a high incidence of prolonged or permanent bladder dysfunction (Figure 2.2).
  ○ Class IV radical hysterectomy is reserved for larger bulky lesions. This procedure involves completely transecting the cardinal and uterosacral ligaments at their origin. One half of the vagina is removed; therefore, sexual

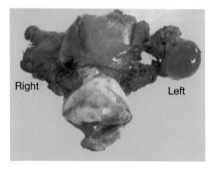

Figure 2.2 Type III radical hysterectomy.

dysfunction occurs from the shortened vagina. The superior vesical artery is sacrificed and all periureteral tissue is removed.

○ Class V radical hysterectomy is reserved for tumors that invade to the lower urinary tract. It involves the removal of involved portions of the bladder as well as the distal ureters.

• There are data to suggest for early-stage (IB–IIA) cervix cancer that there is no difference in recurrence rate or survival rate between class II or III radical hysterectomy. Surgeries took longer for the type III hysterectomies (6).

• A scalene LND is done if there is a question about distant metastasis. There are data to suggest that 10.7% of patients with positive para-aortic LNs have positive scalene nodes. PET scanning may be a reasonable alternative to a scalene LND (20).

○ The boundaries of the neck are the anterior and posterior triangles.

■ The anterior triangle is bordered by the sternocleidomastoid, the mandible, and the midline of the neck.

■ The posterior triangle is bordered by the sternocleidomastoid, the clavicle, and the trapezius. This is the larger triangle of the neck in which the scalene triangle lies.

■ The boundaries of the scalene triangle are the inferior belly of the omohyoid muscle, the sternocleidomastoid, and the subclavian vein. The scalenus anterior muscle lines the floor of the triangle. The phrenic nerve runs through the scalene triangle, as does the thoracic duct. If the duct is transected, it must be ligated at both ends to prevent a fistula.

• Other surgical techniques and indications:

○ Radical vaginal hysterectomy (Schauta–Amreich procedure) is performed in two stages. The first stage involves a retroperitoneal pelvic LND, most commonly via laparoscopy. The second step is to perform a vaginal radical hysterectomy.

○ Laparoscopic radical hysterectomy: this can also be approached with robotic assistance.

○ Radical trachelectomy:

■ This procedure is indicated in patients who desire fertility with tumors that are stage IB1 or lower, low grade histology, and that are less than 2 cm in maximum diameter. There are some feasibility data for tumors up to

4 cm. Of note, 60.7% of these patients had adjuvant therapies based on pathologic high pathologic risk factors to include XRT, chemotherapy, or both (21). Care should be taken with the larger and more aggressive histologic types. Neuroendocrine and adenoma malignum histologies fall into this category. Please refer to Chapter 6 for further fertility discussion.

- A radical trachelectomy involves the radical dissection and removal of the uterine cervix. This can be performed by either an abdominal, laparoscopic (with robotic assistance) or via the Schauta–Amreich vaginal approach. The cervix is amputated from the uterine corpus about 1 cm below the isthmus. An ECC is performed and sent for frozen pathology. If the ECC is positive, the radical hysterectomy is performed. If it is negative, a McDonald's or Shirodkar cerclage is usually placed at the time of surgery due to the risk of preterm labor from creating a shortened cervix. A Saling procedure, which advances the vaginal mucosa to cover the external os, can be performed at 14 weeks intrauterine pregnancy to reduce the risk of ascending infection. A separate LND can be accomplished via extraperitoneal laparoscopic or transperitoneal laparoscopic approaches. Only the parametrial nodes can be removed during the vaginal portion of the surgery.

- Specific indications for surgical therapy and not XRT include a current pelvic abscess, the presence of a pelvic kidney, or a history of prior XRT for other indications.
- Ovarian transposition can be considered in some patients who wish to preserve their fertility or preserve their ovarian function. Studies have shown 41% to 71% of patients maintained their ovarian function after XRT with ovarian transposition (22). Ovaries can migrate down and contraceptive therapy should still be encouraged if a salpingectomy is not performed.

RADIATION THERAPY

- Total dosing is prescribed to defined anatomical points. Please refer to Chapter 5 for an involved discussion. The point A total dose should be at least 80 to 90 Gy. The point B dose is at least 50 to 60 Gy. WP EBXRT is usually dosed at 45 to 50.4 Gy. Brachytherapy provides a dose with LDR of 40 Gy, or with HDR of 30 Gy. The HDR rates are $0.6 \times$ the LDR rate.
- The duration of treatment with XRT affects outcomes in cervical cancer. As treatment time lengthens, the OS decreases. The goal is completion of treatment within 56 days. There is a 1% per day decrease in survival if treatment goes beyond 56 days (Table 2.3).
- Chemotherapy is usually given concurrently with XRT. It can be given as cisplatin monotherapy dosed weekly at 40 or 50 mg/m² with a maximum of 70 mg, or as combination chemotherapy with cisplatin dosed at 40 or 50 mg/m² on day 1 and 5-fluorouracil (5-FU) dosed at 1,000 mg/m²/day as a continuous infusion for 4 days every 3 weeks. For neuroendocrine tumors, etoposide should be added to cisplatin: cisplatin dosed at 25 mg/m² IV days 1-3 and etoposide 100 mg/m² IV days 1-3 of a 21 day cycle.
- There is a 25% chance of needing adjuvant XRT following radical hysterectomy for intermediate risk factors in patients with stage IB1 disease. For stages IB2

Table 2.3 Radiation Therapy Outcomes for Cervical Cancer and Treatment Time Delay

Stage	Treatment time, (wk)	10-year pelvic failure, (%)	10-year disease-specific survival (%)
Stage IB	≤7	5	86
	7.1–9	22	78
	>9	36	55
Stage IIA	≤7	14	73
	7.1–9	27	41
	>9	36	43
Stage IIB	≤7	20	72
	7.1–9	28	60
	>9	34	65

and IIA disease, this possibly increases to about 80%. There are data to suggest that 54% of patients with a tumor less than 4 cm will need adjuvant XRT (7). For those with lesions greater than 4 cm in size, approximately 84% will need adjuvant XRT. Adjuvant XRT recommendations were based on pathological data to include: positive LNs, positive parametria, close margins, and less than 3 mm uninvolved stroma.

- The rate of XRT complications increases in dual therapy patients. In GOG 92, there was a 7% incidence of grade 3 to 4 hematologic, GI, or GU complications in patients who had pelvic XRT after radical hysterectomy versus 2% who received no further treatment (NFT) after radical hysterectomy (23). In the Landoni study, there was a 28% complication rate after radical hysterectomy with adjuvant XRT compared to 12% for definitive XRT alone.

ADJUVANT POSTHYSTERECTOMY TREATMENT

Adjuvant therapies are initiated by 6 weeks postoperatively. Risk factors are based on observational data from GOG 49 (24).

- **Intermediate risk factors** GOG 92 (23): XRT is recommended for intermediate risk factor patients. Please refer to Table 2.4 for risk factor combination that would lead to adjuvant therapies.
- **High-risk factors** GOG 109 (25): Combination chemotherapy (every-3-weeks cisplatin and 5-FU, or weekly cisplatin alone) and XRT are indicated for patients following primary surgical treatment with high-risk factors to include: one or more of the following risk factors: LN metastasis, positive (or close, 0.5 cm) margins, or positive parametria.
- A hemoglobin (Hg) goal of at least 9.4 g/dL has been shown to increase the 5 YS by 9% for patients undergoing XRT (26) but the use of red cell stimulants has been associated with a two times higher risk of DVT. Use of transfusion can increase the Hg but this can be associated with immunosuppression, in addition to the TACO or TRALI reactions. In head, neck, and breast cancers,

Table 2.4 Intermediate Risk Factors for Cervical Cancer Treatment Stratification

LSVI	Stromal invasion	Tumor size
Positive	Deep one-third	Any
Positive	Middle one-third	≥2 cm
Negative	Deep or middle one-third	≥4 cm
Positive	Superficial one-third	≥5 cm

LSVI, Lymphovascular space involvement.

Source: Adapted from Ref. (23). Sedlis A. A randomized trial of pelvic radiation therapy vs. no further therapy in selected patients with stage IB carcinoma of the cervix after radical hysterectomy and pelvic lymphadenectomy: a Gynecologic Oncology Group study. *Gynecol Oncol.* 1999;73(2):177–183.

the aggressive use of transfusion and growth factors has been associated with a poorer survival. GOG 191 (27) randomized patients to aggressive transfusion or red cell stimulation for patients undergoing concurrent chemotherapy and XRT to maintain Hg at or above 12 g/dL compared to the standard level of 10 g/dL. This study was closed early due to higher DVT/VTE complications.

ADVANCED DISEASE

Treatment options for stage IVB cervical cancer are limited. Chemotherapy alone or chemotherapy with palliative pelvic XRT are the two main options. Chemotherapy can include cisplatin in combination with a taxane, topotecan, gemcitabine, vinorelbine, and/or bevacizumab.

RECURRENT DISEASE

A full metastatic workup should be performed. If local recurrence alone is demonstrated, different surgical options exist. If there is extensive recurrent pelvic disease or distant metastasis, patients are often treated with chemotherapy and/or palliative XRT.

- Most recurrences are diagnosed within the first 2 years: 50% in the first year; 75% in the second year; 95% of recurrences are diagnosed in the first 5 years.
- "Triad of Trouble": signs of recurrence which indicate that a mass has reached the pelvic sidewall are:
  - Sciatica (compression/invasion of the sciatic nerve)
  - Lower extremity edema (compression of pelvic lymphatics)
  - Costovertebral angle (CVA) tenderness (hydronephrosis from compression/invasion of the ureter)
- Management is based on location, prior therapies given, and patient comorbidities.
  - Surgery:
    - Radical hysterectomy: can be considered if the recurrent tumor is less than 2 cm and limited to the cervix. The rate of complications is high, however, with fistula occurring at 50%, and patients having a 5 YS of 62%.

- Pelvic exenteration with/without intraoperative radiation therapy (IOXRT): total, anterior, or posterior. The 5 YS with positive pelvic LNs is 15% to 20% and this must be weighed with the morbidity of the procedure. There are certain patient selection factors that are important when considering exenteration: local extension, positive LNs, peritoneal disease, or malignant ascites are adverse factors related to decreased survival. One study found the following three risk factors predicted survival at 18 months: time to recurrence, size, and preoperative pelvic sidewall fixation.
  - Some protocols include consideration of resection of disease at site of failure in noncentral recurrent disease patients with/without IOXRT. This should be followed by systemic or tumor-directed (or both) therapy in most cases.
- Chemotherapy: cisplatin and paclitaxel showed an improved response rate compared to cisplatin alone (GOG 169). Topotecan and cisplatin also showed an improvement in PFS but not OS over cisplatin alone (GOG 170). The addition of bevacizumab to cisplatin and paclitaxel has shown further improvement in PFS and OS (GOG 240) (28).
- Radiation:
  - For radiotherapeutic curative-intent retreatment, patients can be broken down into three categories: central disease, limited peripheral disease, and massive peripheral disease. The central and limited peripheral disease patients are good candidates for curative intent, having a 30% to 70% chance for extended survival.
  - Patients who are candidates for salvage reirradiation include those who are medically inoperable, those who refuse surgery, or in whom surgery is not feasible.
  - External beam doses of 39 to 72 Gy, brachytherapy doses of 60 to 89 Gy, or combination XRT doses up to 90 Gy can be used. This yields 57% control for external beam, 67% for brachytherapy, and 44% for combination therapy (29). For recurrence in the para-aortic region, EBXRT can be delivered, but success rates for adenopathy greater than 2 cm are low. Therefore, resection with combination chemotherapy and XRT can be considered (30).
  - Interstitial XRT implants placed via laparotomy guidance have been reported to yield a 71% rate of local control with 36% of patients having no evidence of disease at follow-up.
  - In the palliative setting, Radiation Therapy Oncology Group (RTOG) protocols have given 3.7 Gy twice daily for two consecutive days at 3- to 6-week intervals repeated up to three times.
  - For palliative intent retreatment, the response rates are low and have a short duration. Combined modality retreatment with chemotherapy in addition to XRT can be considered. Platinum compounds, taxanes, and ifosfamide have a response rate of 20% with a median duration of 4 to 6 months.

Fertility sparing approaches: see Chapter 6 for algorithms.

SURVIVAL

- 5 YS by stage and histology:
  - Stage I: squamous 65% to 90%; adenocarcinoma 70% to 75%
  - Stage II: squamous 45% to 80%; adenocarcinoma 30% to 40%

- o Stage III: squamous 60%; adenocarcinoma 20% to 30%
- o Stage IV: squamous less than 15%; adenocarcinoma less than 15%

PROGNOSTIC FACTORS FOR SURVIVAL

- Stage I:
  - o LVSI (predicts LN metastasis)
  - o Size of tumor
  - o Depth of invasion (greater than half the thickness of cervix)
  - o Tumor volume (>500 mm^3)
  - o Presence of LN metastasis (decreases survival by 50%)
- Stages II to IV:
  - o Stage
  - o LN metastasis (decreases survival by 50%)
  - o Tumor volume
  - o Age
  - o Performance status

FOLLOW-UP

- Every 3 months for the first 2 years
- Every 6 months for years 3 to 5
- Annually thereafter
- The follow-up visit should include:
  - o A directed physical and pelvic examination
  - o An annual Pap smear without HPV testing is considered adequate surveillance
  - o A Pap smear is not performed within the first 3 months following XRT due to XRT-associated changes
  - o Consideration can be given to CT scan of the abdomen and pelvis every 6 to 12 months
  - o PET scanning can be considered

NOTABLE TRIALS IN CERVICAL CANCER

- GOG 49: was a prospective surgical pathological study of stage I squamous carcinoma of the cervix. 1,120 patients with stage IA2 or IB tumors were evaluated, 940 patients were eligible, 732 squamous cell tumors were investigated, and 645 patients underwent pelvic and para-aortic LND (PP-LND). Four risk factors were found on multivariate analysis as independently associated with a higher risk of pelvic LN metastasis: greater than one-third cervical stromal invasion, LVSI, tumor size greater than 4 cm, and age ≤ 50 years. On univariate analysis, parametrial involvement and grade were also found to be significant (31).
- GOG 71: showed that there is no improvement in survival with the addition of hysterectomy after XRT. This study evaluated 256 patients with exophytic or barrel-shaped tumors, measuring ≥ 4 cm, who were randomized to EBXRT and brachytherapy, or attenuated EBXRT followed by extrafascial hysterectomy. 25% of the patients had tumors greater than 7 cm. There was a 27% versus 14% decrease in the local recurrence rate, but there was no difference in the OS. The 5Y PFS was 53% for the XRT arm versus 62% for the XRT with adjuvant hysterectomy arm ($p = 0.09$). Disease progression occurred in 46% of

patients in the XRT arm versus 37% for the XRT with adjuvant hysterectomy arm ($p = 0.07$). XRT dosing was 80 Gy to point A in the XRT arm, whereas the adjuvant hysterectomy arm received 75 Gy to point A. The primary criticism of this study was that the adjuvant hysterectomy arm was underdosed. The study was powered for OS, with PFS as a secondary endpoint. For the subgroup with cervical lesions of 4, 5, or 6 cm, there was a borderline significance for PFS and OS in the adjuvant hysterectomy arm. Paradoxically, cervical tumors of 7 cm or greater had a worse survival when treated with adjuvant hysterectomy (32).

- GOG 92: with 12 years of follow-up, researchers looked at 277 patients with at least two of the following intermediate risk factors: greater than one-third stromal invasion, positive lymphovascular space invasion, or large clinical tumor diameter. These were all stage IB patients who underwent radical hysterectomy with LND and who had negative LNs and negative margins. 70% had tumors greater than 3 cm. 137 patients were randomized to adjuvant XRT (50.4 Gy) and 140 patients received no further therapy. Patients with any combination of two or more risk factors who were treated with XRT were found to have a decreased risk of recurrence. The recurrence rate was 15% with XRT versus 28% for those who were observed over 2 years, yielding a 47% decrease in recurrence risk. At 12 years follow-up, essentially the same decrease in recurrence was seen except for those patients with adenocarcinoma who had a significantly different recurrence of 9% versus 44%. There was no significant difference in OS (Table 2.4) (23,33)

- GOG 123: evaluated 369 bulky stage IB (at least 4 cm) patients who were randomized to XRT followed by hysterectomy versus XRT and concurrent chemotherapy followed by hysterectomy. XRT dosing was 45 Gy EBXRT followed by brachytherapy to a total dose of 75 Gy to point A for both groups. An extrafascial hysterectomy was performed 3 to 6 weeks after XRT. Chemotherapy was dosed with cisplatin at 40 mg/m² weekly for a maximum of six doses. With a median follow-up of 36 months, the 3 YS was 79% versus 83% with concurrent chemotherapy. The OS was 74% versus 83% with concurrent chemotherapy. The relative risk (RR) of death was 0.54. The recurrence rate was 37% versus 21% for the concurrent chemotherapy arm with a RR of recurrence of 0.51, favoring chemoradiation. Fewer patients in the concurrent chemotherapy arm had residual disease in the uterus (34).

- GOG 85: evaluated 388 patients with stages IIB to IVA disease. Patients were randomized to either XRT with hydroxyurea at 80 mg/kg twice weekly during XRT, or XRT with cisplatin at 50 mg/m² and 5-FU at 1,000 mg/m² × 96 hr infusion every 28 days. All had negative para-aortic LNDs. The RR of progression or death was 0.79 (95% CI: 0.62–0.99) in the cisplatin/5-FU (CF) group. There was also a decreased incidence of lung metastasis from 9% to 6% when platinum therapy was given. Survival was significantly better for the patients randomized to CF ($p = 0.018$) (35).

- GOG 120: evaluated 526 patients with stages IIB to IVA with negative para-aortic LNs who were randomized to three arms. XRT was administered concurrently with either hydroxyurea alone, hydroxyurea–5-FU–cisplatin, or cisplatin alone. The dose of hydroxyurea was 2 g/m² twice weekly when in combination and 3 g/m² twice weekly when given alone. The dose of cisplatin when used alone was 40 mg/m² weekly, and the dose of cisplatin with 5-FU was 50 mg/m² days 1 and 29. 5-FU was dosed as a 96-hour infusion of 1,000 mg/m². The RR of PFS or death was 0.55 to 0.57 for the cisplatin-containing groups. There was also a lower rate of lung metastasis with a rate of 3% to 4% versus 10% favoring the cisplatin-containing arms. The OS rate was significantly higher in the cisplatin groups than in the hydroxyurea alone group with RR of death of 0.61 and 0.58, respectively (36).

- GOG 109: evaluated 243 patients staged as IA2 or IB. All were status-post radical hysterectomy and had high-risk factors to include: positive nodes (85%) and/or, positive margins (15%), and/or or positive parametria (15%). Patients were randomized to pelvic EBXRT dosed at 49.3 Gy or pelvic EBXRT with concurrent chemotherapy consisting of cisplatin at 70 mg/m² and 5-FU of 1,000 mg/m²/day for 4 days every 3 weeks for four cycles, two cycles of which were given after completion of XRT. The projected 4Y PFS was 80% versus 63% favoring concurrent chemotherapy, yielding a hazard ratio of 2.01 for PFS and 1.96 for OS. The projected OS rate at 4 years was 71% with XRT alone and 81% with chemoradiation. The toxicity was higher (22% vs. 4%) in the concurrent chemotherapy arm. A reappraisal of the data suggested that concurrent chemotherapy was beneficial specifically for cervical lesions ≥2 cm and for patients with two or more positive LNs. The absolute improvement in 5 YS for adjuvant chemoradiation in patients with tumors ≤2 cm was only 5% (77% vs. 82%), while for those with tumors greater than 2 cm it was 19% (58% vs. 77%). Similarly, the absolute 5 YS benefit was less evident among patients with one nodal metastasis (79% vs. 83%) than when at least two nodes were positive (55% vs. 75%). Furthermore, this study also found that there was a significant difference with respect to histologies. Adenocarcinoma subtypes had a better PFS when treated with combination chemotherapy and XRT (25,37).

- GOG 136: evaluated 86 patients with confirmed para-aortic LN metastases clinically staged I to IVA. Radiation doses were WP-XRT 39.6 to 48.6 Gy, point A intracavitary doses of 30 to 40 Gy, and point B doses 60 Gy combined with a para-metrial boost. Extended field XRT was dosed at 45 Gy given with concomitant chemotherapy consisting of 5-FU 1,000 mg/m²/day for 96 hours and cisplatin 50 mg/m² weeks 1 and 5. The 3Y OS was 39% and the 3Y PFI was 34%. Extended field RT with concomitant chemotherapy is feasible with a 3Y PFI of 33%. 90% of the patients completed the study (38).

- GOG 165: evaluated clinically staged IIB, IIIB, and IVA cervical cancer patients who were treated with 45 Gy WP-XRT with a parametrial boost of 5.4 to 9 Gy using HDR or LDR. Standard therapy was weekly cisplatin 40 mg/m², and experimental therapy was prolonged venous infusion of 5-FU (PVI-FU) at 225 mg/m²/day for 5 d/wk for six cycles concurrent with XRT. The study was closed prematurely when an analysis indicated that PVI-FU/XRT had a higher treatment failure rate (35% higher) (RR unadjusted, 1.29) and a higher mortality rate (RR unadjusted, 1.37). There was an increase in the failure rate at distant sites in the PVI-FU arm. The 4Y PFS for the cisplatin group was 57% compared to 50% with the PVI-FU group (NS). The 4Y pelvic failure rate was 16% and 14% in the cisplatin and PVI-FU arms. The distant failure rate (including abdominal, para-aortic region, bone, liver, and lung) was higher in the PVI-FU group (29% vs. 18%). The PVI-FU group had a higher failure rate for lung metastases (9% vs. 5%) and abdominal failures (11% vs. 3%). Para-aortic failure occurred in only 7% and 5% of patients in the PVI-FU and cisplatin arms, respectively, despite the fact that only 18% of patients were surgically staged in the para-aortic region (39).

- RTOG-79–20: evaluated 337 patients with stages IB, IIA, and IIB disease without clinically or radiologically involved para-aortic LN who were randomized to external beam WP-XRT dosed at 45 Gy or WP-XRT at 45 Gy plus extended field XRT dosed at 45 Gy. Patients who received WP-XRT alone had a 44% 10Y OS compared to a 55% 10Y OS for patients who had pelvic and PA-XRT. Though not statically significant, the difference between the disease specific survival for the pelvic only XRT arm versus the pelvic and PA-XRT arm were 40% and 42%, respectively. 10 year locoregional failure rate was similar (35% for pelvic only and 31% for pelvic and PA). 10 year incidence of grade 4/5 toxicity in the WP-XRT only arm versus the pelvic and PA arm was 4% and 8%, respectively (40).

- RTOG-90–01: evaluated 380 surgically staged patients (IIB–IVA or IB–IIA > 5 cm in size, or those with positive LN) and randomized them to WP and para-aortic XRT with brachytherapy versus WP-XRT and brachytherapy with concurrent cisplatin and 5-FU (75 mg/m²/day 1 and 1,000 mg/m²/day on days 2–5, every 21 days for two cycles). The RR was 0.48 for recurrence favoring cisplatin-based chemoradiotherapy. Total dosing was 85 Gy to point A. The patients in the chemotherapy arm had an improved 8Y OS of 67% versus 41%, and a DFS rate of 61% versus 46%. The chemotherapy arm had a decreased locoregional recurrence rate of 18% versus 35% and distant metastasis of 2% versus 35%. The chemotherapy arm had a nonsignificant increase in PA-LN failures at 7% versus 4% (41,42).

- NCIC cervical cancer trial: this is the only trial to show no difference in survival with concurrent chemotherapy and XRT. 253 patients staged IB greater than 5 cm to stage IVA were included. This trial evaluated XRT versus weekly concurrent XRT and cisplatin (40 mg/m²) for 4 to 6 weeks. Criticisms of this study were that patients had a lower Hg level and longer treatment times. WP-XRT was dosed at 45 Gy with LDR at 35 Gy × 1 or HDR at 8 Gy 3 × versus the same XRT doses with weekly cisplatin at 40 mg/m² × 6. The 5 YS was 62% versus 58% NS (43).

- GOG 169: was a randomized phase III clinical trial with 264 eligible patients. It compared single-agent cisplatin at 50 mg/m² in patients with stage IVB, persistent, or recurrent cervical cancer to combination cisplatin and paclitaxel dosed at 50 mg/m² and 135 mg/m² every 21 days. The addition of paclitaxel improved the response rate (36% vs. 19%, $p = 0.002$) and PFS (4.8 months vs. 2.8 months, $p = 0.001$), but did not impact the median OS (9.7 vs. 8.8 months, $p = $ NS) (44).

- GOG 179: randomized patients with stage IVB, persistent, or recurrent cervical cancer to cisplatin 50 mg/m² q21d versus doublet therapy with topotecan 0.75 mg/m² days1,2,3 and cisplatin 50 mg/m² on day1, q21d. The PFS was 2.9 versus 4.6 months, favoring the topotecan–cisplatin combination. The OS was 6.5 versus 9.4 months ($p = 0.017$), favoring the platinum doublet. The response rate was 13% for cisplatin alone versus 27% for the combination. Febrile neutropenia occurred more often with the topotecan–cisplatin arm with 17% versus 8% of patients having complications. Grade 3/4 neutropenia occurred in 70% of patients on the topotecan–cisplatin arm. QOL measures were not significantly different between the two arms. The platinum/paclitaxel regimens were less toxic and easier to administer so these regimens are favored instead (45).

- GOG 204: evaluated 513 patients with stage IVB or recurrent cervical cancer. Four platinum doublets were evaluated. The control arm was cisplatin-paclitaxel. The experimental-to-cisplatin-paclitaxel HRs of death were 1.15 (95% CI: 0.79–1.67) for vinorelbine–cisplatin (VC), 1.32 (95% CI: 0.91–1.92) for gemcitabine–cisplatin (GC), and 1.26 (95% CI: 0.86–1.82) for TC. The HRs for PFS were 1.36 (95% CI: 0.97–1.90) for VC, 1.39 (95% CI: 0.99–1.96) for GC, and 1.27 (95% CI: 0.90–1.78) for TC. Response rates (RRs) for PC, VC, GC, and TC were 29.1%, 25.9%, 22.3%, and 23.4%, respectively. The trends for RR, PFS, and OS (12.9 vs. 10 months) lead to cisplatin/paclitaxel as the standard/preference with less anemia and thrombocytopenia (46).

- Gemcitabine–cisplatin concurrent chemotherapy for locally advanced cervical cancer. 515 patients with stage IIB to IVA disease were randomly assigned to arm A (cisplatin 40 mg/m^2 and gemcitabine 125 mg/m^2 weekly for 6 weeks with concurrent EBXRT dosed to 50.4 Gy in 28 fractions, followed by brachytherapy dosed 30 to 35 Gy and then two additional 21-day cycles of cisplatin, 50 mg/m^2 on day 1, plus gemcitabine, 1,000 mg/m^2 on days 1 and 8) or to arm B (cisplatin at 40 mg/m^2 weekly and concurrent EBXRT followed by brachytherapy). The PFS at 3 years was 74.4% in arm A versus 65% in arm B. The OS (log-rank $p = 0.0224$; hazard ratio [HR], 0.68; 95% CI: 0.49–0.95) and time to progressive disease (log-rank $p = 0.0012$; HR, 0.54; 95% CI: 0.37–0.79) were both better for arm A. Grade 3/4 toxicities were 86.5% in arm A versus 46.3% in arm B. Problems with this study: the primary endpoint was changed mid-study to PFS; the sample size of approximately 500 evaluable patients was based on the original OS primary endpoint of 436 deaths out of 500 patients at an 80% power (47).

- A second study evaluating cisplatin versus cisplatin–gemcitabine was performed in Asia. 74 patients with II–IVA cervical cancer or stage I–II with positive pelvic/para-aortic LN were included. Of these, 37 were randomized to weekly cisplatin at 40 mg/m^2 and 37 were randomized to weekly cisplatin at 40 mg/m^2 with gemcitabine at 125 mg/m^2 for six cycles. The 3Y PFS was 65.1% for cisplatin alone versus 71% for cisplatin-gemcitabine. ($p = 0.71$) favoring. The 3Y OS was 74.1% for cisplatin versus 85.9% for double therapy but crossed over at 5 years ($p = 0.89$) (48).

- GOG 191: studied 109 eligible patients with stage IIB to IVA cervical cancer with an Hg level less than 14 g/dL. Patients were assigned to concurrent weekly cisplatin and XRT with or without recombinant human erythropoietin (40,000 units SQ weekly) to keep the Hg level at standard levels of 10 g/dL versus ≥ 12 g/dL. Venous thromboembolism (VTE) occurred in 4 of 52 patients receiving chemotherapy and XRT compared to 11 of 57 patients treated with chemotherapy and XRT and erythropoietin, not all considered treatment related. No deaths occurred from VTE. The study closed prematurely, with less than 25% of the planned accrual, due to potential concerns for VTE events with erythropoietin (27).

- GOG 240: a total of 452 evaluable patients with advanced or recurrent cervical cancer were randomly assigned in a 2 × 2 factorial design to cisplatin 50 mg/m^2 and paclitaxel 135 to 175 mg/m^2 or topotecan 0.75 mg/m^2 days 1 to 3, plus paclitaxel 175 mg/m^2 on day 1. Patients were also randomized to bevacizumab 15 mg/kg. Cycles were repeated every 21 days until disease progression or toxicity. The primary endpoint was OS. The topotecan–paclitaxel doublet was not superior to the cisplatin–paclitaxel doublet. The HR for death was 1.20. The addition of bevacizumab to chemotherapy was associated with an increased OS of 3.7 months (17 vs. 13.3 months; HR for death 0.71; 95% CI 0.54–0.95; $p = 0.004$). and higher response rates (48% vs. 36%; $p = 0.008$). The addition of bevacizumab was associated with HTN grade 2 or higher: 25 versus 2%, VTE: 8 versus 1%, and GI fistula grade 3 or higher: 3 versus 0%. As a supplement, a QOL assessment was performed. The FACT-Cx TOI scores for the 309 completed questioners did not differ significantly between patients who received bevacizumab versus those who did not with a $p = 0.27$ (28,49).
- GOG 263/RTOG-1171: adjuvant XRT versus adjuvant chemoradiation in intermediate risk, stage I–IIA cervical cancer after primary radical hysterectomy and pelvic LND: comparator study is GOG 92. The primary objective was the effect of treatment on recurrence-free survival (RFS) with a secondary objective of OS. An estimated 534 patients were randomized to one of two treatment arms after radical hysterectomy and pelvic LND. Arm I: patients underwent pelvic EBXRT or intensity-modulated radiation therapy (IMXRT) 5 days a week for 5.5 weeks. Arm II: patients received cisplatin IV over 1 to 2 hours on day 1 and XRT as in Arm I. Treatment with cisplatin was once every 7 days at 40 mg/m^2 for up to six courses in the absence of disease progression or unacceptable toxicity. Inclusion criteria: pathologically proven primary cervical cancer I to IIA with squamous cell carcinoma, adenosquamous carcinoma, or adenocarcinoma initially treated with a standard radical hysterectomy with pelvic lymphadenectomy and the following pathological characteristics: positive capillary-lymphovascular space involvement and one of the following: deep third penetration; middle third penetration, clinical tumor ≥2 cm; superficial third penetration, clinical tumor ≥5 cm; negative capillary-lymphatic space involvement; middle or deep third penetration, clinical tumor ≥4 cm. Results pending (50).
- GOG 265: ADXS 11–001 Lovaxin C: advaxis consists of a recombinant strain of *Listeria monocytogenes* that secretes HPV 16 E7 protein, which has been attenuated by partial complementation of prfA, the transcriptional factor needed for expression of *Listeria* virulence. ADXS 11–001 (azalimogene filolisbac) uses a multi-copy episomal expression system to secrete a 76kDa fusion protein consisting of the first 417 amino acids of *Listeria* protein Listerolysin O (LLO) followed by the HPV 16 E7 protein. This induces an immune response that promotes a potent antitumor response targeting the E7 protein. The final results of 50 reviewed patients showed a 38% 12 month survival, which is a 52% improvement over the expected survival rate. The mean CR was 18.5 months ranging from 12.2 to 40.6 months. (51).
- JCOG0505: a phase III trial of 253 women with recurrent or metastatic cervical cancer showed that carboplatin/paclitaxel was not inferior to cisplatin/paclitaxel. The OS was 18.3 months for the cisplatin arm versus 17.5 months for the carboplatin doublet (HR = 0.994; 90% CI 0.79–1.25; $p = 0.32$). For patients who had not received cisplatin previously, the OS for the carboplatin doublet

compared to the cisplatin doublet was 13 versus 23.2 months (HR 1.57; 95% CI 1.06–2.32). Thus, carboplatin may be used in place of cisplatin as an equally effective alternative (52).

- Veliparib for persistent or recurrent cervical cancer: twice-daily oral veliparib (10 mg) was administered during once-daily IV topotecan (0.6 mg/m^2) on days 1 to 5 of each treatment cycle every 21 days until disease progression or toxicity. 27 women were enrolled: there were two partial responses (7% [90% CI: 1%–22%]), there were four with disease progression. Patients with low ICH expression (0–1+) of PARP-1 in their primary uterine cervix cancer were more likely to have a longer PFI (HR = 0.25; p = 0.02) and survival (HR = 0.12; p = 0.005) after veliparib-topotecan therapy. Clinical activity of a veliparib–topotecan combination was minimal in persistent or recurrent uterine cervix cancer patients (53).

- GOG 274/RTOG-1174: the OUTBACK Trial: this randomized phase 3 trial evaluated radiosensitizing cisplatin therapy with or without supplemental carboplatin and paclitaxel chemotherapy after definitive XRT in patients with locally advanced cervical cancer. The primary objective was OS with secondary endpoints of PFS, toxicities, and patterns of recurrence. Arm I: patients received cisplatin IV over 60 to 90 minutes on days 1, 8, 15, 22, and 29. Patients also underwent EBXRT once daily, 5 days a week, for 5 weeks. Patients then underwent high-dose rate, pulsed-dose rate, or low-dose rate intracavitary brachytherapy. Arm II: patients received cisplatin and underwent EBXRT and brachytherapy as in Arm I. Beginning 4 weeks later, patients also received adjuvant chemotherapy comprising paclitaxel IV over 3 hours and carboplatin IV over 1 hour on day 1 for four courses in the absence of disease progression or unacceptable toxicity. Eligible patients were diagnosed with FIGO 2009 stage IB1 and node positive, IB2, II, IIIB, or IVA disease suitable for primary treatment with chemoradiation with curative intent. Results pending (54).

- GOG/RTOG-724: a phase III randomized study of concurrent chemotherapy and pelvic XRT with or without adjuvant chemotherapy in high-risk patients with early-stage (1A2, IB, or IIA) cervical carcinoma following radical hysterectomy with high-risk pathologic features including positive pelvic LN, completely resected positive PA-LN, or positive parametria. Results pending.

- GOG 127v: phase II trial of nab-paclitaxel (Abraxane®) in the treatment of recurrent or persistent advanced cervix cancer. Nanoparticle, albumin-bound paclitaxel (nab-paclitaxel) was administered at 125 mg/m^2 IV over 30 minutes on days 1, 8, and 15 of each 28-day cycle to 37 women with metastatic or recurrent cervix cancer that had progressed or relapsed following first-line cytotoxic drug treatment. 35 eligible patients were enrolled, all patients had one prior chemotherapy regimen and 27 had prior XRT with concomitant cisplatin. The median number of nab-paclitaxel cycles was four (range 1–15). Ten (28.6%; CI 14.6%–46.3%) of the 35 patients had a PR and 15 patients (42.9%) had SD. The median PFS and OS were 5.0 and 9.4 months, respectively. The only NCI CTCAE grade 4 event was neutropenia in two patients (5.7%). Grade 3 neurotoxicity was reported in one (2.9%) patient. Nab-paclitaxel has considerable activity and moderate toxicity in the treatment of drug-resistant, metastatic, and recurrent cervix cancer (55).

- GOG 263: 534 patients with stage I–IIA cervical cancer were reviewed. All had ≥2 intermediate risk adverse pathologic factors (Sedlis criteria from GOG 92) after radical hysterectomy and pelvic LND. Patients were randomized to WP-XRT vs cisplatin at 40 mg/m^2 weekly and WP-XRT; Outcomes pending (56).

- Senticol 1: 133 patients with FIGO stage IA–IB1 cervical cancer were evaluated between 2005 and 2007 in this prospective feasibility study. All underwent laparoscopic radical hysterectomy and SLN identification. If the frozen section on the SLN was negative they were randomized to completion full pelvic and para-aortic LND or no further dissection. SLN identification was via combined technetium and patent blue injections. Histology included squamous, adeno, and adenosquamous carcinoma. 14% of patients had nodal micrometastasis. 9% of patients had adjuvant chemoradiation due to adverse prognostic factors. Five year results include: 8% recurred, 5% died of disease progression, there was no difference in PFS or OS, there were no false negatives (57).

- Senticol 2: 206 were patients randomized to radical hysterectomy with SLND with or without completion LND: 105 patients were in the SLN alone group and 101 were in the complete pelvic LND group. No false negatives were identified in the complete LND arm. 3 year follow up reviewed surgical morbidity and showed a 51.5% rate of morbidity compared to a 31.4% rate with SLND alone (morbidities not specified) (58).

- Laparoscopic Approach to Cervical Cancer (LACC) trial: a randomized phase II trial comparing outcomes in radical hysterectomy patients via laparotomy versus laparoscopy. Results pending (59).

- SHAPE Trial: a randomized trial comparing radical hysterectomy and pelvic node dissection versus simple hysterectomy and pelvic LND in patients with low-risk early stage cervical cancer. To demonstrate that simple hysterectomy and LND is not inferior to radical hysterectomy and LND in terms of pelvic relapse rate and is associated with better quality of life/sexual health. Results pending.

- INTERLACE Trial: INduction ChemoThERapy in Locally Advanced CErvical Cancer. A randomized controlled trial of carboplatin AUC 2 and paclitaxel 80 mg/m^2 weeks 1–6 followed by standard cisplatin-based chemotherapy at 40 mg/m^2 weekly with XRT weeks 7 to 13, versus standard cisplatin-based chemotherapy with XRT. Results pending.

- TAKO trial: a randomized controlled trial of weekly cisplatin at 40 mg/m^2 versus every 3 week cisplatin at 75 mg/m^2 in combination with XRT in locally advanced stage IIB to IVA cervical cancer. Results pending.

- TACO trial: is a randomized controlled trial of tri-weekly cisplatin at 75 mg/m^2 for 3 cycles with concurrent XRT in locally advanced cervical cancer compared to weekly cisplatin at 40 mg/m^2 for 6 cycles with XRT in patients staged IB2, IIB-IVA. Results pending.

REFERENCES

1. Massad LS. Assessing disease extent in women with bulky or clinically evident metastatic cervical cancer: yield of pretreatment studies. *Gynecol Oncol.* 2000;76(3):383-387.
2. Havrilesky LJ. FDG-PET for management of cervical and ovarian cancer. *Gynecol Oncol.* 2005;97(1):183-191.
3. Amit A. The role of hybrid PET/CT in the evaluation of patients with cervical cancer. *Gynecol Oncol.* 2006;100(1):65-69.

4. Roma AA, Diaz de Vivar A, Park KJ, et al. Invasive endocervical adenocarcinoma: a new pattern-based classification system with important clinical significance. *Am J Surg Pathol.* 2015 May;39(5):667-72.

5. Roma AA, Mistretta T, Diaz De Vivar A, et al. New pattern-based personalized risk stratification system for endocervical adenocarcinoma with important clinical implications and surgical outcome. *Gynecol Oncol.* 2016;141:36-42.

6. Landoni F. Class II vs. class III radical hysterectomy in stage IB–IIA cervical cancer: a prospective randomized study. *Gynecol Oncol.* 2001;80(1):3-12.

7. Landoni F. Randomised study of radical surgery vs. radiotherapy for stage Ib–IIa cervical cancer. *Lancet.* 1997;350(9077):535-540.

8. Wolf JK. Adenocarcinoma in situ of the cervix: significance of cone biopsy margins. *Obstet Gynecol.* 1996;88(1):82-86.

9. Greer BE. Stage IA2 squamous carcinoma of the cervix: difficult diagnosis and therapeutic dilemma. *Am J Obstet Gynecol.* 1990;162(6):1409-1411.

10. Delgado G. Ovarian metastasis in stage IB carcinoma of the cervix: a Gynecologic Oncology Group study. *Gynecol Oncol.* 1992;166(1):50-53.

11. Whitney CW. The abandoned radical hysterectomy: a Gynecologic Oncology Group study. *Gynecol Oncol.* 2000;79(3):350-356.

12. Ziebarth AJ. Completed vs. aborted radical hysterectomy for node-positive stage IB cervical cancer in the modern era of chemo-radiation therapy. *Gynecol Oncol.* 2012;126(1):69-72.

13. Potter ME. Early invasive cervical cancer with pelvic lymph node involvement: to complete or not to complete radical hysterectomy? *Gynecol Oncol.* 1990;37(1):78-81.

14. Magrina JF. The prognostic significance of pelvic and aortic lymph node metastasis. *CME J Gynecol Oncol.* 2001;6(3):302-306.

15. Goff BA. Impact of surgical staging in women with locally advanced cervical cancer. *Gynecol Oncol.* 1999;74(3):436-442.

16. Cosin JA. Pretreatment surgical staging of patients with cervical carcinoma: the case for lymph node debulking. *Cancer.* 1998;82(11):2241-2248.

17. Smith KB. Postoperative radiotherapy for cervix cancer incidentally discovered after a simple hysterectomy for either benign conditions or noninvasive pathology. *Am J Clin Oncol.* 2010;33(3):229-232.

18. Rose PG. Impact of hydronephrosis on outcome of stage IIIB cervical cancer patients with disease limited to the pelvis, treated with radiation and concurrent chemotherapy: a Gynecologic Oncology Group study. *Gynecol Oncol.* 2010;117(2):270-275.

19. Piver MS. Five classes of extended hysterectomy for women with cervical cancer. *Obstet Gynecol.* 1974;44:265-272.

20. Boran N. Scalene lymph node dissection in locally advanced cervical carcinoma: is it reasonable or unnecessary? *Tumori.* 2003;89(2):173-175.

21. Li J, Wu X, Li X, Ju X. Abdominal radical trachelectomy: Is it safe for IB1 cervical cancer with tumors ≥ 2 cm? *Gynecol Oncol.* October 2013;131(1):87-92.

22. Chambers SK. Sequelae of lateral ovarian transposition in irradiated cervical cancer patients. *Int J Radiat Oncol Biol Phys.* 1991;20(6):1305-1308.

23. Sedlis A. A randomized trial of pelvic radiation therapy vs. no further therapy in selected patients with stage IB carcinoma of the cervix after radical hysterectomy and pelvic lymphadenectomy: a Gynecologic Oncology Group study. *Gynecol Oncol.* 1999;73(2): 177-183.

24. Delgado G. Prospective surgical–pathological study of disease free interval in patients with stage IB squamous cell carcinoma of the cervix: a Gynecologic Oncology Group study. *Gynecol Oncol.* 1990;38(3):352-357.

25. Peters WA. Concurrent chemotherapy and pelvic radiation therapy compared with pelvic radiation therapy alone as adjuvant therapy after radical surgery in high-risk early-stage cancer of the cervix. *J Clin Oncol.* 2000;18(8):1606-1613.

26. Obermair A. Anemia before and during concurrent chemoradiotherapy in patients with cervical carcinoma: effect on progression-free survival. *Int J Gynecol Cancer.* 2003;13(5):633-639.

27. Thomas G. Phase III trial to evaluate the efficacy of maintaining hemoglobin levels above 12.0 g/dL with erythropoietin vs. above 10.0 g/dL without erythropoietin in anemic patients receiving concurrent radiation and cisplatin for cervical cancer. *Gynecol Oncol.* 2008;108(2):317-325.

28. Tewari KS, Sill MW, Long HJ III, et al. Improved survival with bevacizumab in advanced cervical cancer. *N Engl J Med.* February 20, 2014;370(8):734-743.

29. Russell AH. Radical reirradiation for recurrent or second primary carcinoma of the female reproductive tract. *Gynecol Oncol.* 1987;27(2):226-232.

30. Monk BJ. Open interstitial brachytherapy for the treatment of local-regional recurrences of uterine corpus and cervix cancer after primary surgery. *Gynecol Oncol.* 1994;52(2):222-228.

31. Delgado D. A prospective surgical pathological study of stage I squamous carcinoma of the cervix: a Gynecologic Oncology Group study. *Gynecol Oncol.* 1989;35(3):314-320.

32. Keys HM. Radiation therapy with and without extrafascial hysterectomy for bulky stage IB cervical carcinoma: a randomized trial of the Gynecologic Oncology Group. *Gynecol Oncol.* 2003;89(3):343-353.

33. Rotman M. A phase III randomized trial of postoperative pelvic irradiation in stage IB cervical carcinoma with poor prognostic features: a follow-up of a Gynecologic Oncology Group study. *Int J Radiat Oncol Biol Phys.* 2006;65(1):169-176.

34. Keys HM. Cisplatin, radiation, and adjuvant hysterectomy compared with radiation and adjuvant hysterectomy for bulky stage IB cervical carcinoma. *N Engl J Med.* 1999;340(15):1154-1161.

35. Whitney CW. Randomized comparison of fluorouracil plus cisplatin vs. hydroxyurea as an adjunct to radiation therapy in stage IIB–IVA carcinoma of the cervix with negative para-aortic lymph nodes: a Gynecologic Oncology Group and Southwest Oncology Group study. *J Clin Oncol.* 1999;17(5):1339-1348.

36. Rose PG. Concurrent cisplatin-based radiotherapy and chemotherapy for locally advanced cervical cancer. *N Engl J Med.* 1999;340(15):1144-1153.

37. Monk BJ, Wang J, Im S. Rethinking the use of radiation and chemotherapy after radical hysterectomy: a clinical-pathologic analysis of a Gynecologic Oncology Group/ Southwest Oncology Group/Radiation Therapy Oncology Group trial. *Gynecol Oncol.* 2005;96(3):721-728.

38. Varia MA. Cervical carcinoma metastatic to para-aortic nodes: extended field radiation therapy with concomitant 5-fluorouracil and cisplatin chemotherapy: a Gynecologic Oncology Group study. *Int J Radiat Oncol Biol Phys.* 1998;42(5):1015-1023.

39. Lanciano R. Randomized comparison of weekly cisplatin or protracted venous infusion of fluorouracil in combination with pelvic radiation in advanced cervix cancer: a Gynecologic Oncology Group study. *J Clin Oncol.* 2005;23(33):8289-8295.

40. Rotman M. Prophylactic extended-field irradiation of para-aortic lymph nodes in stages IIB and bulky IB and IIA cervical carcinomas. Ten-year treatment results of RTOG 79-20. *JAMA.* 1995;274(5):387-393.

41. Morris M. Pelvic radiation with concurrent chemotherapy compared with pelvic and para-aortic radiation in high-risk cervical cancer. *N Engl J Med.* 1999;340(15):1137-1143.

42. Eifel PJ. Pelvic irradiation with concurrent chemotherapy vs. pelvic and para-aortic irradiation for high-risk cervical cancer: an update of Radiation Therapy Oncology Group trial (RTOG) 90–01. *J Clin Oncol.* 2004;22(5):872-880.

43. Pearcey R. Phase III trial comparing radical radiotherapy with and without cisplatin chemotherapy in patients with advanced squamous cell cancer of the cervix. *J Clin Oncol.* 2002;20(4):966-972.

44. Moore DH. Phase III study of cisplatin with or without paclitaxel in stage IVB, recurrent, or persistent squamous cell carcinoma of the cervix: a Gynecologic Oncology Group study. *J Clin Oncol.* 2004;22(15):3113-3119.

45. Long HJ 3rd, Bundy BN, Grendys EC Jr. Randomized phase III trial of cisplatin with or without topotecan in carcinoma of the uterine cervix: a Gynecologic Oncology Group Study. *J Clin Oncol.* 2005 July 20;23(21):4626-4633. Epub 2005 May 23.

46. Monk BJ. Phase III trial of four cisplatin-containing doublet combinations in stage IVB, recurrent, or persistent cervical carcinoma: a Gynecologic Oncology Group study. *J Clin Oncol.* 2009;27(28):4649-4655.

47. Duenas-Gonzales A. Phase III, open-label, randomized study comparing concurrent gemcitabine plus cisplatin and radiation followed by adjuvant gemcitabine and cisplatin vs. concurrent cisplatin and radiation in patients with stage IIB to IVA carcinoma of the cervix. *J Clin Oncol.* 2011;29(13):1678-1685.

48. Wang CC, Chou HH, Yang LY, et al. A randomized trial comparing concurrent chemoradiotherapy with single-agent cisplatin versus cisplatin plus gemcitabine in patients with advanced cervical cancer: an Asian Gynecologic Oncology Group study. *Gynecol Oncol.* June 2015;137(3):462-467.

49. Penson RT, Huang HQ, Wenzel LB, et al. Bevacizumab for advanced cervical cancer: patient-reported outcomes of a randomised, phase 3 trial (NRG Oncology–Gynecologic Oncology Group protocol 240). *Lancet Oncol.* March 2015;16(3):301-311.

50. Gynecologic Oncology Group. Randomized phase III clinical trial of adjuvant radiation versus chemoradiation in intermediate risk, stage I/IIA cervical cancer treated with initial radical hysterectomy and pelvic lymphadenectomy. Available at: https://clinicaltrials.gov/ct2/show/NCT01101451. NLM identifier: NCT01101451.

51. Huh W, Brady W, Moore KN, et al. A phase 2 study of live-attenuated *Listeria* monocytogenes immunotherapy (ADXS11-001) in the treatment of persistent or recurrent cancer of the cervix (GOG-0265). *J Clin Oncol.* 2013;31(suppl; abstr TPS3121). DOI: 10.1200/jco.2012.30.15_suppl.tps5115

52. Kitagawa R, Katsumata N, Shibata T, et al. Paclitaxel plus carboplatin versus paclitaxel plus cisplatin in metastatic or recurrent cervical cancer: the open label randomized phase III trial JCOG0505. *J Clin Oncol.* 2015;333:2129-2135.

53. Kunos C, Deng W, Dawson D, et al. A phase I–II evaluation of veliparib (NSC #737664), topotecan, and filgrastim or pegfilgrastim in the treatment of persistent or recurrent carcinoma of the uterine cervix: An NRG Oncology/Gynecologic Oncology Group study. *Int J Gynecol Cancer.* March 2015;25(3):484-492.

54. GOG 274: A phase III trial of adjuvant chemotherapy following chemoradiation as primary treatment for locally advanced cervical cancer compared to chemoradiation alone: the OUTBACK TRIAL.

55. Alberts DS, Blessing JA, Landrum LM, et al. Phase II trial of nab-paclitaxel in the treatment of recurrent platinum-sensitive advanced cervix cancer: a gynecologic oncology group study. *Gynecol Oncol Dec.* 2012;127(3):451-455.

56. Ryu HS, Sugiyama T. 9th Korea-Japan Gynecologic Cancer Joint Meeting. *J Gynecol Oncol.* 2012; 23(1):3-4.

57. Mathevet et al SGO Annual Meeting National Harbor Maryland March 2017.

58. Mathevet, Lecuru et al. SGO Annual Meeting National Harbor Maryland March 2017

59. Queensland Centre for Gynaecological Cancer. Laparoscopic approach to cervical cancer (LACC). Available at: https://clinicaltrials.gov/ct2/show/NCT00614211. NLM identifier: NCT00614211.

Tubo-Ovarian Cancers: Ovarian, Fallopian Tube, and Primary Peritoneal

CHARACTERISTICS

- Upon review of pathogenesis for high-grade serous adnexal cancers and reflecting standard clinical practice, ovarian, fallopian tube, and primary peritoneal cancers have now been classified uniformly as high-grade serous tubo-ovarian cancers (HGSTOC). Sex cord stromal and germ cell tumors (GCT) are classified separately and considered to originate from the ovary itself. The more uncommon epithelial subtype origin is undetermined. One in 70 women will develop tubo-ovarian cancer in their lifetime. In 2017, 22,440 new cases are approximated with 14,080 deaths. As awareness has increased regarding the possible origin of HGSTOC, close histolopathologic review can identify the transition within the fallopian tubes from benign to serous carcinoma (Figure 2.3).

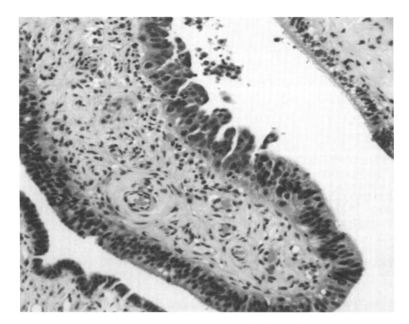

Figure 2.3 Serous tubal intraepithelial carcinoma (STIC) identified in a patient surgically staged as 3C HGSTOC.

- Serous tubo-ovarian cancer (STOC) is most commonly found in advanced stage: 84% of women present with stage IIIC and 12% to 21% present with stage IV disease. Most women die from bowel complications/obstruction.
  - ○ Symptoms include abdominal fullness, dyspepsia, constipation, tenesmus, pelvic fullness or pressure, bloating, and anorexia. Many of these make up the ovarian cancer symptom index.
  - ○ The route of spread for tubo-ovarian cancer is primarily transcoelomic. Cancer cells flake off the ovarian/fallopian tube surface and implant throughout the abdomen and pelvis. Other routes of spread are lymphatic and hematogenous.

PRE-TREATMENT WORKUP

- The pre-treatment workup includes a history and physical examination, lymph node (LN) survey, and laboratory tests, including a CBC, CMP, coagulation profile, CA-125, and other indicated tumor markers. A CXR is recommended in addition to abdominal/pelvic imaging (CT/MRI). Colonoscopy and esophagoduodenoscopy can be considered based on symptoms. Specific attention should be given to pain elicited during the pelvic exam, the presence of a mass that is fixed or solid, the presence of nodularity, and the overall mobility of the rectosigmoid colon and parametrium (Figures 2.4 and 2.5).

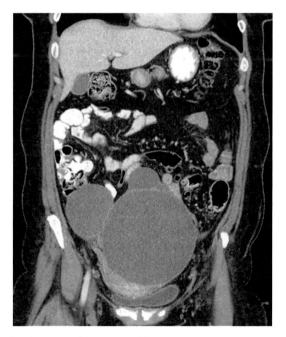

Figure 2.4 Ovarian cancer/pelvic mass CT.

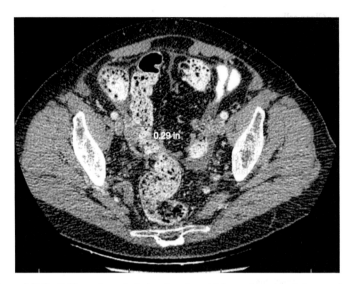

Figure 2.5 Partial large bowel obstruction from high-grade serous tubo-ovarian cancer (HGSTOC).

TREATMENT

- Primary treatment can be surgical (PDS-primary surgical debulking) or with neoadjuvant chemotherapy (NACT).
- Surgery usually consists of an exploratory laparotomy, abdominal cytology, hysterectomy, bilateral salpingo-oophorectomy, omentectomy, and cytoreduction.
- Patients with evidence of up to stage IIIB cancer should be surgically staged to include peritoneal biopsies and a pelvic and para-aortic lymph node dissection (LND). Three-fourths of advanced-stage cancers will have positive retroperitoneal LN. LN drainage tends to follow the ovarian vessels. Dissection around the high precaval and para-aortic regions is important.
- The definition of complete debulking is removal of all gross tumor to no residual visible disease (microscopic status): R0. Optimal debulking is removal of all gross tumor to less than 1 cm visible macroscopic disease: R1. Suboptimal resection is defined as remaining visible tumor with a diameter greater than 1 cm: R2.
- Surgical staging is often inadequate when performed by general surgeons (68%) or general gynecologists (48%), compared to gynecologic oncologists (3%).
- If neoadjuvant chemotherapy is chosen as primary treatment, surgical debulking should follow after 2–3 cycles of chemotherapy.

HISTOLOGY

- World Health Organization (WHO) classification of tubo-ovarian tumors:
  - Common epithelial
    - Serous: high grade and low grade
    - Mucinous
    - Seromucinous
    - Endometrioid

- Clear cell
- Brenner
- Mixed epithelial
- Undifferentiated
- Mixed mesodermal
- Unclassified
- ○ Sex cord stromal ovarian tumors
  - Granulosa stromal cell
    - □ Granulosa cell
    - □ Thecoma–fibroma
  - Androblastoma: Sertoli–Leydig cell tumors
    - □ Well-differentiated Pick's adenoma (Sertoli cell tumor)
    - □ Intermediate differentiation
    - □ Poorly differentiated
    - □ Heterologous elements
  - Lipid cell tumors
  - Gynandroblastoma
  - Unclassified
- ○ Germ cell ovarian tumors
  - Dysgerminoma
  - Endodermal sinus tumor
  - Embryonal carcinoma
  - Polyembryoma
  - Choriocarcinoma
  - Teratoma
    - □ Immature
    - □ Mature: dermoid cyst
    - □ Monodermal: carcinoid, struma ovarii
  - Mixed
  - Gonadoblastoma
- ○ Soft tissue tumors
- ○ Unclassified
- ○ Metastatic secondary tumors: 5% to 6% of adnexal masses are metastases from the breast, gastrointestinal tract, or urinary tract.

STAGING

FIGO staging was last amended in 2014. Staging is surgical (Table 2.5)

Table 2.5A AJCC 8th Edition: T Category		
T	FIGO	T criteria
TX		Primary tumor cannot be assessed
T0		No evidence of primary tumor
T1	I	Tumor limited to ovaries (one or both) or fallopian tube(s)
T1a	IA	Tumor limited to one ovary (capsule intact) or fallopian tube surface; no malignant cells in ascites or peritoneal washings

(continued)

Table 2.5A AJCC 8th Edition: T Category (*continued*)		
T	FIGO	T criteria
T1b	IB	Tumor limited to one or both ovaries (capsules intact) or fallopian tubes; no tumor on ovarian or fallopian tube surface; no malignant cells in ascites or peritoneal washings
T1c	IC	Tumor limited to one or both ovaries or fallopian tubes, with any of the following
T1c1	IC1	Surgical spill
T1c2	IC2	Capsule ruptured before surgery or tumor on ovarian or fallopian tube surface
T1c3	IC3	Malignant cells in ascites or peritoneal washings
T2	II	Tumor involves one or both ovaries or fallopian tubes with pelvic extension below the pelvic brim, or primary peritoneal cancer
T2a	IIA	Extension and/or implants on the uterus and/or fallopian tube(s) and/or ovaries
T2b	IIB	Extension to and/or implants on other pelvic tissues
T3	III	Tumor involves one or both ovaries or fallopian tubes, or primary peritoneal cancer, with microscopically confirmed peritoneal metastasis outside the pelvis, and/or metastasis to the retroperitoneal (pelvic and/or para-aortic) LNs
T3a	IIIA2	Microscopic extrapelvic (above the pelvic brim) peritoneal involvement, with or without positive retroperitoneal LNs
T3b	IIIB	Macroscopic peritoneal metastasis beyond the pelvis, 2 cm or less in greatest dimension, with or without metastasis to the retroperitoneal LNs
T3c	IIIC	Macroscopic peritoneal metastasis beyond the pelvis, more than 2 cm in greatest dimension, with or without metastasis to the retroperitoneal LNs (includes extension of tumor to capsule of liver and spleen without parenchymal involvement of either organ)
LN, lymph nodes.		

Table 2.5B AJCC 8th Edition: N Category		
N	FIGO	N criteria
NX		Regional LNs cannot be assessed
N0		No regional LN metastasis
N0(i+)		Isolated tumor cells in regional LN(s) not greater than 0.2 mm
N1	IIIA1	Positive retroperitoneal LN only (histologically confirmed)
N1a	IIIA1i	Metastasis up to 10 mm in greatest dimension
N1b	IIIA1ii	Metastasis more than 10 mm in greatest dimension
LN, lymph nodes.		

Table 2.5C AJCC 8th Edition: M Category

M	FIGO	M criteria
M0		No distant metastasis
M1	IV	Distant metastasis, including pleural effusion with positive cytology; liver or splenic parenchymal metastasis; metastasis to extra-abdominal organs (including inguinal LNs and LNs outside the abdominal cavity); and transmural involvement of intestine
M1a	IVA	Pleural effusion with positive cytology
M1b	IVB	Liver or splenic parenchymal metastases: metastases to extra-abdominal organs (including inguinal LNs and LNs outside the abdominal cavity); transmural involvement of intestine

LN, lymph nodes.

Table 2.5D AJCC 8th Edition: Stage Grouping

When T is	And N is	And M is	Then the stage group is:
T1	N0	M0	I
T1a	N0	M0	IA
T1b	N0	M0	IB
T1c	N0	M0	IC
T2	N0	M0	II
T2a	N0	M0	IIA
T2b	N0	M0	IIB
T1/T2	N1	M0	IIIA1
T3a	N0/N1	M0	IIIA2
T3b	N0/N1	M0	IIB
T3c	N0/N1	M0	IIIC
Any T	Any N	M1	IV
Any T	Any N	M1a	IVA
Any T	Any N	M1b	IVB

Source: From Amin MB, Edge SB. (2017). *AJCC Cancer Staging Manual* 8th Edition. Chicago, IL: American Joint Committee on Cancer. With permission.

EPITHELIAL TUBO-OVARIAN CANCER

CHARACTERISTICS

- Risk factors for epithelial ovarian cancer (EOC) include age (median age of 61 years), low or nulliparity, infertility, and genetic risk.
- Genetic mutations: the *BRCA 1* and *2* genes are located on chromosome 17q21 and 13q12-13, respectively. Mutations in these genes can cause autosomal

dominant inherited forms of familial cancer and yield a combined 80% overall risk of tubo-ovarian cancer; 11% to 25% of patients of serous TOCs harbor one of these mutations: Rad50/51C/51D, BRIP1, BARD1, CHEK2, MRE11A, MSH2, MLH1, MSH6, PMS2, PPM1Df, POLE, POL-D1, PALB2, 17SNPs, NBN, PALB2, TP53. Hereditary nonpolyposis colon cancer (HNPCC) yields a 10% risk of tubo-ovarian cancer and can present with other cancers such as endometrial cancer (60% risk), colon cancer (60% risk), and urothelial cancers.

- The use of oral contraceptive pills and pregnancy reduce the overall risk (relative risk [RR] = 0.66). OCPs also reduce risk for HGSTOC in carriers of genetic mutations.
- 10% to 14% of apparent early-stage ovarian cancers are staged IIIA1i/ii (based exclusively on retroperitoneal LN involvement).
- The ovaries can be "fertile soil" for metastatic disease. Metastatic disease can be distinguished from a primary ovarian tumor by the following: metastatic tumors to the ovaries are bilateral in 77% of cases, have multifocal and nodular implants, and often smaller in size. Primary tumors are commonly larger than 17 cm and usually unilateral (bilateral only in 13%).
- Terminology has been suggested to distinguish between low-grade and high-grade tubo-ovarian cancers. It is not universally adopted.
  - Type I tumors are the low-grade serous tumors. This is distinct from low malignant potential (LMP)/borderline tumors.
    - The annual incidence is 3.8%, with an overall survival (OS) of 99 months. Diagnosis is with low mitotic activity (below 12 mitosis/per 10 HPF [high power field]). 99% are found at stage III. Even with six cycles of chemotherapy, 88% of patients had stable disease (a 5% ORR). Nine percent respond to hormonal treatment. Bevacizumab has been shown to provide a sustained complete response (CR) in recurrent disease (1).
    - Type I tumors respond to chemotherapy, although not as vigorously as type II because chemoresistance is due to the low growth fraction. In an in vitro chemoresponse profile: 86% of tumors demonstrated a sensitive chemoresponse assay result to at least one agent, 35.7% were pan-sensitive to all seven standard cytotoxic agents: carboplatin, cisplatin, docetaxel, doxorubicin, gemcitabine, paclitaxel, topotecan (2). 23% of low grade (LG) STOC responded in an arbeitsgemeinschaft gynaekologische onkologie (AGO) database (3).
  - Type II tumors are the most common type of tubo-ovarian-type cancers, namely high-grade serous. 80% to 90% of HGSTOC respond to standard chemotherapies (Figure 2.6A and B).

PRE-TREATMENT WORKUP

Workup follows the general preoperative/staging workup as described earlier.

HISTOLOGY (Table 2.6)

- Serous carcinoma is the most common type of EOC. Serous cancers are graded in a two-tiered fashion: low grade and high grade. **Immunohistochemistry Profiling for STOC**: p53+, WT-1 positive, PAX-8 positive, ER/PR indeterminate, CK7+ (see Figures 2.6A and B)

- Clear cell carcinoma: these tumors are difficult to treat; 63% are refractory to primary platinum chemotherapy. There is an increased risk of deep vein thrombosis (DVT): 42% versus 18% when compared to serous histologies in one study (4). There is a 15% rate of venous thromboembolism (VTE) during primary treatment, and 9% occurrence at the time of recurrence in another study (5). The OS is approximately 12 months for patients with advanced-stage disease.
- Mucinous carcinoma tumors are often large and serum CEA can be positive. They have a higher rate of discordance between frozen and final pathology at 34%: 11% were downgraded and 23% were upgraded. This is due in part to their larger size. LN metastases are rare in apparent stage I cancers and an LND can potentially be omitted in these cases without adverse effect on progression-free survival (PFS) or OS (6). Appendectomy is still recommended to ensure primary tumor site identification.
- Brenner tumors: Brenner tumors of the ovary are relatively uncommon neoplasms, constituting 1.4% to 2.5% of all ovarian tumors. Histologically a Brenner tumor is characterized by varying numbers of rounded nests of transitional or squamous-like epithelium and glandular structures of cylindrical cells within

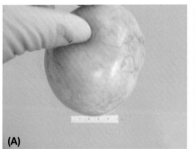 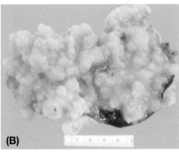

(A)   **(B)**

Figure 2.6 (A) Exterior of pelvic mass. (B) Gross bivalve of same pelvic demonstrating papillary projections of HGSTOC.

Table 2.6 Epithelial Ovarian Cancer Histological Subtypes

Histologic subtypes	Percent of malignant epithelial ovarian tumors	Percent bilaterality
Serous	46	73
Mucinous	36	47
Endometrioid	8	33
Clear cell	3	13
Transitional	2	
Mixed	3	
Undifferentiated	2	
Unclassified	1	
Brenner	1.5	

abundant fibrous nonepithelial tissue. Most Brenner tumors are benign, only 2% to 5% being malignant. Malignant components of the tumor show heterogeneous epithelial growth and atypia with intervening stroma, consist of transitional cells, squamous or undifferentiated carcinoma, or a mixture of these types. The criteria proposed by Hull and Campbell in 1973 are as follows (a): frankly malignant histologic features must be present (b), there must be intimate association between the malignant element and a benign Brenner tumor (c), mucinous cystadenomas should preferably be absent or must be well separated from both the benign and the malignant Brenner tumor (d), and stromal invasion by epithelial elements of the malignant Brenner tumor must be demonstrated.

STAGING

Follows FIGO and AJCC surgical staging protocols.
- Upstaging based on LN metastasis has been reviewed in 14 studies. The mean incidence of LN metastases in clinical stages I to II EOC was 14.2% (range 6.1%–29.6%) of which 7.1% were only in the para-aortic region, 2.9% only in the pelvic region, and 4.3% in both the para-aortic and pelvic regions (7). Grade 1 tumors had a mean incidence of LN metastases of 4.0%, grade 2 tumors 16.8%, and grade 3 tumors 20.0%. According to histologic subtype, the highest incidence of LN metastases was found in the serous subtype (23.3%), the lowest in the mucinous subtype (2.6%). Patterns of LN metastases were largely independent of laterality: among those with unilateral lesions and positive nodes, 50% had ipsilateral LN involvement, 40% had bilateral involvement, and 7% to 13% had isolated contralateral positive LN (8).

TREATMENT

Treatment is usually primary surgical staging with debulking if indicated, followed by adjuvant chemotherapy for all tumors staged greater than IA grade 1. Neoadjuvant chemotherapy followed by surgery can be considered for patients who are poor surgical candidates (large pleural effusions with poor ventilation capacity, severe congestive heart failure (CHF), recent myocardial infarction (MI), recent pulmonary embolus) or who have extensive disease that is potentially unresectable (based on operative skill, patient comorbidities, or risk scoring). Optimal debulking to no visible residual disease is the primary goal. Adjuvant chemotherapy treatment should start within 25 days of surgery. Each additional 10% cytoreduction of disease yields a 5.5% increase in median survival (9).
- Cytoreductive surgery for stage IV TOC can be attempted with 30% achieving optimal cytoreduction; 30% of patients can be expected to have complications (mostly infectious or wound). The preoperative performance status should be two or lower. Bristow et al (10) demonstrated that survival depended on location of the stage IV disease: the median survival for patients with a pleural effusion was 19 months, lung metastasis was 12 months, parenchymal liver metastasis was 18 months, and other extraperitoneal sites were 26 months. If patients had liver metastasis and had optimal intra- and extrahepatic cytoreduction to less than 1 cm, the median OS was 50 months; if there was optimal extrahepatic and suboptimal hepatic resection, the median OS was 27 months; and if there was suboptimal resection at all sites, there was an OS of 8 months.

- Removal of LNs for advanced-stage disease has been studied (11); 427 patients with stage IIB, IIIC, or IV all underwent optimal surgery, including removal of bulky LNs greater than 1 cm in diameter. Intraoperative randomization was performed and the control arm completed optimal surgery, whereas the treatment arm underwent additional retroperitoneal lymphadenectomy to remove pelvic (at least 25 nodes) and para-aortic (at least 15 nodes) LNs. After surgery, all patients received platinum-based chemotherapy. The 5Y progression free interval (PFI) was 31.2% for the LND group compared to 21.6% for those in the control arm. The LND group was more likely to require blood transfusions, had a longer surgery, and had more postoperative complications. At 68.4 months, 202 of the 427 patients had died. There was no difference in the risk of death: 48.5% of the LND group and 47% of the control group were alive 68.4 months after surgery.
- Predictive models for optimal surgical cytoreduction
  - Different presurgical models have attempted to stratify predictive values of various findings for optimal debulking versus candidacy for neoadjuvant therapy (ascites, carcinomatosis, tumor size, CA-125 level) but the proposed models usually fail with validation sets. False-positive criteria range from 10% to 68% for laboratory, clinical, or radiologic criteria. If there is progressive disease (refractory disease) while on NACT, a change in chemotherapy regimen should be considered. If the tumor has regressed, it is appropriate to surgically assess the patient and attempt surgical debulking.
  - A surgical assessment algorithm has been proposed with the potential to categorize patients by location and bulk of disease into theoretically optimally resectable versus not resectable, called: "scope and score" based on the Fagotti score. Care should be taken with this approach as surgeons are passionate about their surgical skill but can vary differently in their opinions and skill sets (12).
    - Fagotti score (seven parameters). Laparoscopic evaluation for feasibility of primary debulking surgery (PDS) versus unresectable to optimal disease status. If patients are deemed not optimally resectable, they are thus dispositioned to neoadjuvant chemotherapy (NACT). It was externally validated and modified by Brun (13) (Table 2.7)

Table 2.7 Scoring System for HGSTOC

Laparoscopic feature	Score 0	Score 2
Peritoneal carcinomatosis	Carcinomatosis involving a limited area (along the paracolic gutter or the pelvic peritoneum) and surgically removable by peritonectomy	Unresectable massive peritoneal involvement as well as with a military pattern of distribution
Diaphragmatic disease	No infiltrating carcinomatosis and nodules confluent with the most part of the diaphragmatic surface	Widespread infiltrating carcinomatosis or nodules confluent with the most part of the diaphragmatic surface

(continued)

Table 2.7 Scoring System for HGSTOC (*continued*)

Laparoscopic feature	Score 0	Score 2
Mesenteric disease	No large infiltrating nodules and no involvement of the root of the mesentery as would be indicated by limited movement of the various intestinal segments	Large infiltrating nodules or involvement of the root of the mesentery indicated by limited movement of the various intestinal segments
Omental disease	No tumor diffusion observed along the omentum up to the large stomach curvature	Tumor diffusion observed along the omentum up to the large stomach curvature
Bowel infiltration	No bowel resection was assumed and no military carcinomatosis on the ansae observed	Bowel resection assumed or military carcinomatosis on the ansae observed
Stomach infiltration	No obvious neoplastic involvement of the gastric wall	Obvious neoplastic involvement of the gastric wall
Liver metastasis	No surface lesions	Any surface lesion

HGSTOC, high grade serous tubo-ovarian cancers.

- If tubo-ovarian cancer is diagnosed incidentally after a TH-BSO without staging, surgical staging should be considered within 3 weeks. The risk of undiagnosed higher-stage disease is 22% to 29% (14); 4% to 25% of unstaged clinical stage I ovarian cancers have positive LNs, and the incidence of isolated contralateral positive LNs ranges from 7% to 13%.

- The timing of ovarian cyst rupture can make a difference. According to one study (15), preoperative cyst rupture had a larger influence on PFS than intraoperative cyst rupture. For preoperative cyst rupture, the hazard ratio (HR) for OS was 2.65 versus 1.64 for intraoperative cyst rupture (16).

- Tumor biology: the impact of disease distribution in stage III ovarian cancer patients was evaluated (17): 417 patients from three randomized Gynecologic Oncology Group (GOG) trials who were microscopically cytoreduced and given adjuvant IV platinum/paclitaxel were reviewed. Patients were divided into three groups based on preoperative disease burden: minimal disease (MD) was defined by pelvic tumor and retroperitoneal metastasis; abdominal peritoneal disease (APD) was considered disease limited to the pelvis, retroperitoneum, lower abdomen, and omentum; and upper abdominal disease (UAD) was considered disease affecting the diaphragm, spleen, liver, or pancreas. The median OS was not reached in MD patients, 80 months in the APD group, and 56 months in the UAD group ($p < 0.05$). The 5Y survival (YS) was 67% for MD group, 63% for APD and 45% for UAD. In multivariate analysis, the UAD group had a significantly worse prognosis than MD and APD both individually and combined (PFS HR 1.44; $p = 0.008$ and OS HR 1.77; $p = 0.0004$). Thus, it is suggested that there is a biological difference in ovarian cancer patients proportional to the amount of disease at presentation.

CHEMOTHERAPY FOR EPITHELIAL TUBO-OVARIAN CANCER

- **First-line chemotherapy** involves platinum-based chemotherapy regimens with a taxane. Single-agent platinum regimens can be considered in older or compromised patients.
- **Second-line agents** are used when cancer recurs after first-line therapy has been given.
  - **Platinum-sensitive and platinum-resistant disease**. This is defined based on disease recurrence in relation to the 6 month time period following completion of first-line platinum-based chemotherapy.
    - Platinum sensitive disease: tumor has recurred but more than 6 months has elapsed since primary treatment with platinum-containing regimens. Second line chemotherapy with platinum-based regimens should be used.
    - Platinum resistance is defined as: disease recurrence occurring less than 6 months after completion of primary platinum-based treatment. If recurrence occurs at less than 6 months, non–platinum-based salvage therapies should be used.
    - Platinum refractory is defined as: patients who have progressive disease while on chemotherapy.
    - Response rates for second-line chemotherapy depend on the time to recurrence after primary chemotherapy. The longer the interval from primary therapy, the better the response rate: 6 to 12 months, 27%; 13 to 24 months, 33%; greater than 24 months, 59%
- **Neoadjuvant chemotherapy** is chemotherapy given prior to surgery. Surgery is usually attempted after two to three cycles of chemotherapy. This has been shown to reduce the radical nature of surgery with a decreased risk of colostomy and hemorrhage.
- **Consolidation:** chemotherapy that is used after primary or adjuvant chemotherapy to decrease the chance of cancer recurrence in patients with complete clinical remission (CCR). This is usually a short duration of treatment.
- **Maintenance:** chemotherapy that is used after primary or adjuvant chemotherapy to decrease the chance of cancer recurrence in patients with CCR. This is usually of a longer duration than consolidation therapy.
- **Intraperitoneal (IP) chemotherapy:** chemotherapy is administered directly into the abdominal cavity. IP chemotherapy using platinum and taxane regimens is indicated for optimally debulked patients stage II or higher.
- **Intraoperative hyperthermic intraperitoneal chemotherapy (HIPEC):** heated cytotoxic regimens are administered at the time of primary or recurrent debulking surgery and circulated intraperitoneally for a specific amount of time.
  - Benefits:
    - A high volume of chemotherapy can be delivered, and a homogeneous distribution can be achieved. This is often not practical in conventional IP therapy, because of abdominal distension and pain, but it is feasible in HIPEC, since the patient is under anesthesia.

- There is no interval between cytoreduction and chemotherapy. The cytotoxic therapy is applied at the time of minimal disease manifestation, and there are no adhesions that might alter the distribution of the drug.
- Hyperthermia (>41°C) has a pharmacokinetic benefit. Several studies have convincingly shown that hyperthermia can increase both the tumor penetration of cisplatin as well as DNA crosslinking.
- High concentrations of chemotherapy can be achieved in the IP compartment with low systemic exposure—in a single intraoperative treatment.
- There is the mechanical continuous flow of perfusion solution.
  - Many combinations of cytotoxic agents have been used:
    - Single agents to include: carboplatin 800 mg/m^2 for 60 to 120 minutes at 41°C to 43°C; oxaliplatin 460 mg/m^2 for 30 minutes; cisplatin 100 mg/m^2 for 90 minutes at 41°C to 43°C.
    - Cisplatin 350 mg/m^2 and alpha-interferon 5 million IU/m^2 and for 90 minutes at 43°C to 44°C; cisplatin 100 mg/m^2 and mitomycin C 15 mg/m^2 for 60 minutes at 41°C to 43°C; paclitaxel 60 to 75 mg/m^2 and cisplatin 100 mg/m^2 or doxorubicin 0.1 mg/kg (if platinum resistant) for 120 minutes at 40°C to 43°C.
  - However, the absence of sufficient levels of scientific evidence to support the use of HIPEC in patients with tubo-ovarian cancer with peritoneal dissemination does not allow a general recommendation outside of clinical trials.

TREATMENT BY STAGE

- Stage IA grade 1 tumors: surgery is definitive. If fertility preservation is a concern, consider leaving the uterus and contralateral tube and ovary.
- Stage IA, grade 2 or 3 and stage IB and IC, any grade: primary treatment is surgery. If fertility is a concern, consider leaving the uterus and contralateral tube and ovary. Adjuvant chemotherapy is platinum based with a taxane for three to six cycles.
- Stages II, III, IV: either NACT or PDS may be offered. NACT has been shown to offer lower peri- and postoperative morbidity but PDS may offer superior survival (18).
  - Primary treatment is surgery (PDS). Adjuvant chemotherapy is platinum based with a taxane for six cycles. This can be administered IV or IP/IV.
  - Consideration can be given to neoadjuvant chemotherapy for:
    - The medically unfit or high perioperative risk patient.
    - Per surgical risk assessment score (Fagotti).

SECOND-LOOK LAPAROTOMY

- Second-look laparotomy is the pathological surgical assessment for residual disease after primary adjuvant chemotherapy in a patient with a clinical complete response. It is used to guide decisions for either continuing chemotherapy, changing chemotherapy, or discontinuing chemotherapy. It can also be used to guide treatment in patients who were suboptimally debulked, or who were primarily unstaged. Routine second-look laparotomy is not the current standard of care; 40% of second-look patients are pathologically positive, and of those who are negative, 50% will recur (see Table 2.8) (19).

Table 2.8 Second-Look Laparotomy for HGSTOC 5 YS Outcomes	
Second-look laparotomy disease status	**5Y survival (%)**
No evidence of disease	50
Microscopic	35
Macroscopic	5

RECURRENCE

- Most recurrences occur within the first 2 years. The risk of recurrence for a grade 1, stage I ovarian cancer is less than 10%. The risk of recurrence for stage III ovarian cancer is much higher, over 50%.

SECONDARY CYTOREDUCTION

- Secondary cytoreduction is the removal of gross recurrent disease after primary or secondary chemotherapy. There are some criteria attributed to Chi, which help stratify patients as appropriate surgical candidates. These are based on time, location, and number of recurrent tumor sites. If the recurrence occurs at greater than 30 months from primary chemotherapy, secondary cytoreduction can be attempted regardless of number of involved sites. If the interval is less than 30 months, and there are one to two sites of recurrence, cytoreduction can again be attempted. If there is carcinomatosis, ascites, or the patient is platinum resistant, it is often not wise to attempt secondary cytoreduction. For those who had less than 0.5 cm of residual disease after secondary cytoreduction, an improvement in OS to 56 months was seen versus 27 months for those who were suboptimally debulked. The overall success at secondary optimal cytoreduction ranges between 24% and 84% (20).

CEREBELLAR DEGENERATION

- Cerebellar degeneration can occur from antibodies to ovarian cancer. This is called **paraneoplastic cerebellar degeneration.** The incidence is 2:1,000 patients with gynecologic cancers. There are two main antibodies: the anti-Yo antibody reacts against the Purkinje cells and the anti-Hu antibody reacts against all neurons.

SURVIVAL

- Relative survival
- 2 YS: 65%; 5 YS: 44%; 10 YS: 36% (21) (Tables 2.9 and 2.10)
- 10 YS: 31% of women survive more than 10 years. Younger age, early stage, low grade, and nonserous histology are significant predictors of long-term survival. One third of those who survived to 10 years had stages III or IV per 1989 staging, 16% of patients with late-stage serous cancer survived more than 10 years (22).

Table 2.9 HGSTOC 5Y Survival by Stage

Stage	Relative 5Y survival (%)
I	90
IA	94
IB	92
IC	85
II	70
IIA	78
IIB	73
III	39
IIIA	59
IIIB	52
IIIC	39
IV	17

HGSTOC, high grade serous tubo-ovarian cancer.

Table 2.10 5Y Survival by Residual Disease

Residual disease	5 YS
Microscopic	40%–75%
Optimal	30%–40%
Suboptimal	5%

YS, year survival.

SURVIVAL CARE

- Follow-up:
  - Every 3 months for 2 years
  - Every 6 months up to 5 years
  - Annually for subsequent visits
- At each visit:
  - Physical and pelvic examination
  - Symptom review
  - Consider CA-125: discussion should be held with the patient regarding surveillance with tumor markers. Rustin et al demonstrated no improvement in survival when tumor markers were followed. Patients had a poorer quality of life with additional unsuccessful cycles of chemotherapy given based on laboratory data. Assessment of symptoms, along with physical examination, can guide the clinician regarding when to order lab tests, imaging, and when to initiate second-line chemotherapy (23).
- CT imaging: CT cannot often detect subcentimeter disease.

EPITHELIAL TUBO-OVARIAN CANCER NOTABLE TRIALS

- **Primary Adjuvant Chemotherapy Trials**
  - ○ ICON 1: this trial evaluated 477 patients who had early ovarian cancer "staged" with hysterectomy, bilateral salpingo-oophorectomy, and recommended omentectomy. Eligibility was if the treating physician was uncertain whether the patient required chemotherapy. 93% of patients were "stage I." Patients were randomized between no further treatment (NFT) and single-agent carboplatin (AUC 5); cisplatin, doxorubicin, cyclophosphamide (CAP); or another platinum regimen. Histology was: 32% serous, 15% clear cell, 23% mucinous. Most patients were apparent stage I; however, there were 7% of patients with stage II or III disease; 70% were grade 2 or 3. At 51 months, the OS was 79% in the chemotherapy arm versus 70% in the NFT arm. The 5Y PFS was 73% in the chemotherapy group versus 62% in the NFT group. For clinical stage I disease that did not get staged, there was a 38% recurrence rate without further treatment and a 30% death rate. Chemotherapy had an HR of 0.66 for survival (24).
  - ○ ACTION: this trial ran concurrently with ICON 1. 30% of 448 patients were comprehensively staged. Patients were randomized to observation or to chemotherapy. Chemotherapy consisted of four to six cycles of single-agent platinum or a platinum-containing regimen. 40% of patients were stage IA or IB and 60% had grade 1 or grade 2 disease. The 5 YS in the observation and adjuvant chemotherapy arms were 75% and 85%. Patients who received chemotherapy had a better recurrence-free survival (RFS; HR 0.63). In nonoptimally staged patients, the adjuvant chemotherapy group had an improved OS and RFS (HR 1.75 and HR 1.78, respectively). Among patients in the observation arm, optimal staging provided an improvement in OS and RFS (HR 2.31 and HR 1.82, respectively). There was no benefit seen from adjuvant chemotherapy in the optimally staged patients. This suggests that in the suboptimally staged group, there were undiagnosed higher-staged patients who benefited when given chemotherapy. A 10Y follow-up found support for most of the original conclusions, except that OS after optimal surgical staging was improved, now among patients who received adjuvant chemotherapy (HR of death 1.89) (25,26).
  - ○ ICON 2: this trial evaluated 1,526 eligible surgically staged patients who needed primary adjuvant chemotherapy. Patients were staged I to IV and were randomized to single-agent platinum-based chemotherapy or CAP. This trial was stopped early due to the availability of taxanes. These patients were then grouped into the control arm of ICON 3 as their outcomes were statistically nonsignificant with an OS HR of 1.0. The median survival in both groups was 33 months and the 2 YS was 60% for both arms. CAP was more toxic (27).
  - ○ ICON 3: this trial evaluated 274 eligible surgically staged patients stages I to IV, 20% of whom were stages I and II. Patients were randomized between a paclitaxel–carboplatin doublet versus the ICON 2 group of single-agent carboplatin or CAP. The OS was 36 months for carboplatin–paclitaxel and 35 months for the control groups of single-agent carboplatin and CAP. The PFS were 17 months versus 16 months for the control arm. There were a lot of confounding factors in this study: a large number of patients were deemed

to have recurrent disease based on elevated CA-125 levels prior to showing clinical recurrence. In addition, 30% of those who did not get paclitaxel as primary treatment received paclitaxel as second-line treatment (28).

○ ICON 4: this trial evaluated 802 eligible patients with recurrent platinum-sensitive ovarian cancer; 75% recurred more than 12 months following initial therapy. Patients were randomized to paclitaxel 175 to 185 mg/m² and cisplatin 50 mg/m² or carboplatin AUC 5 versus single-agent cisplatin 75 mg/m² or carboplatin AUC 5. The doublet therapy showed a statistically significant improvement over the single-agent group with a median PFS of 13 months versus 10 months (HR 0.76; $p = 0.0004$). The doublet therapy showed an improvement in median survival by 5 months (29 months versus 24 months; HR of 0.82, $p = 0.02$). This translated to a 2 YS of 57% versus 50% and a 1Y PFS of 50% versus 40%. Criticisms of this trial were that 75% of patients were in a good prognosis group. This is essentially a trial of platinum-sensitive disease (28).

○ ICON 5/GOG 182 EORTC 55012: this trial evaluated 4,312 surgically staged stage III and IV patients for primary adjuvant therapy. The control arm was the doublet of carboplatin AUC 6 and paclitaxel 175 mg/m² administered for eight cycles. The experimental arms consisted of carboplatin–paclitaxel–gemcitabine as sequential doublets or in triplicate, for a total of eight cycles, or carboplatin–paclitaxel–topotecan as sequential doublets for a total of eight cycles, and carboplatin–paclitaxel–liposomal doxorubicin as a triplicate regimen for eight cycles. There was no difference in median PFS or OS with the PFS in the control arm being 16 months and the OS being 44 months, both in the optimally and suboptimally debulked patients. The median PFS for patients with suboptimal, gross optimal (<1 cm residual), and microscopic residual disease were 13, 16, and 29 months, respectively, and the median OS rates were 33, 40, and 68 months, respectively (29).

○ ICON 7/AGO-OVAR 11: this trial evaluated 1,528 eligible patients stages I to IV, of whom 26% were suboptimally debulked. The control arm was carboplatin AUC 5 or 6 and paclitaxel 175 mg/m² IV every 3 weeks for six cycles. The experimental arm consisted of carboplatin and paclitaxel at the same doses with the addition of bevacizumab at 7.5 mg/kg IV every 3 weeks for six cycles, with maintenance bevacizumab continued for an additional 12 cycles or until progression of disease. Median follow-up was 48.9 months. At 42 months, PFS was 22.4 months without bevacizumab versus 24.1 months with bevacizumab ($p = 0.04$ log rank). In high-risk patients, the PFS was 14.5 months versus 18.1 months with bevacizumab and median OS was 28.8 versus 36.6 months with bevacizumab. At 48.9 months though, no difference in PFS was seen. For the entire population at 48.9 months, the restricted mean survival time (RMST; OS) demonstrated an improvement of only 0.9 months from 44.6 to 45.5 months (95% confidence interval [CI] log rank $p = 0.85$, pH test $p = 0.02$) with bevacizumab—not significant (NS). In a subgroup analysis, RMST for the poor prognosis group (stage IV, inoperable stage III [6%], and suboptimally debulked >1 cm stage III) demonstrated a 4.8-month RMST improvement from 34.5 to 39.3 months (log rank $p = 0.03$ PH test = 0.007). In the average prognosis group, the RMST was 49.7 months versus 48.4 months

(p = 0.2) in the bevacizumab group. No benefit from bevacizumab was seen in low-grade serous tumors, clear cell tumors, or low-stage high-risk patients (stage I–IIA clear cell or G3). Hypertension attributed to bevacizumab was seen in 18% of patients who received bevacizumab versus 2% of patients in the control arm. Bowel perforation was seen in 10 patients in the bevacizumab group versus three patients in the control arm (30,31).

○ GOG 1: 86 evaluable surgical stage I patients were randomized to observation, whole pelvic radiation therapy (WP-XRT), or melphalan chemotherapy. Recurrence was 17% in the observation group, 30% in those irradiated, and 6% in those who received chemotherapy. Recurrence was related to grade: grade 1, 11%; grade 2, 22%; grade 3, 27% (32).

○ GOG 111: this trial evaluated 386 eligible suboptimally debulked stage III and IV patients. Patients with greater than 1 cm residual disease were randomly assigned to receive cisplatin 75 mg/m^2 and cyclophosphamide 750 mg/m^2 or cisplatin 75 mg/m^2 and 24-hour paclitaxel 135 mg/m^2. Overall response rate in the first arm was 73% compared to 60%. PFS was longer in the paclitaxel-containing arm at 17.9 months versus 12.9 months. OS was longer in the paclitaxel arm at 37.5 months compared to 24.4 months (33).

○ OV-10: this trial evaluated cyclophosphamide and cisplatin versus 3-hour paclitaxel and cisplatin in 680 eligible patients with stage IIB, IIC, III, or IV disease, who were optimally and suboptimally debulked. The ORR was 58.6% in the cisplatin and paclitaxel arm versus 44.7% in the cyclophosphamide and cisplatin arm. The PFS was 15.5 months versus 11.5 months favoring the paclitaxel arm and the OS was 35.6 months versus 25.8 months, again, all favoring paclitaxel (34).

○ GOG 132: this trial evaluated 648 suboptimal stage III and any stage IV patients. There were three arms: a doublet of cisplatin and paclitaxel dosed at 75 and 135 mg/kg; single-agent paclitaxel dosed at 200 mg/kg; and single-agent cisplatin dosed at 100 mg/kg. The PFS, respectively, were 14 months, 11 months, and 16 months. The OS, respectively, were 26 months, 26 months, and 30 months. The response rates were, respectively, 67%, 67%, and 47% (35).

○ GOG 157: this trial evaluated three versus six cycles of paclitaxel and carboplatin in 427 eligible patients staged IAG3, IBG3, IC, and II. The primary endpoint was recurrence rate. 457 patients were registered, 213 in each arm. Of these, 70% were stage I, 30% were stage II, and there were 30% clear cell cancers in each arm. The recurrence rate was 27.4% for three cycles versus 19% for six cycles (95% CI: 0.53–1.13). The probability of surviving 5 years was 81% for three cycles versus 83% for six cycles (95% CI: 0.66–1.57). The HR for recurrence was 0.74, p = 0.18 (NS). Criticisms of the study were: insufficient power to detect a difference, and only 29% (126) of patients were staged appropriately. Chan updated the data in 2006 and found a benefit to six cycles of chemotherapy specifically for serous tumors with a 5Y RFS of 83% compared to 60% in those who received six versus three cycles of chemotherapy, respectively (p = 0.007). Those with serous tumors had a significantly lower risk of recurrence after six versus three cycles of chemotherapy (HR 0.33; 95% CI: 0.14–0.77; p = 0.04) in contrast to nonserous tumors (HR 0.94; 95% CI: 0.60–1.49) (36,37).

○ GOG 158: this trial compared 792 optimally cytoreduced stage III ovarian cancer patients to 24-hour paclitaxel and cisplatin versus 3-hour paclitaxel and carboplatin. This was designed as a noninferiority study and there was provision for second-look laparotomy, which about 50% chose to do (Greer et al subset analysis proved that second-look laparotomy was not beneficial). 85% were able to receive all six cycles. The PFS was 19 months for paclitaxel and cisplatin and 20 months for paclitaxel and carboplatin. The OS was 48 months for paclitaxel cisplatin and 57 months for paclitaxel carboplatin. The RR of recurrence was 0.88 (95% CI: 0.75–1.03), and the RR for the OS was 0.84 (95% CI: 0.7–1.02) favoring carboplatin and paclitaxel. The carboplatin arm had less myelotoxicity and electrolyte problems, with similar neurotoxicity (19,38).

○ GOG 218: this randomized trial evaluated 1,873 staged III or IV suboptimally debulked patients with a control arm of carboplatin and paclitaxel. The investigational arms consisted of carboplatin and paclitaxel with either bevacizumab for 5 months during primary therapy or an extended dosing of bevacizumab after six initial cycles of carboplatin, paclitaxel, and bevacizumab for a total of 18 cycles. The PFS was, respectively, 10.3, 11.2, and 14.1 months; the PFS HR was 0.91/0.72. The OS, respectively, was 39.9, 38.7, and 39.7 months; OS HR was 1.036/0.92. Maximum separation of the PFS occurred at 15 months and the curves merged 9 months later. The degree of neutropenia was associated with a greater PFS and OS (HR 0.76 and 0.73, respectively) (39).

○ SCOTROC 1: this trial evaluated 1,077 patients with stage IC to IV disease and randomized them to docetaxel 75 mg/m^2 versus paclitaxel at 175 mg/m^2 each with carboplatin at an AUC of 5 for six cycles. The PFS was 15 months versus 14.8 months. Docetaxel was found to not be inferior. The OS was 64.2% versus 68.9%, respectively (40).

○ OCTAVIA: this single-arm study evaluated 189 patients treated with primary adjuvant bevacizumab plus weekly paclitaxel and every 21 days carboplatin. For patients with stage IIB to IV or grade 3/clear-cell stage I/IIA, bevacizumab was dosed at 7.5 mg/kg on day 1; paclitaxel at 80 mg/m^2 on days 1, 8, 15; and carboplatin at an AUC 6 on day 1 IV every 21 days for six to eight cycles, followed by single-agent maintenance bevacizumab to total 1 year. 74% of the patients had stage IIIC/IV disease. The primary objective was PFS. Patients received a median of six chemotherapy and 17 bevacizumab cycles. At the predefined cutoff 24 months after last patient enrollment, 99 patients (52%) had progressed and 19 (10%) had died, all from ovarian cancer. The median PFS was 23.7 months (95% CI: 19.8–26.4 months), 1Y PFS rate was 85.6%, response evaluation criteria in solid tumors (RECIST) response rate was 84.6%, and median response duration was 14.7 months. Most patients (≥90%) completed at least six chemotherapy cycles. Grade ≥3 peripheral sensory neuropathy occurred in 5% and febrile neutropenia in 0.5%. There was one case of gastrointestinal perforation (0.5%) and no treatment-related deaths (41).

○ AGO-OVAR 9: This was a randomized phase III front-line chemotherapy trial by the Gynecologic Cancer InterGroup (GCIG) for previously untreated patients with stages I to IV epithelial ovarian cancer. 1,742 patients were randomly allocated to receive a combination of paclitaxel, carboplatin, and gemcitabine (TCG) or paclitaxel and carboplatin (TC). TC was given day 1 every

21 days for a planned minimum of six courses. Gemcitabine was given on days 1 and 8 of each cycle in the TCG arm. The median PFS for the TCG arm vs TC arm was 17.8 months and 19.3 months, respectively (HR 1.18; 95% CI: 1.06–1.32; $p = 0.0044$). The median OS for TCG and TC arm was 49.5 months and 51.5 months, respectively. Patients on the TCG arm experienced more grade 3 to 4 hematologic toxicity and fatigue compared to patients treated on the TC arm. Quality of life analysis showed a disadvantage in the TCG arm (42).

o AGO-OVAR 10/MIMOSA study: abagovomab is an anti-idiotypic antibody produced by mouse hybridoma and generated against OCA-125. Abagovomab maintenance therapy or placebo was administered as a 2 mg 1 mL suspension once every 2 weeks for 6 weeks then once every 4 weeks until recurrence for up to 21 months after primary surgery with adjuvant platinum–taxane chemotherapy in 888 EOC patients randomized in a 2:1 ratio. A robust immune response was seen but the HR for RFS and OS were 1.099 (95% CI: 0.919–1.315; $p = 0.301$) and 1.15 (95% CI: 0.872–1.518; $p = 0.322$), respectively. A prior phase I/II trial of 119 patients showed prolonged survival in those who demonstrated an immune response to vaccination (23.5 vs. 4.9 months) contrary to this phase III trial (43).

o AGO-OVCAR 12/LUME-Ovar1: (Nintedanib) 1,366 women with stage IIB to IV with EOC underwent PDS to R1/R0 status. Patients were randomly assigned (2:1) to receive six cycles of carboplatin (AUC 5 mg/mL/min or 6 mg/mL/min) and paclitaxel (175 mg/m^2) in addition to either 200 mg of nintedanib (nintedanib group) or placebo (placebo group) twice daily on days 2 to 21 of every 3-week cycle for up to 120 weeks. The primary endpoint was PFS. Addition of antiangiogenic to standard chemotherapy increased median PFS in the nintedanib group versus the placebo group (17.2 months [95% CI: 16.6–19.9] vs. 16·6 months [95% CI: 13.9–19.1]; HR 0.84 [95% CI: 0.72–0.98]; $p = 0·024$). The most common adverse events (AEs) were: diarrhea in the nintedanib group at 22% versus in the placebo group at 3%: and neutropenia in the nintedanib group (42%) versus placebo (36%). Serious AEs were reported in 42% of the nintedanib group and 34% of the placebo group; 2% of patients in the nintedanib group experienced serious AEs associated with death compared with 3% in the placebo group. Nintedanib in combination with carboplatin and paclitaxel prolonged the PFS in first-line treatment of ovarian cancer patients with a higher impact in patients with low postoperative tumor burden (44).

o AGO-OVAR 15: this was randomized phase II study that compared carboplatin, paclitaxel and lonafarnib to carboplatin and paclitaxel alone as frontline treatment in 105 EOC patients FIGO stages IIB to IV. Lonafarnib was dosed at 100 mg PO BID during chemotherapy and increased to 200 mg for up to 6 months after chemotherapy for maintenance therapy. PFS was 11.5 months in the lonafarnib, carboplatin and paclitaxel taxol (LTC) arm versus 16.4 months in the TC arm ($p = 0.0141$) and the median OS was 20.6 months versus 43.4 months in the TC arm ($p = 0.012$). For those with R1–R2 disease, lonafarnib was inferior treatment, thus, further investigation was not recommended (45).

o AGO-OVAR-17 (**B**evacizumab **O**varian **O**ptimal **S**tandard **T**reatment [BOOST]) Trial: a prospective randomized phase III trial to evaluate optimal treatment duration of first-line bevacizumab in combination with carboplatin and paclitaxel in patients with primary epithelial ovarian, fallopian tube, or peritoneal cancer. 927 patients with FIGO stages IIB to IV EOC were randomized 1:1 to paclitaxel 175 mg/m^2 and carboplatin AUC 5 q21 days with bevacizumab 15 mg/kg q21 days with an additional 22 cycles of bevacizumab: versus paclitaxel 175 mg/m^2 and carboplatin AUC 5 q21 days with bevacizumab 15 mg/kg q21 days with maintenance bevacizumab for an additional 44 cycles. NCT01462890: results pending.

o GOG 241: carboplatinum/paclitaxel ± bevacizumab versus oxaloplatin–capacetabine ± bevacizumab as first-line therapy in advanced or recurrent chemonaive mucinous EOC. NCT01081262: results pending.

- **Dose Density Trials**
  o GOG 97: this study investigated four cycles versus eight cycles of cyclophosphamide and cisplatin in 458 eligible patients. The four-cycle regimen dosed the chemotherapy doublets at 1,000/100 mg/m^2 whereas the eight-cycle doublet dosed the chemotherapy at 500/50 mg/m^2 given every 3 weeks. This provided no difference in OS, and the total dosing was the same (46).

  o Fruscio weekly cisplatin: this trial evaluated 285 eligible patients and randomized them to weekly cisplatin at 50 mg/m^2 for 9 weeks versus cisplatin at 75 mg/m^2 for six cycles every 3 weeks. At 16.8 years follow-up, no difference in PFS was seen (17.2 months vs. 18.1 months, HR 1.08) and no difference in OS was seen (35 months vs. 32 months, HR 0.97) for the dose dense weekly cisplatin versus standard treatment (47).

  o The Scottish Dose Dense Trial: this trial evaluated six cycles of cyclophosphamide at 750 mg/m^2 and cisplatin at doses of either 50 or 100 mg/m^2 q21 days in 159 patients. The OS for the 100 and 50 mg/m^2 patients was 32.4% and 26.6%, and the overall relative death rate was 0.68 ($p = 0.043$). From this trial, the standard 75 mg/m^2 dose was chosen for its modest toxicity (48).

  o The Dutch/Danish Study: this trial randomized 222 patients between different doublet doses of carboplatin and cyclophosphamide. Carboplatin was dosed at an AUC of either 4 or 8 q28 days for six cycles in combination with cyclophosphamide at a constant dose of 500 mg/m^2. There was no difference in OS (2 YS 45%) or complete pathologic response (32% and 30%) (49).

  o Gore et al. randomized 227 patients to single-agent carboplatin at either an AUC of 6 for six courses or an AUC of 12 for four courses every 4 weeks. There was no difference in PFS or OS at 5 years at 31% and 34%, respectively. There was more toxicity in the AUC 12 arm (50).

  o GOG 134: this trial included 271 eligible patients with persistent, recurrent, or progressive disease who were evaluated with paclitaxel dosed at 135 mg/m^2/24 hr, paclitaxel at 175 mg/m^2/24 hr, or paclitaxel at 250 mg/m^2/24 hr. The 135 mg/m^2 arm was closed early. The partial and complete response to paclitaxel at 250 mg/m^2 (36%) was higher than those receiving 175 mg/m^2 (27%, $p = 0.027$). The median duration for OS was 13.1 months and 12.3 months for paclitaxel 175 and 250 mg/m^2, respectively. Thus, paclitaxel exhibited a dose effect with regard to response rate, but there was no survival benefit (51).

  o European–Canadian randomized trial of paclitaxel in relapsed ovarian cancer: this trial evaluated infusion length of paclitaxel in recurrent ovarian cancer in 391 eligible patients. This was a 2×2 study design of 3-hour versus 24-hour infusion and 135 mg/m^2 versus 175 mg/m^2. The high-dose group had a longer PFS at 19 weeks versus 14 weeks ($p = 0.02$). The 175 mg/m^2 dose was found to have a better response rate at 19% versus the 135 mg/m^2 dose with a response rate of 16% (NS). There was no difference in survival (52).

○ NOVEL Trial: New Ovarian Elaborate Trial JGOG 3016: this phase III trial evaluated 631 patients with stages II, III, and IV EOC patients, stratified by residual disease less than 1 cm or greater than 1 cm as well as by histology (clear cell/mucinous vs. serous/others) to carboplatin AUC 6 q21 days for six to nine cycles versus dose dense weekly paclitaxel 80 mg/m^2 on days 1, 8, 15 with carboplatin AUC 6 day 1 q21 days for six to nine cycles. Carboplatin was dosed at an AUC 6 and given every 3 weeks with either: weekly paclitaxel at 80 mg/m^2 or standard 3-week dosing at 180 mg/m^2. The median follow-up was 76.8 months. The median PFS was 28.2 months (95% CI: 22.3–33.8) versus 17.5 months ([15.7–21.7]; HR 0.76; 95% CI: 0.62–0.91; $p = 0.0037$). The median OS was 100.5 months (95% CI: 65.2–∞) in the dose-dense treatment group and 62.2 months (95% CI: 52.1–82.6) in the conventional treatment group (HR 0.79; 95% CI: 0.63–0.99; $p = 0.039$). The HR for progression was 0.71 (95% CI: 0.58–0.88; $p = 0.0015$). The 3Y OS was 72% versus 65% ($p = 0.03$), respectively. The 5Y OS was 58.6% versus 51.0%, respectively, with an HR of 0.79 (53,54).

○ GOG 262: 692 patients were enrolled in a phase III randomized trial in which 84% elected to receive bevacizumab in addition to either paclitaxel 175 mg/m^2 every 3 weeks with carboplatin AUC 6 for six cycles, or paclitaxel dosed weekly 80 mg/m^2 plus carboplatin AUC 6 for six cycles. In the intention-to-treat analysis, weekly paclitaxel was not associated with longer PFS than paclitaxel administered every 3 weeks (14.7 months and 14.0 months, respectively; HR for progression or death = 0.89; 95% CI: 0.74–1.06; $p = 0.18$). For those patients who did not receive bevacizumab, weekly paclitaxel was associated with PFS that was 3.9 months longer than that observed with paclitaxel administered every 3 weeks (14.2 vs. 10.3 months; HR 0.62; 95% CI: 0.40–0.95; $p = 0.03$ This is similar to JGOG 3016 outcomes). However, among patients who received bevacizumab, weekly paclitaxel did not significantly prolong PFS, as compared with paclitaxel administered every 3 weeks (14.9 months and 14.7 months, respectively; HR 0.99; 95% CI: 0.83–1.20; $p = 0.60$). A test for interaction that assessed homogeneity of the treatment effect showed a significant difference between treatment with bevacizumab and without bevacizumab ($p = 0.047$). Patients who received weekly paclitaxel had a higher rate of grade 3 or 4 anemia than did those who received paclitaxel every 3 weeks (36% vs. 16%), as well as a higher grade 2 to 4 sensory neuropathy (26% vs. 18%); although lower rates of grade 3 or 4 neutropenia (72% vs. 83%) were observed. Weekly paclitaxel, compared to every 21 day paclitaxel did not prolong PFS (55).

○ MITO7 (dose intense): 810 patients with stages IC to IV EOC were randomized in a 1:1 fashion to carboplatin AUC 6 and Taxol 175 mg/m^2 every 3 weeks for six cycles versus carboplatin AUC 2 and paclitaxel 60 mg/m^2 every week for 18 weeks. Primary endpoints were PFS and quality of life (QOL). The median follow-up was 22.3 months. The median PFS was 17.3 months for every 3 week treatment versus 18.3 months for weekly treatment; HR 0.96; 95% CI: 0.8–1.16; $p = 0.66$. The weekly group had less neutropenia and neuropathy. 25% had neoadjuvant chemotherapy, 24% were not operated on, 23% were suboptimally debulked, 25% were stage IV, and 67% were serous histology. The 2 YS was 79% with every 3-week treatment and 77% with weekly treatment. This was not a dose-dense study so is not a parallel to the JGOG study (56).

○ ICON 8: an international phase III randomized trial of dose fractionated chemotherapy compared to standard three weekly chemotherapy, following immediate primary surgery or as part of delayed primary surgery, for women with newly diagnosed epithelial ovarian, fallopian tube, or primary peritoneal cancer. Arm 1 (Control arm): carboplatin and paclitaxel on day 1 of a 21-day cycle for six cycles: carboplatin administered IV at AUC 5 and paclitaxel 175 mg/m² IV. Arm 2: carboplatin AUC 5 on day 1 and dose-fractionated weekly paclitaxel 80 mg/m² on days 1, 8, and 15 of a 21-day cycle for six cycles. Arm 3: dose-fractionated weekly carboplatin AUC 2 and weekly paclitaxel 80 mg/m² on day 1, 8, and 15 of a 21-day cycle for six cycles. Results pending.

- **IP Trials**
  ○ GOG 104: this trial evaluated 546 patients for primary adjuvant chemotherapy after "optimal" debulking to a size of less than 2 cm. IV cyclophosphamide was given at 600 mg/m² for six cycles every 3 weeks with either IP cisplatin or IV cisplatin (both dosed at 100 mg/m²). The median OS was significant favoring the IP arm at 49 months versus the IV group at 41 months. The HR for death was lower in the IP group, 0.76; 95% CI: 0.61 to 0.96; $p = 0.02$ (57).

  ○ GOG 114: this trial evaluated 462 stage III patients who were optimally debulked to less than 1 cm. Patients were randomized to IV cisplatin at 75 mg/m² and IV paclitaxel 135 mg/m² over 24h every 3 weeks for six cycles versus IV carboplatin at an AUC 9 for two cycles q28 days followed by IP cisplatin at 100 mg/m² with IV paclitaxel 135 mg/m² over 24h every 3 weeks for six cycles. Second-look laparotomy was optional. The PFS was 27.6 months versus 22.5 months with $p = 0.01$, the OS was 63.2 months versus 52.5 months with a $p = 0.05$, all favoring IP therapy (58).

  ○ GOG 172: this trial evaluated 415 stage III patients who were optimally debulked to less than 1 cm residual. Patients were randomized to either IV paclitaxel at 135 mg/m² over 24 hours, with cisplatin dosed at 75 mg/m² or to IP cisplatin on day 1 dosed at 100 mg/m² with IV paclitaxel at 135 mg/m² over 24 hours on day 2, and paclitaxel again on day 8 dosed at 60 mg/m² IP. 64% had gross residual disease after primary surgery and 50% of patients chose a second-look surgery. 41% of the IV group versus 57% of the IP group had a pathologic complete response at second-look laparotomy (SLL). Only 42% of the IP group completed all IP cycles whereas 83% of the IV group received all six cycles. The PFS was 18.3 months for the IV arm versus 23.8 months for the IP arm ($p = 0.05$). The OS was 49.7 months for the IV arm versus 65.6 months for the IP arm with a 16-month survival advantage favoring IP therapy ($p = 0.03$). A 5.5-month PFS was seen. Patients with no visible residual disease did well with a 78-month median survival for those on the IV arm and the median survival has not been reached for the IP arm (59).

○ A 10Y follow-up of GOG 114 and 172: a combined review of two IP studies including 876 patients showed the median PFS for IP therapy was 25 months compared to 20 months for IV therapy. The OS was 61.8 versus 51.4 months, respectively. The risk of death decreased by 12% for each cycle of IP chemotherapy completed. The disease-free survival (DFS) for those who received IP therapy with R0 disease (complete cytoreduction) was 60.4 months, with an OS of 127.6 months (60).

○ Prognostic factors for stage III EOC treated with IP chemotherapy: a combined review of surgically debulked patients on GOG IP studies 114 and 172: a second 10Y follow-up of GOGs 114 and 172. IP versus IV OS was 61.8 months versus 51.4 months with risk reduction of death 23%. Those patients with R0 disease who received IP therapy had a PFS of 38 months with a median OS not yet reached and a median follow-up of 53 months. An OS of 127 months with R0 disease after PDS was seen in this subgroup. The OS for those treated on the IV arm with R0 disease was 78 months. The difference in the median OS between the IV and IP arms was 16 months, the difference between RD1 versus RD0 exceeded 39 months. Considering all patients in GOGs 114 and 172: the difference in OS between the IV and IP arms was 11 months, while the difference between RD1 and RD0 for those receiving IP was over 60 months. This then concludes there is huge value in resecting all gross disease with acceptable morbidity. 29% of patients underwent bowel resection, which is a surrogate for surgical effort (61).

○ 205 patients randomized to IP therapy on GOG 172: of these, 58% did not complete treatment, 13% did not receive IP treatment, 57% completed one to two cycles, 29% received three to five cycles. 34% were not able to complete treatment because of catheter-related issues, 38% due to poor tolerance to the treatment, 29% did not have IP treatment because of disease progression of other complications (62).

○ GOG 9921: this was a phase I feasibility study evaluating dose modification of GOG 172. 23 patients were evaluated. IP cisplatin was dosed at 75 mg/m^2 with IV paclitaxel at 135 mg/m^2 over 3 hours on day 1, with IP paclitaxel 60 mg/m^2 administered on day 8, of a 21-day cycle with a 95% rate of adherence for an outpatient regimen (63).

○ **IP catheter outcomes** GOG 172: of the 58% of patients not completing six IP cycles, one third were catheter-related (catheter infection in 20 of 41 cases, blocked catheter in 10 of 41 cases). One third were related to IP treatment (pain, bowel complications, patient refusal, other noncatheter infection). One third of discontinuations were probably unrelated to the catheter (nausea, renal, metabolic). Left colon resection or colostomy related to a decreased ability to tolerate IP chemotherapy. Appendectomy, small bowel resection, or right colon surgery did not appear to affect IP tolerance. Optimal placement is the use of a 9.6-F catheter through a separate incision (not the laparotomy incision), and tunneled at least 10 cm, with 10 cm length left in the peritoneal cavity. A waiting time of 24 hours post-insertion before use was recommended to avoid leakage (64).

○ GOG 252: this was a phase III trial of patients with stage II to IV epithelial tubo-ovarian cancer to include suboptimally debulked patients. 1,560 patients were randomized to one of three arms: Arm 1 (control arm similar to GOG 262): IV paclitaxel at 80 mg/m² weekly with IV carboplatin AUC 6 every 3 weeks and IV bevacizumab 15 mg/kg every 3 weeks continuing with maintenance bevacizumab × 22 weeks. Arm 2: IV paclitaxel 80 mg/m² weekly with IP carboplatin AUC 6 every 3 weeks and IV bevacizumab 15 mg/kg every 3 weeks with maintenance bevacizumab × 22 weeks. Arm 3: IV paclitaxel at 135 mg/m² on day 1 followed by IP cisplatin at 75 mg/m² on day 2, then IP paclitaxel at 60 mg/m² on day 8 and bevacizumab at 15 mg/kg every 3 weeks with maintenance bevacizumab for 22 weeks. The median age was 58, 34% were stage III, 10% stage II, 72% were G3 serous, 57% achieved R0 debulking, 90% in Arm 1 completed platinum therapy, 90% in Arm 2, and 84% in Arm 3. PFS was the primary outcome. Median PFS for the 461 patients in Arm 1 was 26.8 months, for the 464 patients in Arm 2 was 28.7 months (log rank $p = 0.661$), and for the 456 patients in Arm 3, was 27.8 months (log rank $p = 0.122$). Of note: this was not a platinum dose intense trial similar to GOG 172, and bevicuzimab was added as primary therapy and maintenance, similar to GOG 218 (64).

○ iPocc Trial (GOTIC-001/JGOG-3019): the target accrual is 746. In this trial, dose-dense weekly paclitaxel at 80 mg/m² was administered in combination with carboplatin AUC 6 every 3 weeks either IV or IP. Eligible patients had EOC stages II to IV. This study will explore the potential of IP chemotherapy to include suboptimally debulked advanced ovarian cancer (65).

○ OV-21/GCIG study led by the Canadian National Cancer Institute: all patients with stage III EOC will receive neoadjuvant chemotherapy. Those patients who respond to the neoadjuvant chemotherapy will receive interval debulking surgery (IDS), and if the residual disease after IDS becomes the optimal (less than 1 cm), the patient will be randomized to one of the three arms. The control arm is the combination of IV paclitaxel at 135 mg/m² followed by IV carboplatin at AUC 5 on day 1, and then IV paclitaxel at 60 mg/m² will be given on day 8. The second arm is same as the control arm but carboplatin will be given by the IP route. The third arm is the modified GOG 172 winner arm, which is the same as the third arm of GOG 252 trial but in which bevacizumab is not given. One of these two IP arms (Arm 2 or Arm 3) will be chosen, in a randomized phase II manner, and the winner arm will be compared with the control arm as a phase III trial. Results pending.

- **Maintenance/Consolidation Trials**
  ○ GOG 178: this trial evaluated consolidation therapy in 222 eligible stage III and IV patients and randomized patients to 12 versus 3 cycles of paclitaxel at 175 mg/m² after completion of six cycles of platinum/paclitaxel with a clinical complete response. At 50% enrollment, the protocol dictated interim analysis. This showed an improvement in PFS favoring 12 cycles with an HR of 2.31 demonstrating a 28 month versus 21 month PFS ($p = 0.002$ 99% CI: 1.08 to 4.94). The study was closed at this point. Patients were allowed to crossover so all those on the three-cycle arm could complete up to 12 cycles of therapy (66).

o Follow-up study to GOG 178: criticisms cited from this study were the crossover may have masked a difference between study arms, there was insufficient power within the study, and treatment at relapse equalized outcomes. The PFS was 22 versus 14 months favoring the 12-month paclitaxel. OS was 53 versus 48 months ($p = 0.34$ NS) (67).

o Initiation of salvage chemotherapy; a retrospective institutional evaluation of maintenance therapy vs. expectant management in patients with recurrent disesase reviewed 59 eligible patients with a median follow-up of 51 months. The median time from CCR to start of second-line chemotherapy was 21 months; the median time to the start of third-line agents was 43 months. 12 months elapsed between completion of first-line therapy and recurrence in 50% of patients. Thus, a similar time frame of 40 months between clinical complete response and the start of third-line therapies exists, which is comparable to results in GOG 178 (68).

o GOG 175: this trial evaluated 542 eligible patients who were staged IA or IB grade 3 or clear cell, all stage IC and all stage II ovarian cancer. They were all given IV carboplatin AUC 6 and paclitaxel 175 mg/m² for three cycles followed by randomization to either observation or weekly paclitaxel for 24 weeks. The 5Y recurrence probability rate was 23% for those observed, and 20% for those who received maintenance paclitaxel, HR 0.8. The 5 YS was 85.4% versus 86.2% (NS) (69).

o AGO-OVAR16: 940 patients with EOC, FIGO stages II–IV, and no evidence of progression after PDS and ≥5 cycles of platinum–taxane chemotherapy were randomized 1:1 to receive 800 mg pazopanib once daily, or placebo for up to 24 months. Of these, 91% had stage III/IV disease, 58% had no residual disease after surgery and 15% had *BRCA* 1/2 mutations. The primary endpoint was PFS by RECIST. Median follow-up was 24 months. Patients in the pazopanib arm had a prolonged PFS of 5.6 months versus placebo (HR 0.766; 95% CI: 0.64–0.91; $p = 0.0021$; The median PFS was 7.9 vs 12.3 months for pazopanib v placebo respectively). The first interim analysis for OS (only 189 OS events = 20.1% of population) showed no difference between arms. The median PFS was 30.3 in *BRCA* 1/2 carriers vs 14.1 months in the placebo arm (HR 0.48; 95% CI: 0.29–0.78; $p = 0.0031$). The median PFS in the pazopanib arm was 30.1 months vs 17.7 months with a HR of 0.64, (95% CI: 0.4–1.03; $p = 0.069$). Among *BRCA* 1/2 non carriers, the PFS was longer for those treated with pazopanib at 17.7 months compared to 14.1 months in the placebo arm (HR 0.77; 95% CI: 0.62–0.97; $p = 0.024$). Pazopanib mean exposure was shorter versus placebo (8.9 vs. 11.7 months). Pazopanib treatment was associated with a higher incidence of AEs and serious AEs (26% vs. 11%) versus placebo. The most common AEs were hypertension, diarrhea, nausea, headache, fatigue, and neutropenia. Fatal serious AEs were reported in three patients on pazopanib and one patient on placebo (70).

o Study 19: olaparib maintenance therapy. 256 patients with platinum-sensitive, relapsed, high-grade serous ovarian cancer who had received two or more platinum-based regimens and had had a partial or complete response to their most recent platinum-based regimen were included in this double blind phase II randomized study. *BRCA* 1/2 mutation status was not required but was known in 36.6% of patients at study entry. Olaparib was dosed at 400 mg twice daily. The primary endpoint was PFS. A total of 136 were assigned to the olaparib group and 129 to the placebo group. The PFS was significantly longer with olaparib than with placebo (median, 8.4 months vs. 4.8 months from randomization on completion of chemotherapy; HR for progression or death, 0.35; 95% CI: 0.25–0.49; $p < 0.001$). Subgroup analyses of PFS showed that, regardless of subgroup, patients in the olaparib group had a lower risk of progression. Adverse events reported in the olaparib group versus the placebo group were nausea (68% vs. 35%), fatigue (49% vs. 38%), vomiting (32% vs. 14%), and anemia (17% vs. 5%); the majority of AEs were grade 1 or 2. An interim analysis of OS (38% maturity, meaning that 38% of the patients had died) showed no significant difference between groups (HR with olaparib, 0.94; 95% CI: 0.63–1.39; $p = 0.75$). A subset analysis showed patients with mutations were most likely to benefit. There was an 82% reduction in risk of disease progression or death in mutation patients, translating to a median PFS of 11.2 months with drug compared to 4.3 months on placebo. OS data for mutation patients were 34.9 versus 31.9 months (NS). The highest benefit was seen in *BRCA*-mutation carriers with platinum sensitive disease (71).

o Solo-1: this is a phase III study testing olaparib as maintenance therapy following response to frontline platinum-based treatment in g*BRCA*-mutated FIGO stage III to IV surgically debulked ovarian cancer patients. This is a double-blind multicenter study in which patients are randomized (2:1) to receive olaparib (300 mg [2 × 150 mg tablets] BID) or placebo. Patients must have high-grade serous or endometrioid ovarian type cancer, including primary peritoneal and/or fallopian tube cancer, who have a known deleterious (or suspected deleterious) *BRCA*m and who are in complete or partial response following the completion of platinum-based chemotherapy. The primary objective is PFS by blinded independent central review using RECIST v1.1. Radiologic scans will be performed at baseline and every 12 weeks for 120 weeks, and every 24 weeks thereafter. Blinded treatment will continue until objective DP. Primary analyses will be performed at approximately 60% maturity using log-rank tests. Other objectives for both trials include: OS; time to earliest progression (RECIST or CA-125); time from randomization to second progression (PFS2); health-related quality of life (HRQOL); tolerability. Target recruitment: n is approximately equal to 344 randomized patients. Results pending.

o ARIEL3: this is a phase III trial designed to evaluate the effect of rucaparib as maintenance treatment following platinum-based therapy in women with platinum-sensitive, relapsed, high-grade serous or endometrioid ovarian, fallopian tube, or primary peritoneal cancer. The biomarker results from the ARIEL2 study will be applied to the analysis of results in this study. NCT01968213: results pending.

o AGO-OVAR 16: a phase III study evaluated the efficacy and safety of pazopanib monotherapy versus placebo in women who have not progressed after first-line chemotherapy for epithelial ovarian, fallopian tube, or primary peritoneal cancer. 940 patients were randomized 1:1 to receive either 800 mg of pazopanib once daily or placebo for up to 24 months. The median follow-up was 24.3 months. The median PFS was 17.9 months in the pazopanib arm and 12.3 months in the placebo arm (HR – 0.77; $p = 0.0021$). The interim survival analysis did not show any significant difference between the two study arms after events in 36.5% of the study population. In an exploratory analysis of ethnicity, pazopanib appeared to have superior benefit in the 78% of patients who were not of East Asian descent (HR – 0.69; median PFS benefit, 5.9 months), compared to 22% of patients of East Asian descent who had an HR of 1.16. Toxicity was high and treatment discontinuation occurred more often in the pazopanib arm: 33% of patients discontinued treatment compared with 5.6% of patients in the placebo arm. The incidence of grade 3 or 4 AEs was higher in the pazopanib arm: hypertension in 30.8%, neutropenia in 9.9%, liver-related toxicity in 9.4%, diarrhea in 8.2%, thrombocytopenia in 2.5%, and palmar–plantar erythrodysesthesia in 1.9%. Three patients in the pazopanib arm had a fatal AE—a myocardial infarction, pneumonia, and posterior reversible encephalopathy syndrome. One patient in the placebo arm had fatal acute leukemia (70).

o MANGO-2/ILIAD: this was a phase IV trial using biomarker data for ovarian cancer patients treated on study 55041 with bevacizumab and carboplatin followed by erlotinib maintenance versus observation in patients with no evidence of DP after first-line platinum-based chemotherapy. Somatic mutations in KRAS, BRAF, NRAS, PIK3CA, EGFR, and PTEN were determined in 318 (38%) and expression of EGFR, pAkt, pMAPK, E-cadherin and Vimentin, and EGFR and HER2 gene copy numbers in 218 (26%) of a total of 835 randomized patients. Biomarker data were correlated with PFS and OS. Only 28 mutations were observed among KRAS, BRAF, NRAS, PIK3CA, EGFR, and PTEN (in 7.5% of patients), of which the most frequent were in KRAS and PIK3CA. EGFR mutations occurred in only three patients. When all mutations were pooled, patients with at least one mutation in KRAS, NRAS, BRAF, PIK3CA, or EGFR had longer PFS (33.1 vs. 12.3 months; HR 0.57; 95% CI: 0.33–0.99; $p = 0.042$) compared to those with wild-type tumors. EGFR overexpression was detected in 93 of 218 patients (42.7%), and 66 of 180 patients (36.7%) had EGFR gene amplification or high levels of copy number gain. 58 of 128 patients had positive pMAPK expression (45.3%), which was associated with inferior OS (38.9 vs. 67.0 months; HR 1.81; 95% CI: 1.11–2.97; $p = 0.016$). Patients with positive EGFR fluorescence in situ hybridization (FISH) status had worse OS (46.1 months) than those with negative status (67.0 months; HR 1.56; 95% CI: 1.01–2.40; $p = 0.044$) and shorter PFS (9.6 vs. 16.1 months; HR 1.57; 95% CI: 1.11–2.22; $p = 0.010$). None of the investigated biomarkers correlated with responsiveness to erlotinib. Conclusion: increased EGFR gene copy number was associated with worse OS and PFS in patients with ovarian cancer (72).

o TRINOVA-3 AGO-OVAR 18: randomized phase III trial evaluating paclitaxel and carboplatin plus trebananib or placebo followed by trebananib or placebo maintenance for 18 months in the front-line therapy. Results pending.

• **Recurrent Disease Trials**

o EORTC 55005: gemcitabine-carboplatin versus carboplatin: this trial evaluated platinum-sensitive relapsed ovarian cancer in 356 eligible patients. Single-agent carboplatin AUC 5 was compared to carboplatin AUC 4 with gemcitabine dosed at 1,000 mg/m^2 given on days 1 and 8, every 21 days. The PFS was improved with the addition of gemcitabine (8.6 months vs. 5.8 months HR 0.72 (95% CI: 0.58–0.90; p = 0.0031)). The study was not powered to detect a difference in OS. The ORR was 47% with the addition of gemcitabine versus 30% with single-agent carboplatin (HR 0.96; 95% CI: 0.75–1.23; p = 0.7349). 60% of patients recurred at greater than 12 months and 40% recurred between 6 months and 12 months (73).

- A randomized phase III study of pegylated liposomal doxorubicin (PLD) versus topotecan in recurrent EOC. This trial evaluated 474 patients with recurrent disease in response to single-agent therapy. Liposomal doxorubicin was dosed at 50 mg/m^2 every 4 weeks, and topotecan was dosed at 1.5 mg/m^2/day for 5 days every 3 weeks. The median survival for patients was 63 weeks for PLD versus 60 weeks for topotecan (HR 1.216; 95% CI: 1–1.478; p = 0.05). For those patients who had platinum-sensitive disease there was a significant difference in time until progression: 108 weeks versus 70 weeks, favoring PLD (HR 1.432; 95% CI: 1.066–1.923; p = 0.017). For patients with platinum resistant disease, OS was similar (74).

- OCEANS: this trial evaluated 484 eligible patients who received carboplatin AUC 4 and gemcitabine 1,000 mg/m^2 on days 1 and 8 with or without the addition of bevacizumab at 15 mg/kg IV every 3 weeks in recurrent platinum-sensitive disease. Six to 10 cycles were given with a median follow-up of 58.2 months in the bevacizumab arm and 56.4 months in the placebo arm. An ORR of 78.5% versus 57.4% was seen. Duration of response was 10.4 months versus 7.4 months (HR 0.534; 95% CI: 0.408–0.698), favoring the bevacizumab arm. The median OS was comparable between arms, with 33.6 months in the bevacizumab arm versus 32.9 months in the placebo arm (HR 0.95 log rank p = 0.65), thus no difference between arms. The PFS demonstrated a HR of 0.48, favoring the bevacizumab arm, with months until progression of 12.4 versus 8.4. Grade 3 HTN occurred in 17.4% of the experimental arm versus 1% with placebo. OS results were possibly confounded by extensive use of subsequent anticancer therapies (75,76).

- CALYPSO EORTC 55051: 976 patients in this international noninferiority trial with recurrent late relapsing (>6 months after first- or second-line platinum- and paclitaxel-based therapies) platinum-sensitive ovarian cancer were treated with the doublets of carboplatin AUC 5 and liposomal doxorubicin dosed at 30 mg/m^2 every 4 weeks (CD) versus the standard of carboplatin AUC 5 and paclitaxel 175 mg/m^2 for at least six cycles every 3 weeks (CP). 40% of patients had received two prior regimens before entering the study. A maximum of nine cycles were administered. The ORR was 63%, including 38% of patients who achieved a complete response. Patients in the CD arm had a better PFS of 11.3 months compared to the CP arm with 9.4 months (HR 0.82 (95% CI: 0.72, 0.94); p = 0.005)). The median survival times were 30.7 months and 33 months for the CD arm versus the CP arm (NS). CD led to delayed progression but similar OS compared to CP in platinum-sensitive ovarian cancer. In a subset analysis: patients with a tumor free interval > 24 months were analyzed separately. A total of 259 very platinum-sensitive patients were included (n = 131, CD; n = 128, CP). The median PFS was 12.0 months for the CD arm and 12.3 months for CP (HR 1.05; 95% CI: 0.79–1.40; p = 0.73 for superiority) and median OS was 40.2 months for CD and 43.9 for CP (HR 1.18; 95% CI: 0.85–1.63; p = 0.33 for superiority). ORRs were 42% and 38%, respectively (p = 0.46). This subset analysis found that CP and CD were equally effective treatment regimens for patients with very platinum-sensitive recurrent ovarian cancer but the favorable risk-benefit profile suggested that carboplatin-PLD should be the treatment of choice for these patients due to better toxicity profiles (77,78).

○ AURELIA trial (Avastin Use in Platinum-Resistant Epithelial Ovarian Cancer) AGO-OVAR 2.15: 361 patients with platinum resistant disease following front line platinum chemotherapy were enrolled and randomly allocated to receive a single nonplatinum chemotherapy agent alone or with bevacizumab (10 mg/kg every 2 weeks or 15 mg/kg every 3 weeks). The nonplatinum chemotherapy agent was selected by the investigator from one of the following options: liposomal doxorubicin (PLD) 40 mg/m^2 q28 days; weekly paclitaxel at 80 mg/m^2; topotecan 1.25 mg/ m^2 on days 1 to 5 q3 weeks, or topotecan 4 mg/m^2 on days 1, 8, 15 q28 days. If patients progressed on the single agent chemotherapy arm, they were allowed to cross over to bevacizumab alone. The primary endpoint was PFS. Patients in the chemotherapy alone arm had a median PFS of 3.4 months vs 6.7 months with bevacizumab (HR 0.48, 95% CI: 0.38–0.60; p < 0.001). The RECIST ORR was 11.8% in the chemotherapy alone arm versus 27.3% in the group with bevacizumab added (p = 0.001). The HR for OS was 0.85 (95% CI: 0.66–1.08; p < 0.174). There was no statistically significant difference in OS between the chemotherapy regimens (HR 0.85; 95% CI: 0.66–1.08 unstratified log-rank p < 0.174). There was no statistically significant difference in OS between the regimens (HR 0.85; 95% CI: 0.66–1.08 unstratified log-rank p < 0.174). Crossover occurred in 40% of patients randomized initially to CT. The median OS was 13.3 months for chemotherapy versus 16.6 months for chemotherapy plus bevacizumab (95% CI: 13.7–19). Gastrointestinal (GI) perforation occurred in 2.2% of bevacizumab-treated patients. The QOL arm showed a greater than 15% improvement in abdominal/GI symptoms at weeks 8/9 with the addition of bevacizumab; 21.9% versus 9.3% difference. In a subset analysis of the chemotherapy alone cohort, there was found to be an extensive crossover from chemotherapy alone to bevacizumab (PLD, 39%; paclitaxel, 38%; topotecan, 41%), which complicated interpretation of the data. The PFS HRs were 0.57 (95% CI: 0.39–0.83) for PLD (median 5.4 vs. 3.5 months, favoring the addition of bevacizumab), 0.46 (95% CI: 0.30–0.71) in the paclitaxel cohort (median 10.4 vs. 3.9 months), and 0.32 (95% CI: 0.21–0.49) for the topotecan cohort (median 5.8 vs. 2.1 months). The overall response rate evaluable by RECIST criteria was greater in regimens that included bevacizumab compared to chemotherapy alone for all cohorts: PLD cohort 13.7% vs. 7.8% (95% CI: –7.2% to 19.0%); paclitaxel cohort 53.3% vs. 30.2% (95% CI: 1.7%–44.5%);

topotecan cohort 17.0% vs. 0.0% (95% CI: 5.1%–28.9%). Gastrointestinal symptoms improved by 15% or more in each group that contained bevacizumab compared to chemotherapy alone: PLD cohort 21.1% versus 6.8%; paclitaxel cohort 25.0% versus 13.0%, and topotecan cohort 20.0% versus 8.8%. The unadjusted HRs for bevacizumab-containing chemotherapy versus chemotherapy alone were: HR 0.91 (95% CI: 0.62–1.36) for the PLD cohort (median 13.7 vs. 14.1 months); HR 0.65 for the paclitaxel cohort (95% CI: 0.42–1.02) (median 22.4 versus 13.2 months); and HR 1.09 (95% CI: 0.72–1.67) for the topotecan cohort (median 13.8 vs. 13.3 months). In the chemotherapy alone arms, progression, median PFS and ORR varied among groups. Topotecan was usually given weekly and seemed less active than weekly paclitaxel, whereas PLD had intermediate results. There was no difference in OS between treatment arms in the PLD and topotecan cohorts, but Kaplan–Meier curves for OS were clearly separated in the paclitaxel cohort; thus, a combination of paclitaxel and bevacizumab may enhance both of their antiangiogenic effects and potentially account for their better HRs in AURELIA (79,80).

○ TRINOVA-1: this was a randomized, double-blind international phase III study in women with recurrent EOC evaluating trebananib in antiangiogenesis. 919 women were enrolled. Patient eligibility criteria included having been treated with three or fewer previous regimens, and a platinum-free interval of less than 12 months. Patients were randomly assigned to weekly IV paclitaxel (80 mg/m^2) plus either weekly masked IV placebo or trebananib (15 mg/kg). Patients were stratified on the basis of platinum-free interval ($\geq$0 and $\leq$6 months vs. >6 and $\leq$12 months), presence or absence of measurable disease, and region. The primary endpoint was PFS. The median PFS in the trebananib arm was 7.4 months (95% CI: 7.0–7.8) versus 5.4 months (95% CI: 4.7–5.5) in the placebo arm (HR 0.70; 95% CI: 0.61–0.80; $p < 0.001$). The ORR was 29.8% versus 38.4% ($p = 0.0071$). The median OS was 19.3 months in the trebananib arm versus 18.3 months in the control arm (NS); (HR 0.95; 95% CI: 0.81–1.11; $p = 0.52$). In a subgroup analysis, trebananib improved the median OS compared with placebo (14.5 vs. 12.3 months; HR 0.72; 95% CI: 0.55–0.93; $p = 0.011$) in patients with ascites at baseline ($n = 295$). In the intent-to-treat population, trebananib significantly improved median PFS-2 compared with placebo (12.5 vs. 10.9 months; HR 0.85; 95% CI: 0.74–0.98; $p = 0.024$). PFS-2 confirmed that the PFS benefit associated with trebananib was maintained through the second DP, independent of the choice of subsequent therapy (81,82).

○ TRINOVA-2 AGO-OVAR 2.19/ENGOT-OV-6: this was a randomized phase III trial evaluating PLD plus trebananib or placebo in patients with recurrent partially platinum-sensitive or -resistant disease that enrolled 223 patients. No subgroup of patients showed a favorable PFS with experimental treatment but those with baseline ascites treated with trebananib showed a trend toward improved PFS (HR 0.6; 95% CI: 0.35–1.04). Trebananib use was associated with an improved response rate but no improvement in OS (83).

○ ICON6: this was a three-arm, double-blind, placebo-controlled randomized trial using the oral VEGFR-1,2,3 inhibitor, cediranib, in relapsed platinum sensitive ovarian cancer. 456 patients were enrolled with a median age of 62 years. Previous treatment interval greater than 12 months (67%) was balanced between arms. The primary endpoint was PFS. Patients were randomized 2:3:3 for up to six cycles of platinum-based chemotherapy with either placebo, cediranib 20 mg/day during chemotherapy (paclitaxel/carboplatin, gemcitabine/carboplatin, or single agent carboplatin) followed by placebo for up to 18 months (concurrent) or cediranib 20 mg/day followed by maintenance cediranib (concurrent + maintenance). Cediranib plus platinum-based chemotherapy followed by maintenance cediranib provided a benefit compared to chemotherapy alone, with an improved PFS from 9.4 to 12.5 months and an improved OS by 2.7 months (17.6–20.3 months HR 0.7; log-rank test $p = 0.0419$). PFS comparing reference and concurrent plus maintenance using a log-rank test gave a p-value of 0.00001 with an associated HR of 0.57 (95% CI: 0.45–0.74). However, because of nonproportional hazards ($p = 0.0237$ for PFS and $p = 0.0042$ for OS) the HR can be difficult to interpret, and instead survival time was estimated using restricted means (RM) and HRs were given for completeness. The RM estimates an increased time to progression of 3.2 months from 9.4 to 12.6, during 2 years. Similarly using RM, OS increased by 2.7 months from 17.6 to 20.3 (HR 0.70; log-rank test $p = 0.0419$). PFS using RM for the reference versus concurrent arms saw an increase of 2.0 months from 9.4 to 11.4 months (HR 0.68; log-rank test $p = 0.0022$). AEs significantly more common in the cediranib-maintenance arm were: hypertension, diarrhea, hypothyroidism, hoarseness, hemorrhage, proteinuria, and fatigue (84).

○ NOVA trial: Niraparib OVArian trial (MK-4827): this was a double blind, placebo-controlled phase III trial of niraparib. 490 patients with high-grade serous, platinum-sensitive, relapsed ovarian cancer were enrolled into one of two independent cohorts based on germline *BRCA* mutation status. Cohort 1 was germline *BRCA* mutation carriers (g*BRCA*mut), and cohort 2 was those who were not germline *BRCA* mutation carriers (non-g*BRCA*mut). The non-g*BRCA*mut cohort included patients with homologous recombination deficiency (HRD)-positive tumors, including those with somatic *BRCA* mutations and other HR defects, and patients with HRD-negative tumors. Within each cohort, patients were randomized 2:1 to receive niraparib or placebo and were treated continuously with placebo or 300 mg of niraparib until progression. Among patients who were germline *BRCA* mutation carriers, the niraparib arm successfully achieved statistical significance over the control arm for the primary endpoint of PFS, with an HR of 0.27. The median PFS for patients treated with niraparib was 21.0 months, compared to 5.5 months for control ($p < 0.0001$). For patients who were not germline *BRCA* mutation carriers but whose tumors were determined to be HRD positive using the Myriad myChoice® HRD test, the niraparib arm successfully achieved statistical significance over the control arm for the primary endpoint of PFS, with an HR of 0.38. The median PFS for patients with HRD-positive tumors who were treated with niraparib was 12.9 months, compared to 3.8 months for control ($p < 0.0001$).

A statistical significance in the overall nongermline *BRCA* mutant cohort was also seen for niraparib, which included patients with both HRD-positive and HRD-negative tumors. The niraparib arm successfully achieved statistical significance over the control arm for the primary endpoint of PFS, with an HR of 0.45. The median PFS for patients treated with niraparib was 9.3 months, compared to 3.9 months for control ($p < 0.0001$). The most common grade 3/4 AEs were thrombocytopenia (28.3%), anemia (24.8%), and neutropenia (11.2%). The discontinuation rate was 14.7% for niraparib-treated patients and 2.2% for control. The rates of myelodysplastic syndrome/acute myelogenous leukemia in the niraparib (1.3%) and control (1.2%) arms were similar. There were no deaths among patients during study treatment (85).

○ OVA-301: in a phase III randomized trial, trabectedin plus PLD in recurrent ovarian cancer resulted in a 35% risk reduction of disease progression or death (HR 0.65, 95% CI: 0.45–0.92; $p = 0.0152$). 337 patients were randomized to the combination trabectedin/PLD arm vs 335 patients randomized to the PLD arm. The median PFS was 7.4 versus 5.5 months. There was a 41% decrease in the risk of death (HR 0.59; 95% CI: 0.43–0.82; $p = 0.0015$). The median survival was 23.0 versus 17.1 months favoring the trabectedin arm. Similar proportions of patients received subsequent therapy in each arm (76% vs. 77%), although patients in the trabectedin/PLD arm had a slightly lower proportion of further platinum (49% vs. 55%). Importantly, patients in the trabectedin/PLD arm survived significantly longer after subsequent platinum (HR 0.63; $p = 0.0357$; median 13.3 vs. 9.8 months). This hypothesis-generating analysis demonstrates that superior benefits with trabectedin/PLD in terms of PFS and survival in the overall population appear particularly enhanced in patients with partially sensitive disease (PFI 6–12 months) (86).

○ MITO 11: this was an open-label, randomized phase II trial addressing the effect of adding pazopanib to paclitaxel for patients with platinum-resistant or platinum-refractory advanced ovarian cancer. Patients previously treated with a maximum of two lines of chemotherapy, ECOG PS 0–1, and no residual peripheral neurotoxicity were randomly assigned (1:1) to receive weekly paclitaxel 80 mg/m^2 with or without pazopanib 800 mg daily, and stratified by center, number of previous lines of chemotherapy, and platinum-free interval status. The primary endpoint was PFS, assessed in the modified intention-to-treat population. 74 patients were enrolled: 37 were assigned to receive paclitaxel and pazopanib and 37 assigned to paclitaxel only. The median follow-up was 16.1 months (IQR 12.5–20.8). The PFS was significantly longer in the pazopanib plus paclitaxel group than in the paclitaxel only group (median 6.35 months [95% CI: 5.36–11.02] vs. 3.49 months [2.01–5.66]; HR 0.42 [95% CI: 0.25–0.69]; $p = 0.0002$). No unexpected toxic effects or deaths were recorded. AEs were more common in the pazopanib and paclitaxel group to include neutropenia (30% vs. 3%], fatigue (11% vs. 6%), leucopenia (11% vs. 3%), and hypertension (8% vs. 0%). One patient in the pazopanib group had a small bowel perforation. The PFS was 6.3 versus 3.5 months (HR 0.42, 95% CI: 0.25–0.69). The RR was 50% versus 21% ($p = 0.03$) (87).

○ GOG 26FF: this phase II study evaluated single-agent paclitaxel at 170 mg/m^2 IV over 24 hours every 3 weeks in 43 refractory or platinum-resistant ovarian cancer patients. The ORR was 37%. The median PFI was 4.2 months, the median survival was 16 months. PFS was 4 months (88).

○ GOG-186F: this was a phase II study that estimated the activity of docetaxel 60 mg/m^2 IV over 1 hour followed by trabectedin 1.1 mg/m^2 over 3 hours with filgrastim, pegfilgrastim, or sargramostim every 3 weeks. 71 patients with recurrent and measurable disease, PS ≤ 2, and ≤3 prior regimens were eligible. A historical GOG taxane control study was used for direct comparison. The goal of this study was to determine if the trabectedin regimen had an RR of ≥36% with 90% power. The median number of cycles given was six (438 total cycles, range 1–22). The number of patients responding was 21 (30%; 90% CI: 21%–40%). The OR for responding was 2.2 (90% 1-sided CI: 1.07–∞). The median PFS and OS were 4.5 months and 16.9 months, respectively. The median duration of response was 6.2 months (89).

○ GOG 186i: 107 women with recurrent platinum sensitive or resistant EOC treated with one to three prior chemotherapy lines were randomized to bevacizumab or bevacizumab with fosbretabulin (a vascular disrupting agent). PFS was improved to 7.3 versus 4.8 months (HR 0.69; 95% CI: 0.47–1 at 90%). Response rates were 36% versus 28%. Although not a statistically significant result, patients receiving the combination had an ORR of 35.7% ($n = 42$) compared to 28.2% for patients on bevacizumab alone ($n = 39$). The study achieved its primary endpoint and demonstrated a statistically significant increase in PFS for the combination as compared to bevacizumab alone ($p = 0.049$; HR 0.685). In a post-hoc subgroup analysis, data showed that in patients who were platinum resistant, the addition of fosbretabulin to bevacizumab increased the ORR to 40% ($n = 10$) compared to 12.5% ($n = 8$) for bevacizumab. Among those patients, the median PFS was 6.7 months for those on bevacizumab and fosbretabulin compared to 3.4 months for those receiving bevacizumab alone ($p = 0.01$; HR 0.57). Patients in the combination arm experienced an increased incidence of G3 HTN compared to the control arm (90).

○ GOG186j: this phase II trial evaluated weekly paclitaxel ± pazopanib in women with recurrent EOC and one to three lines of prior chemotherapy. 100 women were analyzed and PFS was the primary endpoint. Compared to weekly paclitaxel there was no significant difference in PFS: the median was 7.5 versus 6.2 months (HR 0.84; 90% CI: 0.57–1.22) in the combination versus single-agent group. The RR was 32% versus 23%, respectively. HTN was more common in the combination arm and lead to treatment discontinuation in 37% versus 10% of the paclitaxel-only arm. More patients progressed on the control arm at 65% versus 32% (91).

○ Veliparib in *BRCAm* relapsed ovarian cancer patients. In this phase II study, 50 patients were evaluated of whom 60% were platinum resistant. The median number of cycles was six. Veliparib was administered at 400 mg BID with a cycle length of 28 days. The ORR was 26%; 3 patients had a CR, and 11 patients had a partial response (PR). Platinum-resistant patients had a 20% RR, and platinum-sensitive patients had a 35% RR. The median PFS was 8.2 months (92).

○ AGO-OVAR 2.20: PENELOPE trial: a two-part randomized phase III double blind trial evaluating pertuzumab in combination with standard chemotherapy in women with recurrent platinum-resistant EOC and low HER3 mRNA expression. 156 patients were randomized to pertuzumab or placebo. Pertuzumab was administered at 840 mg IV loading dose followed by q21 day dosing at 420 mg IV in combination with either paclitaxel at 80 mg/m² on days 1, 8, 15 every 3 weeks or gemcitabine 1,000 mg/m² on days 1, 8 every 3 weeks, or topotecan 1.25 mg/m² on days 1 to 5 every 3 weeks. PFS was 4.3 months for pertuzumab plus chemotherapy versus 2.6 months for placebo for chemotherapy. PFS was extended in the paclitaxel (most pronounced) and gemcitabine cohorts specifically and further exploration of this agent in combination regimens can be explored. A longer PFS was also seen in those with no prior antiangiogenic therapy (93).

○ Combination cediranib and olaparib versus olaparib alone; this was a randomized phase II study of women with recurrent platinum-sensitive ovarian cancer. 46 women received olaparib at 400 mg PO BID and 44 received combination therapy with olaparib dosed at 200 mg PO BID with cediranib 30 mg PO daily. The median PFS was significantly longer with cediranib/olaparib compared with olaparib alone (17.7 vs. 9.2 months; HR 0.42; $p = 0.005$). In a subset analysis of gBRCA mutation status, a significant improvement in PFS in gBRCA wild-type or unknown patients receiving cediranib–olaparib compared with olaparib alone (16.5 vs. 5.7 months; $p = 0.008$) with no significant improvement in PFS observed in the gBRCA patients (19.4 vs. 16.5 months; $p = 0.16$) (94,95).

○ Cediranib in recurrent or persistent ovarian, peritoneal, or fallopian tube cancer: this was a phase II trial of cediranib dosed at 30 mg daily. 74 patients were evaluated: 39 were platinum sensitive (Pl-S) and 35 were platinum resistant (Pl-R). For those who were Pl-S, 26% had a PR and 51% had stable disease (SD). In the Pl-R arm there were no PR but 66% had SD. The median PFS for all patients was 4.9 months, for the Pl-S patients the PFS was 7.2 months and for the Pl-R patients, the PFS was 3.7 months. The median OS was 18.9 months, 27.7 for the Pl-S and 11.9 for the Pl-R patients (96).

○ SOLO-2: 295 germline BRCA 1/2 mutant patients with platinum sensitive (2 or more prior platinum therapies in PR or CR) relapsed EOC were randomized 2:1 in a phase III trial to treatment with olaparib 300 mg BID compared to placebo maintenance therapy. The olaparib arm had a 19 month DFS compared to the placebo arm at 5.5 months (HR 0.3, 95% CI: 0.22–0.41, $p < 0.0001$). PFS in the olaparib arm was 30.2 months compared to 5.5 months in the placebo arm (HR 0.25, 95% CI: 0.18–0.35, $p < 0.0001$). A benefit in time to second progression or death was also seen (HR 0.50 95% CI: 0.34-0.72, $p = 0.0002$) with the median not reached compared to 18.4 months. Grade 3 Adverse events were identified in 36.9% of patients on the olaparib arm compared to 18.2% in the placebo arm. 75.6% had nausea compared to 2.6% in the placebo arm (136).

○ ARIEL2 (Assessment of Rucaparib In Ovarian Cancer Trial): this phase II study for patients with relapsed, high-grade, platinum-sensitive ovarian cancer evaluated the clinical activity of rucaparib dosed at 600 mg BID in

3 pre-determined HRD subgroups: *BRCA* mutated (germline or somatic), *BRCA* wild-type/ loss of heterozygosity (LOH) high and *BRCA* wild-type/ LOH low. The primary endpoint for the study was progression free survival. Median PFS was 12.8 months (95% CI: 9.0-14.7) in the *BRCA* mutated group, 5.7 months (5.3–7.6) in the *BRCA* wild-type/LOH high group, and 5.2 months (3.6-5.5) in the *BRCA* wild-type/LOH low subgroup. *BRCA* mutated (HR 0.27, 95% CI: 0.16–0.44, $p < 0.0001$) and *BRCA* wild-type/ LOH high (0.62, 0.42–0.90, $p = 0.011$) groups had a significantly longer progression free survival than the *BRCA* wild-type/LOH low subgroup. Anemia (22% patients) and elevated liver enzymes (12%) were the 2 most common grade 3 side effects. Interim results identified robust activity with a 65% ORR in patients with a germline *BRCA* mutation and improved RR of 36% in *BRCA* wild type patients with homologous recombination deficiency measured by high loss of heterozygosity in tumors (97).

o DESKTOP I (Descriptive Evaluation of Preoperative Selection KriTeria for OPerability): 267 platinum-sensitive recurrent ovarian cancer patients were retrospectively reviewed for predictability of secondary cytoreduction. Complete secondary resection was associated with longer survival compared to any residual postoperative disease (45.2 vs. 19.7 months). Variables associated with complete resection were: performance status, early-stage FIGO disease (I/II), residual disease left after primary surgery (none vs. any), absence of ascites, and less than 500 mL of ascites. A combination of good PS, early FIGO stage, no residual disease, and absent ascites predicted complete resection in 79% of patients (98).

o DESKTOP II AGO-OVAR OP.2: This trial evaluated 516 recurrent platinum-sensitive ovarian cancer patients. Patients were screened with the DESKTOP I prediction factors for operability for recurrent disease: (a) complete resection at first surgery, (b) good performance status, and (c) absence of ascites. The DESKTOP II trial was intended to verify the DESKTOP I trial. 51% were classified as score positive; of these 261 patients, 129 were operated on. The rate of complete resection was 76%, confirming score validity and; 11% had second operations for complications (99).

o GOG 254: sunitinib evaluation in the treatment of persistent or recurrent clear cell ovarian cancer: 30 patients were treated in this phase II trial of sunitinib 50 mg per day for 4 weeks administered in repeated 6-week cycles until DP or toxicity. 6.7% had a PR or CR. The median PFS was 2.7 months. The median OS was 12.8 months. There was minimal activity in second- and third-line treatment in recurrent clear cell ovarian cancer (100).

o Volasertib in platinum resistant or refractory ovarian cancer: 109 patients were randomized to single agent investigator chosen nonplatinum chemotherapy (PLD, topotecan, paclitaxel, or gemcitabine) or volasertib (an inhibitor of Polo-like kinases) at 300 mg IV q21 days until disease progression or toxicity. The primary endpoint was 24-week disease control rates. The disease control rate for volasertib was 30.6% versus 43.1% for chemotherapy. Median PFS was 13.1 versus 20.6 weeks favoring chemotherapy. 11% of patients receiving volasertib had a durable response rate with PFS more than 1 year, and none had that response rate with chemotherapy. Thus, single agent volasertib has shown antitumor activity in this ovarian cancer patient population (101).

○ FANG vaccine: this was a phase II trial consisting of 331 women who achieved a CCR with standard adjuvant chemotherapy. Patients were randomized 2:1 to receipt of an autologous tumor-based vaccine product incorporating a plasmid encoding granulocyte-macrophage colony-stimulating factor (GMCSF) and a novel bifunctional short hairpin ribonucleic acid (bi-shRNAi) targeting furin convertase, thereby downregulating endogenous immunosuppressive transforming growth factors (TGF) $\beta1$ and $\beta2$. Patients with advanced cancer received up to 12 monthly intradermal injections of FANG vaccine (1×10^7 or 2.5×10^7 cells/mL injection). GMCSF, TGFβ1, TGFβ2, and furin proteins were quantified by enzyme-linked immunosorbent assay (ELISA). PFS was 19.3 in the vaccine group versus 12.4 months in the observation group and saw an improved 3Y recurrence rate of 90% versus 60%. The researchers harvested cells from the tumor removed during the initial surgery to develop the personalized immunotherapy. Patients assigned the vaccine then received 1×10^7 cells/intradermal injection monthly for up to 12 doses. Researchers evaluated T-cell activation per interferon-gamma enzyme-linked immunospot assay (ELISPOT). A greater proportion of patients who were chemotherapy-naive achieved interferon-gamma ELISPOT response in the current analysis compared with the previous phase I trial (92% vs. 50%) (102).

○ **INOVATYON trial:** a phase III clinical trial of recurrent platinum-sensitive ovarian cancer [identifier: NCT01379989] comparing Arm A: PLD 30 mg/m² with carboplatin AUC 5 to Arm B: PLD 30 mg/m² and trabectedin 1.1 mg/m². Accruing.

• **Interval Debulking Trials**
○ EORTC 44865: this trial randomized 319 patients with stage III and IV after suboptimal surgery to chemotherapy with cyclophosphamide and cisplatin for six cycles or to chemotherapy with cyclophosphamide and cisplatin for three cycles with interval debulking followed by three more cycles. The interval debulking group had a significantly better median PFS of 18 months versus 13 months. The median OS was 26 months versus 20 months, favoring the interval debulking group. The risk of death decreased by 33%, $p = 0.008$ (103).

○ GOG 152: this trial randomized 424 eligible patients stage III and IV after suboptimal surgery to chemotherapy with cisplatin and paclitaxel for six cycles or to chemotherapy for three cycles with interval debulking, followed by three more cycles of chemotherapy. The median PFS was 10.5 months versus 10.7 months (HR 1.07; 95% CI: 0.869 to 1.31; $p = 0.54$). The OS was 33.7 in the chemotherapy alone group compared to 33.9 months in the IDS group. The RR for death was 0.99 (95% CI: 0.786–1.24; $p = 0.92$) (104).

There were differences between the two preceding interval debulking studies. Namely, there was a more effective second-line therapy (paclitaxel) in the GOG study, the chemotherapy regimens were different, residual disease was 5 cm or less for fewer than two thirds of patients in GOG 152 versus one third of patients in the EORTC study, and generalists did a majority of the primary surgery in the EORTC study. Furthermore, residual disease after three cycles of chemotherapy was greater than 1 cm in 65% of patients in the EORTC study, thus there was an increased chance of optimal cytoreduction in the EORTC study, compared to only 45% who were converted to optimal debulking in the GOG study.

- o GOG 213: this was a phase III randomized study with two primary objectives: (a) to examine the role of bevacizumab at 15 mg/kg in combination with paclitaxel at 175 mg/m^2 and carboplatin AUC 5 followed by bevacizumab maintenance, and (b) to examine the role of secondary cytoreduction before initiation of chemotherapy in recurrent patients. The primary endpoint was OS. Secondary endpoints were safety toxicity, allergy, PFS, and QOL. 674 patients were randomized. Prior bevacizumab was received in 67/606 patients. The median age was 60. For the chemotherapy arm: CTB combination chemotherapy improved the HR of death by 18.6% (HR 0.827; 95% CI: 0.683–1.005; $p = 0.056$) with a median OS of 42.2 versus 37.3 months. The PFS was improved with CTB with an HR 0.614 (95% CI: 0.522–0.722; $p < .0001$) with median PFS 13.8 versus 10.4 months. It extended the OS to 42.2 months versus 37.3 months but the p-value was NS at 0.056. Estimated completion for the surgical debulking arm is March 2019 (105).

- o DESKTOP III AGO-OVAR OP.4: a randomized multicenter study to compare the efficacy of additional tumor surgery versus chemotherapy alone in recurrent platinum-sensitive ovarian cancer. The AGO-score was used to select patients with a less than 30% risk of ending with residual tumor after surgery for recurrent disease to avoid including patients who would not benefit from an operation. The goal of this study was to evaluate whether maximum effort of cytoreductive surgery followed by platinum-based combination chemotherapy improved OS compared to platinum-based combination chemotherapy alone in AGO-score positive patients. Primary outcome was OS in patients with platinum-sensitive recurrent ovarian cancer with a positive AGO-score. Secondary outcome measures: QOL and PFS. Results pending.

- o SOCceR-1 trial: this is a multicenter randomized trial for women with first recurrence of FIGO stage IC to IV platinum-sensitive epithelial ovarian, fallopian tube, or primary peritoneal cancer. First line treatment must have consisted of optimal (≤1 cm) cytoreductive surgery and (neoadjuvant) platinum/taxol-based chemotherapy. Inclusion criteria are: ascites < 500 mL (pocket < 8 cm on ultrasound examination), and the potential for R0 status after secondary cytoreduction, and a ECOG PS 0–1. First recurrence is defined as clinical and radiological signs of recurrence (RECIST 1.1 criteria) or elevated CA 125 (GCIG criteria). Participants were randomized between the standard of at least six cycles of IV platinum-based chemotherapy without secondary debulking surgery or versus the experimental treatment of secondary cytoreductive surgery followed by at least six cycles of IV platinum-based chemotherapy. The primary outcome measure was PFS. Results pending (106).

- o Surgery in Ovarian Cancer Quality of life Evaluation Research study (SOCQER 1): SOCQER 1 was a single institution prospective evaluation of QOL following primary PDS or IDS in 93 women, 24 of whom had extensive ovarian cancer surgery, 32 who had standard ovarian cancer surgery (based on Aletti Surgical Complexity Score of 3 or lower) compared to 32 patients who had surgery for benign indications. These were reviewed at sequential time points. The cohort undergoing extensive surgery had deterioration in the immediate and short term QOL measures. But by 9 months scores in all three cohorts were equal (107).

- **Neoadjuvant Therapy Trials**
  - EORTC 55971: this trial evaluated 632 eligible patients who were staged IIIC or IV. They were randomized to upfront debulking surgery versus three cycles of neoadjuvant platinum-based chemotherapy followed by interval surgery and subsequent chemotherapy. Inclusion criteria were biopsy-proven ovarian cancer, in combination with a pelvic mass, the presence of metastases of ≥2 cm outside the pelvis, and a CA-125:CEA ratio ≥25. The median follow-up was 4.8 years. Baseline characteristics for Arms A and B were, respectively: median largest metastasis, 80/80 mm; FIGO stage IIIC, 76%/76%. The largest residual tumor was ≤1 cm in 48% after PDS (Arm A) and 83% after IDS (Arm B). Complications of PDS and IDS were: postoperative mortality 2.7%/0.6%; sepsis 8%/2%; grade 3/4 and hemorrhage 7%/4%. The PFS was 11 months in both arms (HR 0.99; 95% CI: 0.87–1.13). An OS of 29 and 30 months was seen for Arms A and B (HR 0.98; 95% CI: 0.85–1.14) (95).

    Some critics suggest that this OS is still less than the 36 months seen in the carboplatin/paclitaxel arm of GOG 111 evaluating suboptimally debulked ovarian cancer. Regarding neoadjuvant therapy versus PDS: the overall PFS was similar for both arms, approximately 12 months. OS was 30 versus 29 months overall. For those with R0 disease, OS was 38 versus 45 months, R1 disease 27 versus 32 months, R2 disease 25 versus 26 months.

  - MRC CHORUS trial: this study attempted to confirm the results of EORTC 55971. In this study, 550 patients with clinical FIGO stages III to IV ovarian cancer were randomized to surgery followed by six cycles of chemotherapy or NACT. The median age was 65, the median tumor size was 8 cm, 25% were stage IV, and 19% had a WHO PS of 2. There was a well-balanced randomization. In the intent-to-treat analysis, a median OS of 22.8 months for PDS was observed versus 24.5 months for NACT (HR 0.87; 95% CI: 0.76–0.98) favoring NACT. The median PFS was 10.2 versus 11.7 months (HR 0.91; 95% CI: 0.81–1.02) (108).

  - Which patients benefit most from primary surgery or neoadjuvant chemotherapy in stage IIIC or IV ovarian cancer? 670 patients from EROTC 55971 were reviewed. These patients had been randomly assigned to PDS or neoadjuvant chemotherapy. Clinical factors were reviewed for those who could benefit more from the differing primary approaches. The size of the largest metastatic tumor and clinical stage were significantly associated with the magnitude of the benefit from treatment in terms of 5 YS. Stage IIIC patients with tumors less than 4.5 cm benefited more from PDS whereas stage IV patients with metastatic tumors greater than 4.5 cm benefited more from neoadjuvant chemotherapy. Primary outcome was OS. The potential 5 YS in the population of treated patients would be 27.3%, 7.8% higher than if all were treated with primary surgery, and 5.6% higher than if all were treated with neoadjuvant chemotherapy (109).

  - A meta-analysis suggests that, for each extra cycle of neoadjuvant chemotherapy, there is a 4.1-month decrease in survival. Within this meta-analysis, each 10% increase in cytoreduction yielded a 5.5% median increase in survival time, which equates to 3 months (10).

○ SCORPION trial: this was a phase III trial evaluating 110 patients randomized to either PDS followed by adjuvant chemotherapy or NACT followed by IDS. Patients were triaged preoperatively to laparoscopic staging to assess tumor load. Tumor load was documented as a Fagotti score. 45.5% of the PDS patients had R0 status postoperatively compared to 57.7% of those who received NACT; $p = 0.206$. 52.7% of the patients in the PDS arm had grade 3–4 complications compared to 5.7% in the IDS arm, $p = 0.0001$ (110–112).

○ Neoadjuvant chemotherapy has also been found to not improve the rate of complete resection or affect the morbidity of IDS in another study. This retrospective study reviewed 200 patients in separate cohorts based on year of diagnosis. Cohort 1 was those diagnosed from 2009 to 2011 with PDS; cohort 2 was those diagnosed after 2011 to 2013 (at publication of EORTC Vergote) and they underwent visceral-peritoneal debulking after three cycles of neoadjuvant chemotherapy. Patients with complete response or progressive disease never underwent surgical resection. Patients had diagnostic laparoscopy before debulking to evaluate for small bowel serosal disease or porta hepatic encasement. If no small bowel or porta hepatic involvement, conversion to laparotomy and debulking was attempted. Debulking was completed in 90% of patients in both groups. There was no difference in operating room times, estimated blood loss, hospital stay, or postoperative complications between cohorts (113).

○ Yet another study shows that PDS should be the primary management approach for advanced EOC. Those who had NACT were more likely to have no residual disease (50.1% vs. 41.5%). The 7 YS for PDS was found to be 41% versus 8.6% if NACT was used. For those who obtained R0 at PDS, the 7 YS was 73.6% versus 21%. Those who had PDS with R0 status and had IP chemotherapy had a 7 YS of 90% (114).

○ Summation of OS and PFS in seminal NACT, IP, and PDS trials.
  ▪ JGOG Dose-dense* paclitaxel versus conventional q21 days dosing:
    □ OS 100.5 versus 62.2 months
    □ PFS 28.2 months versus 17.5 months
  ▪ GOG 172 IP* versus IV dosing
    □ OS 65.5 versus 49.7 months
    □ PFS 23.8 months versus 18.3 months
  ▪ Landrum's review on GOG 114/172 data on R1/R0 patients IP* versus IV
    □ OS 43.2 months versus 20.1 months
    □ PFS 100 months versus 50.9 months
  ▪ Chan's GOG 262 dose dense paclitaxel versus q21 day with bevacizumab
    □ PFS 14.7 months versus 14 months overall. But subgroup analysis:
      – 14.2 months versus 10.3 months dose dense* no bevacizumab
      – 14.9 months versus 14.7 months dose dense plus bevacizumab
  ▪ Vergote's EORTC neoadjuvant versus PDS* both using q21 day dosing
    □ PFS similar: both around 12 months
    □ OS is similar at 30 months neoadjuvant versus 29 months PDS, but see the following for subgroup analysis by R status

- □ R0: 38 months versus 45 months favoring PDS
- □ R1: 27 months versus 32 months favoring PDS
- □ R2: 25 months versus 26 months
- **Translational Studies**:
  - ○ OVCAD study: "Ovarian Cancer—Diagnosis of a Silent Killer" is a study aimed to investigate new predictors for early detection of minimal residual disease in EOC. In this study, 275 consecutive patients with EOC were included and their clinical outcomes with regard to pathology, surgery, and chemotherapy were reviewed. Evaluable patients had stage II to IV cancer who underwent cytoreductive surgery, adjuvant platinum-based chemotherapy and had tissue specimens collected. Characteristics of the patients included the following: median age of diagnosis was 58 years, 94.5% Stage III/IV, 96% grade 2/3, 86% with serous histology, 67.6% with peritoneal implants, 76% with ascites, 52% with positive lymph nodes. The majority of patients underwent a bilateral salpingo-oophorectomy (90.9%) and omentectomy (92.4%); 77.3% underwent hysterectomy. 37.7% patients had a resection of the large bowel while 13.4% of patients had a small bowel resection. 69.5% of patients had a pelvic lymph node dissection and 66.9% underwent para aortic lymph node dissection. "Macroscopic" cytoreduction was achieved in 68.4%. Platinum-based chemotherapy was used in 98.2% of the patients. At the time of median follow up (37 months), 70 patients (25.5%) had platinum resistant recurrent disease. Results from this trial are being used in a myriad of other reviews (115).

OVARIAN TUMORS OF LOW MALIGNANT POTENTIAL (LMP): BORDERLINE TUMORS

CHARACTERISTICS

- LMP tumors represent 5% to 15% of ovarian malignancies. The median age at diagnosis ranges from 39 to 45 years old. 20% of these tumors are diagnosed at stage III or IV. There are no known risk factors.
- Clinical features include a mass, abdominal pain, bloating, abdominal distension, early satiety, dyspepsia, and an elevated CA-125.
- The route of spread is often transcoelomic, and can be lymphatic.
- Prognostic factors are stage, residual tumor, the presence of invasive implants, and micropapillary histology.

HISTOLOGY

- Pathologically, there is the absence of stromal invasion and the tumors have at least two of the following: nuclear atypia, mitotic activity, pseudostratification, and epithelial budding. There are two main histologic types: serous and mucinous. If foci are found of stromal invasion measuring 3 to 5 mm or 10 mm^2, the tumor is considered microinvasive. Outcomes for microinvasive tumors are usually favorable and parallel LMP tumors. If a mucinous borderline tumor is found to have three or more layers of epithelial cell stratification, it is considered a carcinoma. There is guidance from WHO that LMP tumors may represent the early part of the disease spectrum for invasive tubo-ovarian carcinomas.

- Frozen section diagnosis of borderline tumors can be difficult. In one study of patients with a final diagnosis of LMP tumor, 10% were diagnosed as having invasive cancer and 25% were reported to have benign cystadenomas on intra-operative frozen section. Therefore, the sensitivity of the frozen section analysis for LMP's was 65% (95% CI: 55%, 75%) (116). Size greater than 8 cm, micro-papillary, endometrioid, or clear cell carcinoma histologies can contribute to this difficulty.

- The micropapillary subtype is a distinct entity and carries an adverse prognosis. *BRAF* mutations are commonly found in this subtype. The distinguishing architecture is a height-to-width ratio of 5:1. It is often associated with invasive implants. Micropapillary histology has a higher rate of recurrence at 26%.

- Serous LMP tumors represent 62% of all LMP tumors; 30% are diagnosed as stage I, and they are often bilateral; 10% to 20% have invasive implants.

- Mucinous LMP tumors represent about 38% of LMP tumors and 80% to 90% are found as stage I; 5% are bilateral. There is a greater malignant potential with these tumors than with the serous LMP tumors.

- Invasive implants are a major factor in determining whether to treat with adjuvant therapies or not. The 7Y OS for patients with noninvasive implants is 96%, and for those with invasive implants, 66%. The risk of invasive implants accompanies histology: for serous borderline tumors the risk is 6%, but increases to 49% with micropapillary tumors.

PRE-TREATMENT WORKUP

- Workup is the same as for TOC.

STAGING

- Staging is the same as for TOC. Contralateral tubo-ovarian and uterine conservation may be considered in patients considering future fertility with completion surgery after childbearing.

TREATMENT

- Treatment is primarily surgical and follows the same directives as those for malignant ovarian cancer: complete surgical staging with full cytoreduction to microscopic disease status.

- Fertility sparing treatment is a reasonable option if desired. A cystectomy or unilateral salpingo-oophorectomy (USO) can be performed with additional staging LND, biopsies, and omentectomy. The recurrence rate overall is 12%. If a cystectomy is performed, the recurrence rate is 23%, compared to 8% with a USO. The median time to recurrence is 2.6 years after a cystectomy and 4.7 years after a USO.

- If surgical staging was not performed or this was an incidental pathologic finding, there are data to suggest that repeat staging is not beneficial in this patient population, given that no micropapillary histology is present. One series (116) compared early-stage LMP tumors in 31 staged patients to 42 unstaged patients ($p = 0.01$). 17% of patients had their stage upgraded based on surgical staging, but 5Y OS was 93% for all stages. The OS was similar in both groups. LN positivity made no difference in OS. Oftentimes endosalpingiosis is seen in the LN.

- Adjuvant chemotherapy should be considered if there are invasive implants. Treatment usually includes adjuvant chemotherapy that is platinum based. There is an average 25% response rate for LMP tumors to chemotherapy. At second look, the response to chemotherapy was 15% if noninvasive implants were present, versus 57% if invasive implants were present, thus borderline tumors are not completely chemoresistant (117).

RECURRENCE

- Recurrence in a spared contralateral ovary can occur in 16%–23% of patients, but is treated by resection of the tube and ovary. There were no deaths in those managed conservatively.
- Recurrent disease is often indolent. Recommended treatment is repeat cytoreduction. Overall, 5% to 10% of tumors recur. There are data to suggest that 73% recur as low-grade invasive cancers (118).

SURVIVAL (Table 2.11)

Table 2.11 LMP Ovarian Cancer 10Y Survival by Stage

Stage	Relative 10Y survival (%)
I	99
II	98
III	96
IV	77

LMP, low-malignant potential.

SURVIVAL CARE

- Follows the same pattern as that of HGSTOC.

FALLOPIAN TUBE CANCER

CHARACTERISTICS

- The origin of primary ovarian cancer, based on advancing genetic investigations and correlation with histopathologic evidence is most likely metastatic primary fallopian tube cancer (PFTC). Thus, fallopian tube, ovarian, and primary peritoneal cancers are now grouped under the same umbrella for diagnosis, treatment, and management as tubo-ovarian cancers. The incidence of PFTC was stated to be 0.41/100,000 women (119). Bilateral involvement is found in 5% to 30% of patients, and one third of patients have LN metastasis at the time of staging. Route of spread is transcoelomic, lymphatic, and hematogenous.

- Hu's criteria were established to assist in the definitive diagnosis of PFTC (120). This was further modified by Sedlis in 1978 (121) and the criteria are: a) the main tumor is in the tube and arises from the endosalpinx; b) the pattern histologically reproduces the epithelium of fallopian tube mucosa and shows a papillary pattern; c) the transition between benign and malignant tubal epithelium should be demonstrable; d) and the ovaries and endometrium are normal or contain less tumor than the tube.
- There is often a triad of symptoms: pelvic pain, a pelvic mass, and watery vaginal discharge (hydrops tubae profluens). This occurs in 11% of patients. A pelvic mass is diagnosed in 12% to 66% of patients.

PRE-TREATMENT WORKUP

- Workup includes a history and physical examination with lab tests. Tumor markers including a CA-125 are drawn. An abnormal Pap smear has been found to be positive in 18% to 60% of patients. Imaging with ultrasound, CT, or MRI can be helpful.

HISTOLOGY

- Ninety percent of tumors are serous, but other subtypes are found including endometrioid, transitional and mixed mesodermal Müllerian tumor.

STAGING

- Staging follows the same criteria as that for tubo-ovarian cancer.

TREATMENT

- Primary treatment is usually surgical to follow the general TOC protocols.
- Surgery includes full staging with a TH-BSO, LND (if less than stage IIIC), omentectomy, peritoneal biopsies, and debulking to microscopic residual disease.
- Chemotherapy follows the same principles as that of tubo-ovarian cancer with first-line platinum- and paclitaxel-based combination regimens.
- Treatment by stage and grade:
  - Stage I grade 1: definitive surgery
  - Stage I grade 2 or 3: surgery and adjuvant chemotherapy
  - Stage II to IV: surgery and (neo) adjuvant chemotherapy

SURVIVAL (Table 2.12)

Table 2.12 Fallopian Tube Cancer 5Y Survival by Stage	
Stage	Relative 5Y survival (%)
I	87
II	86
III	52
IV	40

SURVIVAL CARE

- Follows the same principles as that of TOC.

PRIMARY PERITONEAL CANCER

- Differentiation between primary peritoneal cancer (PPC) and primary tubo-ovarian carcinomas can be difficult. PPC may be unrecognized metastatic serous tubal intraepithelial carcinoma (STIC) or PFTC. Pathologic criteria previously established to determine a primary peritoneal site are: the bulk of tumor is on the peritoneum rather than on the ovaries; normal-sized ovaries are present or the ovaries are enlarged by a benign process; tumor involves the ovaries to a depth that is less than 5 mm and a width that is less than 5 mm; the tumor is serous by nature. Again, peritoneal, tubal, and ovarian cancers are now grouped under one heading for diagnosis, treatment, and management.
- PPC can be considered an expression of hereditary breast and ovarian cancer syndromes. There is a 2% to 4.3% risk of primary peritoneal cancer after prophylactic oophorectomy in hereditary cancer mutation carriers.
- Workup, staging, treatment, survival, and survival care follow the same principles as that of TOC.

GERM CELL TUMORS

CHARACTERISTICS

- GCTs are hypothesized to arise from an unfertilized ovum. They represent 15% to 20% of ovarian cancers, and 70% of ovarian tumors in women less than 30 years of age. The median age at diagnosis is 19 years, 30% are malignant, 60% to 75% are stage I at diagnosis, and 25% to 30% are stage III at diagnosis.
- Clinical symptoms include a mass, abdominal distension, bloating, pelvic pressure, or pain. Pain can occur from mass effect, torsion, and/or hemorrhage.
- Paraneoplastic syndromes are common: hyperthyroidism can occur from teratomatous thyroid tissue, hypertension from renin-producing teratomas, hypoglycemia from insulin production, as well as autoimmune hemolytic anemia from teratomas.
- 5Y survival (Table 2.13)

Table 2.13 Germ Cell Ovarian Cancer 5Y Survival by Stage

Stage	Relative 5Y survival (%)
I	98
II	94
III	87
IV	69

PRE-TREATMENT WORKUP

- The pre-treatment workup includes a physical examination, CXR, abdominal pelvic imaging to include pelvic ultrasound, CT, or MRI, serum tumor markers, and a karyotype in short or premenarchal females.
- Serum tumor markers specific to histology include:
  - Dysgerminoma: human chorionic gonadotropin (hCG) (5%), lactate dehydrogenase (LDH)
  - Endodermal sinus tumor: alpha fetoprotein (AFP), LDH
  - Immature teratoma (IT): AFP, LDH
  - Embryonal carcinoma: hCG, AFP, LDH
  - Choriocarcinoma: hCG
  - Polyembryoma: hCG, AFP, LDH
  - Mixed: hCG, AFP, LDH

STAGING

- Staging for GCT is per tubo-ovarian cancer FIGO and AJCC protocols.
- Inadequately staged patients can be managed in two ways: with surgical re-exploration and staging; or chemotherapy without re-exploration, especially if the histologic subtype demands chemotherapy regardless of stage.

TREATMENT

- Surgical exploration is advised if a mass greater than 2 cm is found in premenarchal girls, or a mass greater than 6 to 8 cm is found in adolescents or postmenopausal females. If tumor markers such as AFP or hCG are found elevated, and pregnancy is ruled out, exploration should also be considered. Surgical treatment includes: washings, a USO if fertility is desired, along with staging biopsies, omentectomy, LND, and debulking of disease. If fertility is not desired, a hysterectomy with BSO is indicated in addition to the preceding staging procedures.
- The role of optimal cytoreduction is also important with these tumors. In a study of 76 patients, a 28% recurrence rate was seen if they were completely resected, versus a 68% recurrence rate if there was residual disease (122). In another study of patients treated with cisplatin–vinblastine–bleomycin (PVB), those with measurable disease had a 34% DFS versus 65% if optimally debulked (123).
- Adjuvant chemotherapy is recommended for all tumors except for stage IA dysgerminomas and stage IAG1 ITs. Chemotherapy is recommended to be platinum based and consists of bleomycin–etoposide–cisplatin (BEP) for three to four cycles. Total bleomycin dose should be evaluated to ensure it does not surpass 450 mg/m2, which is the toxicity level.
- The number of BEP cycles is debated. Three cycles are recommended for optimally debulked stages I to III disease. Four cycles are given for suboptimally debulked disease or stage IV disease. If tumor markers are still elevated, chemotherapy should continue for two cycles past normalization of these markers.

RECURRENCE

- Recurrence is documented by physical examination, a rise in serum tumor markers, or imaging. 90% of relapses occur within 2 years.
- GCTs are classified as platinum resistant if there is recurrence within 4 to 6 weeks. Patients with elevated tumor markers at presentation and who do not achieve a negative marker status at four cycles are considered to be failure of response. Salvage chemotherapy should be implemented.
- Some clinicians have recommended salvage cytoreduction showing a 61% 5 YS if optimally salvaged versus 14% 5 YS in those not secondarily optimally cytoreduced (124).

FOLLOW-UP

- For nondysgerminomatous tumors, follow-up should occur every 3 months for the first 2 years, every 6 months up to 5 years.
- For dysgerminomas, a 10Y follow-up is recommended. Serum hCG and AFP should be measured for all patients, even if not initially elevated. 10–20% of tumors do relapse.

HISTOLOGIC SUBTYPES AND DIRECTED THERAPIES

- **Dysgerminomas** represent 40% of GCT; 95% are found in stage I. There is greater malignant potential if the tumor is larger than 10 cm, there is an elevated LDH, a high mitotic index, and necrosis. Five percent of tumors produce hCG and placental alkaline phosphatase (PLAP), due to the presence of syncytiotrophoblastic tissue.
  - Adjuvant therapy is indicated for patients staged IB or greater. BEP for three to four cycles is the recommended regimen; alternatively radiation therapy (XRT) can be considered.
  - It is important to check a karyotype because 15% of patients are intersex with XY gonadal dysgenesis. If this is found, a prophylactic bilateral gonadectomy should be considered because of the high risk for contralateral dysgerminoma. Gonadectomy should be performed before puberty except in females with testicular feminization. The gonads should be removed after puberty in these cases.
  - If a dysgerminoma is found incidentally after primary surgery, restaging can be considered but is not always indicated, if there is no bulky disease.
  - For Stage IA patients, there is a 20% recurrence rate. If patients were unstaged, consider surveillance, and salvage therapies initiated at recurrence. If there is recurrent disease, XRT or chemotherapy can be administered.
- Gonadoblastomas are rare benign GCTs. These tumors have up to a 10% chance of malignant transformation. The gonads should be removed if a gonadoblastoma is found in a dysgenic gonad.
- Endodermal sinus tumors represent 22% of GCT.
  - The histologic pearl is the presence of Schiller–Duval bodies. These are hyaline bodies that resemble the glomerulus in the kidney.
  - All patients require adjuvant postoperative chemotherapy, which should begin within 7 to 10 days of surgery due to rapid growth of disease.

Recommended therapy is BEP for three to four cycles, or POMB-ACE every 3 weeks for four cycles. Survival is 2% to 10% without chemotherapy. This is the most virulent of the GCT.

- Embryonal carcinoma is a rare tumor that occurs in younger patients. There are no trophoblastic tissues in this tumor. Adjuvant treatment should consist of BEP chemotherapy regardless of stage.
- Choriocarcinoma is a rare tumor, especially the nongestational type. Adjuvant treatment should consist of BEP chemotherapy regardless of stage.
- Polyembryoma is an extremely rare GCT with fewer than 40 cases reported in the literature. Embryoid bodies are seen at pathology. Adjuvant treatment consists of BEP chemotherapy regardless of stage.
- Mixed GCT constitutes 1% to 15% of all GCT. They most commonly consist of dysgerminomatous and endodermal sinus tumor components. Adjuvant treatment should consist of BEP chemotherapy regardless of stage.
- Mature cystic teratoma, also known as a dermoid, represents 95% of ovarian teratomas. All three germ cell layers are represented. This tumor does not constitute a malignancy. It can present as a mass, and it can cause pain via torsion or rupture (Figure 2.7).
  - The tubercle of Rokitansky is a mural density seen on radiologic imaging.
  - Treatment is surgical with a cystectomy or USO.
  - Malignant degeneration can occur in 1% to 2% of mature cystic teratoma (MCTs). This is usually found in a focus of squamous cell carcinoma from skin lining the cyst. Intraoperative spill of sebaceous contents can cause a chemical peritonitis.
  - Gliomatosis peritonei is the presence of benign peritoneal implants of mature neuroglia. These implants usually undergo remission upon resection of the primary tumor.
- **Immature teratomas** constitute 20% of GCTs. An immature teratoma (IT) is defined as the presence of any immature neural tissue. Immature neural tissue is seen as rosettes or neurotubules within the tumor.

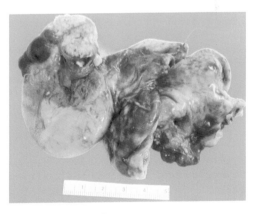

Figure 2.7 Dermoid tumor with teeth.

○ The amount of immature tissue on one low-power slide determines the grade. The grading system for IT is: grade (G) 1, 1 low-power field (LPF 10×) of neural elements in any slide; G2, no greater than a total of 3 LPFs of neural elements in any slide; G3, greater than 3 LPFs full of neural elements in at least one slide.

○ Chemotherapy is indicated for all patients except stage IA grade 1. Recommended therapy is BEP every 3 weeks for three to four cycles.

○ A second-look laparotomy is recommended if there is residual tumor seen on imaging after completion of chemotherapy. This can remove chemoresistant disease or determine if there was conversion to mature teratoma.

GCT TRIALS

- GOG 10: 76 patients with malignant GCTs received vincristine, dactinomycin, and cyclophosphamide (VAC) postoperatively; 54 patients were optimally debulked; 28% of these failed compared to 68% of those who were incompletely resected and failed. Therefore, PVB was trialed for those who were suboptimally resected (122).

- GOG 45: 97 eligible patients with stage II to IV or recurrent disease were treated with three to four cycles of PVB. Of 35 patients with tumors other than dysgerminoma who had clinically measurable disease, 43% had a CR. The OS was 71% and the DFS was 51% (123).

- GOG 78: this study evaluated 93 eligible patients with surgically staged and resected GCTs. Three cycles of BEP were given as primary adjuvant therapy; 89 of the 93 patients were continuously disease free. At second-look laparotomy, two patients were found to have foci of IT but remained CCR. Final conclusions were that 91 of 93 patients were progression free after surgery and three cycles of BEP. Patients with IT may benefit from secondary debulking if residual disease is identified (125).

- GOG 90: 20 patients with incompletely resected ovarian dysgerminoma were treated with cisplatin, bleomycin, and either vinblastine or etoposide. Consolidation chemotherapy with VAC was included for some. 11 patients had clinically measurable disease postoperatively, and 10 responded completely. Fourteen second-look procedures were done, and all were negative; 19 of 20 patients were disease-free with a median follow-up of 26 months (126).

- GOG 116: this study evaluated 39 eligible stage IB to III completely resected dysgerminoma patients. Carboplatin 400 mg/m^2 on day 1 and etoposide 120 mg/m^2 on days 1,2,3 q28 days for three courses were used as primary adjuvant therapy. This doublet therapy was found to be well tolerated for those who needed to reduce chemotoxicity. There were no recurrences. Critics suggest the lack of bleomycin can contribute to an inferior outcome such as that seen in testes cancer (pharmacologic sanctuary), so the doublet should not be used without bleomycin in ovarian GCTs (127).

- A GOG assessment of SLL in GCT evaluated 117 patients from GOG studies 45, 78, and 90. Of the 45 patients treated with BEP after optimal debulking, 38 had a negative SLL. They concluded there was no need for SLL. A subgroup analysis suggested that SLL may be of value in approximately 33% of patients with suboptimal debulking for GCT with teratomatous elements. Of the 24 patients with teratoma in the primary tumor, 16 patients had bulky residual disease; 14 of 16 patients were disease free after secondary debulking (135).

SEX CORD STROMAL TUMORS

CHARACTERISTICS

- Sex cord stromal tumors represent 5% to 8% ovarian malignancies and 5% of childhood tumors. They are bilateral in 2% of patients. 85% of these tumors produce steroid hormones. The route of spread is transcoelomic, lymphatic, and hematogenous.
- 5Y survival (Table 2.14)

Table 2.14 Sex Cord Stromal Ovarian Cancer 5Y Survival by Stage

Stage	5Y survival (%)
I	95
II	78
III	65
IV	35

PRE-TREATMENT WORKUP

- The pre-treatment workup includes serum hormonal evaluation (free testosterone, estradiol, 17-hydroxy-progesterone, serum cortisol, dehydroepiandrosterone sulfate (DHEAS), dehydroepiandrosterone (DHEA), AFP, LDH, inhibin A, inhibin B, and hCG), and imaging including CXR and ultrasound, CT, or MRI.

STAGING

- Staging is the same as TOC. There are data to suggest a primary LND does not often yield positive results (128).

TREATMENT

- Surgical treatment is with washings, a USO if fertility is desired, along with staging biopsies, omentectomy, LND, and debulking of disease. A D&C should be considered if fertility preservation is undertaken especially for granulosa cell tumors. If fertility is not desired, a hysterectomy with BSO is indicated.

HISTOLOGY (Table 2.15)

Table 2.15 Ovarian Stromal Tumor WHO Classification Overview and Risk of Malignancy

Granulosa cell tumors	
Adult	Malignant
Juvenile	Malignant
Thecoma	
Thecomas, typical	Benign

(continued)

Table 2.15 Ovarian Stromal Tumor WHO Classification Overview and Risk of Malignancy (*continued*)

Thecomas, luteinized	Malignant potential
Thecoma with increased mitotic figures	Malignant potential
Fibroma	
Cellular fibroma	Malignant potential
Cellular fibroma with increased mitotic figures	Malignant potential
Fibrosarcoma	Malignant
Stromal tumor with minor sex cord elements	Benign
Sclerosing stromal tumor	Benign
Signet ring stromal tumors	Benign
Unclassified	Malignant potential
Sertoli–Leydig cell tumors	
Well differentiated	Malignant potential
Intermediate differentiation	Malignant
Poorly differentiated	Malignant
Sertoli–Leydig tumors with heterologous elements	Malignant
Sertoli cell tumors	Malignant potential
Leydig cell tumors	Benign
Stromal–Leydig cell tumors	Benign
Sex cord tumors with annular tubules (SCTAT)	Malignant
Microscopic SCTAT associated with Peutz–Jeghers syndrome	Benign
Gynandroblastoma	Malignant/malignant potential
Unclassified sex cord stromal tumors	Malignant potential
Steroid cell tumors	Malignant

Source: Ref. (129). Tavassoeli FA, Devilee P, eds. *WHO Classification of Tumours, Pathology and Genetics: Tumours of the Breast and Female Genital Organs.* Lyon: IARC; 2003.

- **Stromal tumors**
  - **Granulosa cell tumors**
    - Granulosa cell tumors represent 1% to 2% of ovarian tumors.
    - These tumors tend to produce high levels of estrogen that can cause the refeminization of postmenopausal patients, and isosexual precious puberty in prepubertal girls. Patients may experience associated vaginal

bleeding, with up to 50% of patients having endometrial hyperplasia and up to 5% with a concordant uterine cancer.

- The histologic pearls are: the presence of Call–Exner bodies and coffee bean nuclei.
- Most granulosa tumors are of the adult type (95%) and the rest are of the juvenile type.
- The juvenile type is relatively benign in early stages but can be aggressive in advanced stages. Associated syndromes are Ollier's disease (enchondromatosis) and Maffucci's syndrome (hemangiomas and sarcomas). The OS for stage I juvenile tumors is 97% versus 23% for stage III/IV. There are no Call–Exner bodies in the juvenile type.
- It is important to check a serum estradiol (>30 pg/mL in a postmenopausal woman is abnormal) and both the alpha and beta inhibin levels.
- Treatment is surgical with comprehensive staging.
- Adjuvant chemotherapy is considered for stage IC and higher. Recurrence is often indolent at 5 to 20 years. See MITO-9 study.
- Prognostic factors for adverse outcomes are: size greater than 10 cm, rupture, greater than 2 mitosis/10 HPF, LVSI, and nuclear atypia.
- For recurrent or metastatic disease, patients can be retreated with BEP or other regimens to possibly include platinum with paclitaxel, high-dose progestins, gonadotropin-releasing hormone (GnRH) agonists, or XRT. One study demonstrated a 43% CCR with XRT in patients with measurable disease (130). Another study has shown an 86% RR for granulosa cell tumors treated with XRT (131).

○ **Thecomas**
  - Thecomas represent 1% of ovarian tumors and are bilateral in 3%. They are benign tumors. They can produce estrogen.

○ **Fibroma–fibrosarcoma**
  - Fibromas are the most common sex cord stromal tumor and 10% are bilateral. They are benign tumors. They occasionally secrete estrogen. They have an association with Meigs syndrome, which is the presence of an adnexal fibroma, ascites, and a pleural effusion.

○ **Sex-cord Tumors Androblastomas**
  - This tumor is diagnosed at a median age of 30 years. This tumor can cause virilization. It is important to follow the serum AFP and testosterone. Adjuvant chemotherapy is recommended if the tumor contains heterologous elements or is poorly differentiated. Recurrence is usually within the first 2 years.

○ **Sertoli cell tumor**
  - Sertoli cell tumor is also called a Pick's adenoma.
  - It produces estrogen in 65% of patients and can also produce androgens. It rarely produces hyperaldosteronism with associated hyperkalemia and hypertension.
  - The histologic pearl is: the Pick's body.
  - There is an increased risk of malignancy if: hemorrhage, necrosis, a high mitotic count, or poor differentiation is present.

- ○ **Leydig cell tumors**
  - ▪ Leydig cell tumors produce androgens in 80% and estrogen in 10% of patients; 2.5% are malignant. They usually present after the age of 50 years and are associated with thyroid disease.
- ○ **Sertoli–Leydig cell tumor**
  - ▪ Sertoli–Leydig cell tumors can cause virilization in 1/2 to 2/3's of patients. Most tumors produce testosterone and this can cause menstrual irregularities.
  - ▪ The histologic pearl is: the crystals of Reinke.
  - ▪ Ninety percent are found at stage I, and less than 20% are malignant.
  - ▪ For those who are malignant: 10% are grade 2 and 60% are grade 3. Malignant tumors tend to have more necrosis, are larger, and hemorrhage more frequently.
  - ▪ Adjuvant chemotherapy should consist of BEP if malignant.
- **Gynandroblastoma**
  - ○ Gynandroblastoma tumors can produce androgens and estrogens. These tumors can have both granulosa and Sertoli–Leydig components.
- **Sex cord tumor with annular tubules**
  - ○ Sex cord tumors with annular tubules can produce estrogen. Two thirds are bilateral.
    - ▪ These tumors can be associated with Peutz–Jeghers (PJ) syndrome and are benign when they have this association. PJ syndrome has an associated 15% risk of cervical adenocarcinoma (adenoma malignum) and hysterectomy should be considered after fertility is concluded.
    - ▪ If patients are not diagnosed with PJ syndrome, these tumors are considered malignant. Treatment for non-PJ syndrome patients is surgical with a USO, LND, and staging. A D&C, endocervical curettage (ECC), and colposcopy should be performed if fertility is desired, and a TH-BSO otherwise.
- **Unclassified**
  - ○ **Lipid cell tumors**
    - ▪ Lipid cell tumors can be virilizing and produce Cushing's syndrome. They produce estrogen, progesterone, and testosterone.
    - ▪ These are malignant in 20% of cases. Indications of malignancy are: pleomorphism, necrosis, a high mitotic count, and a size greater than 8 cm.
    - ▪ Adjuvant BEP chemotherapy is recommended if found to be malignant.
  - ○ **Sex cord tumors not otherwise specified**
    - ▪ Sex cord tumors not otherwise specified produce a variety of hormones; up to 17% of patients have Cushing's disease.
    - ▪ Forty-three percent of these tumors are malignant. Malignant tumors contain fibrothecomatous areas and/or granulosa cell-like proliferation as well as areas of tubular differentiation.
    - ▪ Adjuvant BEP chemotherapy is recommended if malignant.

5Y SURVIVAL

- Dysgerminoma
  - ○ Stage I: 90% to 95%
  - ○ All stages: 60% to 90%

- Endodermal sinus tumor
  - Stage I and II: 90%
  - Stage III and IV: 50%
- Immature teratoma
  - Stage I: 90% to 95%
  - All stages: 70% to 80%
  - Grade 1: 82%
  - Grade 2: 62%
  - Grade 3: 30%
- Embryonal carcinoma
  - All stages: 39%
- Choriocarcinoma: poor
- Polyembryoma: poor
- Mixed: depends on tumor composition
- Granulosa cell:
  - Stages I, II: 85% to 95%
  - Stages III, IV: 55% to 60%
- Sertoli–Leydig:
  - Grade 3: poor survival

SEX CORD STROMAL TUMOR TRIALS

- GOG 115: this study evaluated 57 eligible patients who had incompletely resected stages II to IV ovarian stromal malignancies. BEP was used as first-line therapy every 3 weeks for four cycles. The endpoint was negative second-look laparotomy: 37% had negative findings. Patients with measurable disease had the highest risk of progression and death. BEP was found to be active in stromal tumors (132).
- GOG 264: a randomized phase II trial of paclitaxel and carboplatin versus bleomycin etoposide and cisplatin for newly diagnosed advanced stage and recurrent chemo-naive sex cord stromal tumors of the ovary. Results pending with estimated completion date 2024.
- MITO-9: 40 patients with stage 1C granulosa cell tumor were retrospectively reviewed. 35% had fertility-sparing treatment, 22.5% received adjuvant BEP or carboplatin/taxol, 35% relapsed, and there was no difference in DFS between those who received and those who did not receive adjuvant chemotherapy. 5Y DFS was 27% compared to 50%, $p = 0.4$. Adjuvant chemotherapy was not predictive for recurrence although incomplete surgical staging was. This study was limited by being a retrospective review and by low power (133).
- Surveillance options after initial surgery for pediatric and adolescent girls with stage I ovarian GCTs are debatable. High-risk histologies or stage IB and higher should be, in our opinion, considered for adjuvant chemotherapy.
  - A report from the Children's Oncology Group states that some girls can be watched rather than treated upfront due to high salvage rates. Careful discussion should be held with patient and family due to this being a small study 48% recurrent with surveillance, and one death was observed. 25 girls were reviewed with a median age of 12 years. Of these, 23 patients

had an elevated AFP at diagnosis. The predominant histology was YST, with embryonal, or choriocarcinoma also represented. The median follow-up was 42 months. Surveillance was: measurement of serum tumor markers and radiologic imaging at defined intervals, AFP and b-HCG every 3 weeks through week 9, monthly from 2 to 6 months, and every 3 months from 6 to 24 months. LND was not required, sparing of fallopian tubes was allowed, and no staging biopsies were needed. In those with residual or recurrent disease, a compressed BEP regimen was initiated every 3 weeks for three cycles. 12 patients had evidence of persistent or recurrent disease. The 4Y event free survival (EFS) was 52%, the median time to recurrence was 2 months. All patients had elevated AFP at recurrence. 11 of 12 patients received successful salvage chemotherapy with a 4Y OS of 96%. There was one death. The compressed regimen of BEP was: cisplatin 33 mg/m^2 on days 1 to 3, etoposide 167 mg/m^2 on days 1 to 3, bleomycin 15 mg/m^2 on day 1; for three cycles (134).

REFERENCES

1. Diaz-Padilla I, Malpica AL, Minig L, et al. Ovarian low-grade serous carcinoma: a comprehensive update. *Gynecol Oncol.* August 2012;126(2):279-285.
2. Previs R, Leath CA III, Coleman RL, et al. Evaluation of in vitro chemoresponse profiles in women with Type I and Type II epithelial ovarian cancers: an observational study ancillary analysis. *Gynecol Oncol.* August 2015;138(2):267-271.
3. Grabowski JP, Harter P, Heitz F, et al. Operability and chemotherapy responsiveness in advanced low-grade serous ovarian cancer. An analysis of the AGO Study Group meta-database. *Gynecol Oncol.* March 2016;140(3):457-462.
4. Duska LR, Garrett L, Henretta M, et al. When "never-events" occur despite adherence to clinical guidelines: the case of venous thromboembolism in clear cell cancer of the ovary compared with other epithelial histologic subtypes. *Gynecol Oncol.* 2010;116(3):374-377.
5. Diaz ES, Walts AE, Karlan BY, Walsh CS. Venous thromboembolism during primary treatment of ovarian clear cell carcinoma is associated with decreased survival. *Gynecol Oncol.* December 2013;131(3):541-545.
6. Schmeler KM, Tao X, Frumovitz M, et al. Prevalence of LN metastasis in primary mucinous carcinoma of the ovary. *Obstet Gynecol.* 2010;116(2, pt. 1):269-273.
7. Kleppe M, Wang T, Van Gorp T, Slangen BF, Kruse AJ, Kruitwagen RF. Lymph node metastasis in stages I and II ovarian cancer: a review. *Gynecol Oncol.* 2011;123(3):610-614.
8. Powless CA, Aletti GD, Bakkum-Gamez JN, et al. Risk factors for LN metastasis in apparent early-stage epithelial ovarian cancer: implications for surgical staging. *Gynecol Oncol.* 2011;122(3):536-540.
9. Bristow RE, Tomacruz RS, Armstrong DK, et al. Survival effect of maximal cytoreductive surgery for advanced ovarian carcinoma during the platinum era: a meta-analysis. *J Clin Oncol.* March 1, 2002;20(5):1248-1259.
10. Bristow RE, Montz FJ, Lagasse LD, et al. Survival impact of surgical cytoreduction in stage IV epithelial ovarian cancer. *Gynecol Oncol.* 1999;72(3):278-287.
11. Panici PB, Maggioni A, Hacker N, et al. Systematic aortic and pelvic lymphadenectomy versus resection of bulky nodes only in optimally debulked advanced ovarian cancer: a randomized clinical trial. *J Natl Cancer Inst.* 2005;97(8):560-566.
12. Fagotti A, Ferrandina G, Fanfani F, et al. Prospective validation of a laparoscopic predictive model for optimal cytoreduction in advanced ovarian carcinoma. *Am J Obstet Gynecol.* December 2008;199(6):642e1-642.e6.

13. Brun JL, Rouzier R, Uzan S, Daraï E. External validation of a laparoscopic-based score to evaluate resectability of advanced ovarian cancers: clues for a simplified score. *Gynecol Oncol.* 2008;110:354-359.
14. Garcia-Soto AE, Boren T, Wingo SN, et al. Is comprehensive surgical staging needed for thorough evaluation of early-stage ovarian carcinoma? *Am J Obstet Gynecol.* 2012;206(3):242.e1–242.e5.
15. Vergote I, De Brabanter J, Fyles A, et al. Prognostic importance of degree of differentiation and cyst rupture in stage I invasive epithelial ovarian carcinoma. *Lancet.* 2001;357(9251):176-182.
16. Van Le L. Stage IC ovarian cancer: the clinical significance of intraoperative rupture. *Obstet Gynecol.* 2009;113(1):4-5.
17. Hamilton CA, Miller A, Miller C, et al. The impact of disease distribution on survival in patients with stage III epithelial ovarian cancer cytoreduced to microscopic residual: a Gynecologic Oncology Group study. *Gynecol Oncol.* 2011;122(3):521-526.
18. Wright A, Bohlke K, Armstrong DK, et al. Neoadjuvant chemotherapy for newly diagnosed, advanced ovarian cancer: Society of Gynecologic Oncology and American Society of Clinical Oncology Clinical Practice Guidelines. *J Clin Oncol.* October 1, 2016; 34(28):3460-3473.
19. Greer BE, Bundy BN, Ozols RF, et al. Implications of second-look laparotomy in the context of optimally resected stage III ovarian cancer: a non-randomized comparison using an exploratory analysis: a Gynecologic Oncology Group study. *Gynecol Oncol.* 2005;99(1):71-79.
20. Chi DS, McCaughty K, Diaz JP, et al. Guidelines and selection criteria for secondary cytoreductive surgery in patients with recurrent, platinum-sensitive epithelial ovarian carcinoma. *Cancer.* 2006;106(9):1933-1939.
21. Baldwin LA, Huang B, Miller RW, et al. Ten-year relative survival for epithelial ovarian cancer. *Obstet Gynecol.* 2012;120(3):612-618.
22. Cress RD, Chen YS, Morris CR, et al. Characteristics of long-term survivors of epithelial ovarian cancer. *Obstet Gynecol.* September 2015;126(3):491-497.
23. Rustin GJ, van der Burg ME, Griffin CL, et al. Early versus delayed treatment of relapsed ovarian cancer (MRC OV05/EORTC 55955): a randomised trial. MRC OV05; EORTC 55955 investigators. *Lancet.* 2010;376(9747):1155-1163.
24. Colombo N, Guthrie D, Chiari S, et al. International Collaborative Ovarian Neoplasm trial 1: a randomized trial of adjuvant chemotherapy in women with early-stage ovarian cancer. *J Natl Cancer Inst.* 2003;95(2):125-132.
25. Trimbos JB, Vergote I, Bolis G, et al. Impact of adjuvant chemotherapy and surgical staging in early-stage ovarian carcinoma: European Organisation for Research and Treatment of Cancer-Adjuvant ChemoTherapy in Ovarian Neoplasm trial. *J Natl Cancer Inst.* 2003;95(2):113-125.
26. Trimbos B, Timmers P, Pecorelli S, et al. Surgical staging and treatment of early ovarian cancer: long-term analysis from a randomized trial PMCID: PMC2911043. *J Natl Cancer Inst.* July 7, 2010;102(13):982-987.
27. ICON2: randomised trial of single-agent carboplatin against three-drug combination of CAP (cyclophosphamide, doxorubicin, and cisplatin) in women with ovarian cancer. ICON Collaborators. International Collaborative Ovarian Neoplasm Study. *Lancet.* 1998;352(9140):1571-1576.
28. Parmar MK, Ledermann JA, Colombo N, et al. Paclitaxel plus platinum-based chemotherapy versus conventional platinum-based chemotherapy in women with relapsed ovarian cancer: the ICON4/AGO-OVAR-2.2 trial. *Lancet.* 2003;361(9375):2099-2106.
29. Bookman MA, Brady MF, McGuire WP, et al. Evaluation of new platinum-based treatment regimens in advanced-stage ovarian cancer: a phase III trial of the Gynecologic Cancer InterGroup (GCIG). *J Clin Oncol.* 2009;27:1419-1425.

30. Perren TJ, Swart AM, Pfisterer J, et al. A phase 3 trial of bevacizumab in ovarian cancer. *N Engl J Med.* 2011;365(26):2484-2496. Erratum in: *N Engl J Med.* 2012;366(3):284.

31. Oza AM, Cook AD, Pfisterer J, et al. Standard chemotherapy with or without bevacizumab for women with newly diagnosed ovarian cancer (ICON7): overall survival results of a phase 3 randomised trial. *Lancet Oncol.* 2015;16:928-936.

32. Hreshchyshyn MM, Park RC, Blessing JA, et al. The role of adjuvant therapy in stage I ovarian cancer. *Am J Obstet Gynecol.* 1980;138(2):139-145.

33. McGuire WP, Hoskins WJ, Brady MF, et al. Cyclophosphamide and cisplatin compared with paclitaxel and cisplatin in patients with stage III and stage IV ovarian cancer. *N Engl J Med.* 1996;334(1):1-6.

34. Piccart MJ, Bertelsen K, James K, et al. Randomized intergroup trial of cisplatin-paclitaxel versus cisplatin-cyclophosphamide in women with advanced epithelial ovarian cancer: three-year results. *J Natl Cancer Inst.* 2000;92(9):699-708.

35. Muggia FM, Braly PS, Brady MF, et al. Phase III randomized study of cisplatin versus paclitaxel versus cisplatin and paclitaxel in patients with suboptimal stage III or IV ovarian cancer: a Gynecologic Oncology Group study. *J Clin Oncol.* 2000;18(1):106-115.

36. Bell J, Brady MF, Young RC, et al. Randomized phase III trial of three versus six cycles of adjuvant carboplatin and paclitaxel in early stage epithelial ovarian carcinoma: a Gynecologic Oncology Group study. *Gynecol Oncol.* 2006;102(3):432-439.

37. Chan JK, Tian C, Fleming GF, et al. The potential benefit of 6 vs. 3 cycles of chemotherapy in subsets of women with early-stage high-risk epithelial ovarian cancer: an exploratory analysis of a Gynecologic Oncology Group study. *Gynecol Oncol.* March 2010;116(3):301-306.

38. Ozols RF, Bundy BN, Greer BE, et al. Phase III trial of carboplatin and paclitaxel compared with cisplatin and paclitaxel in patients with optimally resected stage III ovarian cancer: a Gynecologic Oncology Group study. *J Clin Oncol.* 2003;21(17):3194-3200.

39. Burger RA, Brady MF, Bookman MA, et al. Incorporation of bevacizumab in the primary treatment of ovarian cancer. *N Engl J Med.* December 29, 2011;365(26):2473-2483.

40. Vasey PA, Jayson GC, Gordon A, et al. Phase III randomized trial of docetaxel-carboplatin versus paclitaxel-carboplatin as first-line chemotherapy for ovarian carcinoma. *J Natl Cancer Inst.* 2004;96(22):1682-1691.

41. Gonzalez-Martin A, Gladieff L, Tholander B, et al. Efficacy and safety results from OCTAVIA, a single-arm phase II study evaluating front-line bevacizumab, carboplatin and weekly paclitaxel for ovarian cancer. *Eur J Cancer.* December 2013;49(18): 3831-3838.

42. du Bois A, Herrstedt J, Hardy-Bessard AC, et al. Phase III trial of carboplatin plus paclitaxel with or without gemcitabine in first-line treatment of epithelial ovarian cancer. *J Clin Oncol.* September 20, 2010;28(27):4162-4169.

43. Sabbatini P, Hartner P, Scambia G, et al. Abagovomab as maintenance therapy in patients with epithelial ovarian cancer: A phase II trial of the AGO OVAR, COGI, GINECO, and CEICO—The MIMOSA Study. *J Clin Oncol.* 2013;31:1554-1561.

44. du Bois A, Kristensen G, Ray-Coquard I, et al. Standard first-line chemotherapy with or without nintedanib for advanced ovarian cancer (AGO-OVAR 12): a randomised, double-blind, placebo-controlled phase 3 trial. *Lancet Oncol.* January 2016;17(1):78-89.

45. Meier W, Du Bois QA, Rau J, et al. Randomized phase II trial of carboplatin and paclitaxel with or without lonafarnib in first-line treatment of epithelial ovarian cancer stage IIB-IV. *Gynecol Oncol.* August 2012;126(2):236-240.

46. McGuire WP, Hoskins WJ, Brady MF, et al. Assessment of dose-intensive therapy in suboptimally debulked ovarian cancer: a Gynecologic Oncology Group study. *J Clin Oncol.* 1995;13(7):1589-1599.

47. Fruscio R, Garbi A, Parma G, et al. Randomized phase III clinical trial evaluating weekly cisplatin for advanced epithelial ovarian cancer. *J Natl Cancer Inst.* 2011;103(4): 347-351.

48. Kaye SB, Paul J, Cassidy J, et al. Mature results of a randomized trial of two doses of cisplatin for the treatment of ovarian cancer. Scottish Gynecology Cancer Trials Group. *J Clin Oncol.* 1996;14(7):2113-2119.
49. Jakobsen A, Bertelsen K, Andersen JE, et al. Dose-effect study of carboplatin in ovarian cancer: a Danish Ovarian Cancer Group study. *J Clin Oncol.* 1997;15(1):193-198.
50. Gore M, Mainwaring P, A'Hern R, et al. Randomized trial of dose-intensity with single-agent carboplatin in patients with epithelial ovarian cancer. London Gynaecological Oncology Group. *J Clin Oncol.* 1998;16(7):2426-2434.
51. Omura GA, Brady MF, Look KY, et al. Phase III trial of paclitaxel at two dose levels, the higher dose accompanied by filgrastim at two dose levels in platinum-pretreated epithelial ovarian cancer: an intergroup study. *J Clin Oncol.* 2003;21(15):2843-2848.
52. Eisenhauer EA, ten Bokkel Huinink WW, Swenerton KD, et al. European-Canadian randomized trial of paclitaxel in relapsed ovarian cancer: high-dose versus low-dose and long versus short infusion. *J Clin Oncol.* 1994;12(12):2654-2666.
53. Katsumata N, Yasuda M, Takahashi F, et al. Dose-dense paclitaxel once a week in combination with carboplatin every 3 weeks for advanced ovarian cancer: a phase 3, open-label, randomised controlled trial. *Lancet.* October 17, 2009;374(9698):1331-1338.
54. Katsumata N, Yasuda M, Isonishi S, et al. Long-term results of dose-dense paclitaxel and carboplatin versus conventional paclitaxel and carboplatin for treatment of advanced epithelial ovarian, fallopian tube, or primary peritoneal cancer (JGOG 3016): a randomised, controlled, open-label trial. *Lancet Oncol.* September 2013;14(10):1020-1026.
55. Chan JK, Brady MF, Penson RT. Weekly vs. every-3-week paclitaxel and carboplatin for ovarian cancer. *N Engl J Med.* 2016;374:738-748.
56. Pignata S, Scambia G, Katsaros D, et al. Carboplatin plus paclitaxel once a week versus every 3 weeks in patients with advanced ovarian cancer (MITO-7): a randomised, multicentre, open-label, phase 3 trial. *Lancet Oncol.* April 2014;15(4):396-405.
57. Alberts DS, Liu PY, Hannigan EV, et al. Intraperitoneal cisplatin plus intravenous cyclophosphamide versus intravenous cisplatin plus intravenous cyclophosphamide for stage III ovarian cancer. *N Engl J Med.* 1996;335(26):1950-1955.
58. Markman M, Bundy BN, Alberts DS, et al. Phase III trial of standard-dose intravenous cisplatin plus paclitaxel versus moderately high-dose carboplatin followed by intravenous paclitaxel and intraperitoneal cisplatin in small-volume stage III ovarian carcinoma: an intergroup study of the Gynecologic Oncology Group, Southwestern Oncology Group, and Eastern Cooperative Oncology Group. *J Clin Oncol.* 2001;19(4):1001-1007.
59. Armstrong DK, Bundy B, Wenzel L, et al. Intraperitoneal cisplatin and paclitaxel in ovarian cancer. *N Engl J Med.* 2006;354(1):34-43.
60. Tewari D, Java JJ, Salani R, et al. Long-term survival advantage and prognostic factors associated with intraperitoneal chemotherapy treatment in advanced ovarian cancer: a gynecologic oncology group study. *J Clin Oncol.* May 1, 2015;33(13):1460-1466.
61. Landrum LM, Java J, Mathews CA, et al. Prognostic factors for stage III epithelial ovarian cancer treated with intraperitoneal chemotherapy: a Gynecologic Oncology Group study. *Gynecol Oncol.* July 2013;130(1):12-18.
62. Walker JL, Armstrong D; Huang H, et al. Intraperitoneal catheter outcomes on GOG 172: a gynecologic oncology group study in women with optimally debulked stage III ovarian cancer. *Int J Gynecol Cancer.* September/October 2004;14:19.
63. Dizon DS, Sill MW, Gould SC, et al. Phase I feasibility study of intraperitoneal cisplatin and intravenous paclitaxel followed by intraperitoneal paclitaxel in untreated ovarian, fallopian tube, and primary peritoneal carcinoma: a Gynecologic Oncology Group study. *Gynecol Oncol.* 2011;123:182-186.
64. Walker JL, Armstrong DK, Huang HQ, et al. Intraperitoneal catheter outcomes in a phase III trial of intravenous versus intraperitoneal chemotherapy in optimal stage III ovarian and primary peritoneal cancer: a Gynecologic Oncology Group study. *Gynecol Oncol.* 2006;100(1):27-32.

65. Fujiwara K, Aotani E, Hamano T, et al. A Randomized Phase II/III trial of 3 weekly intraperitoneal versus intravenous carboplatin in combination with intravenous weekly dose-dense paclitaxel for newly diagnosed ovarian, fallopian tube and primary peritoneal cancer. *Jpn J Clin Oncol.* 2011;41:278-282.

66. Markman M, Liu PY, Wilczynski S, et al. Phase III randomized trial of 12 versus 3 months of maintenance paclitaxel in patients with advanced ovarian cancer after complete response to platinum and paclitaxel-based chemotherapy: a Southwest Oncology Group and Gynecologic Oncology Group trial. *J Clin Oncol.* 2003;21(13): 2460-2465.

67. Markman M, Liu PY, Moon J, et al. Impact on survival of 12 versus 3 monthly cycles of paclitaxel (175 mg/m^2) administered to patients with advanced ovarian cancer who attained a complete response to primary platinum–paclitaxel: follow-up of a Southwest Oncology Group and Gynecologic Oncology Group phase 3 trial. *Gynecol Oncol.* 2009;114(2):195-198.

68. McMeekin DS, Tillmanns T, Chaudry T, et al. Timing isn't everything: an analysis of when to start salvage chemotherapy in ovarian cancer. *Gynecol Oncol.* 2004;95(1):157-164.

69. Mannel RS, Brady MF, Kohn EC, et al. A randomized phase III trial of IV carboplatin and paclitaxel 3 × 3 courses followed by observation versus weekly maintenance low-dose paclitaxel in patients with early-stage ovarian carcinoma: a Gynecologic Oncology Group study. *Gynecol Oncol.* 2011;122(1):89-94.

70. du Bois A, Floquet A, Kim JW, et al. Incorporation of pazopanib in maintenance therapy of ovarian cancer. *J Clin Oncol.* October 20, 2014;32(30):3374-3382.

71. Ledermann J, Harter P, Gourley C, Friedlander M. Olaparib maintenance therapy in platinum-sensitive relapsed ovarian cancer. *N Engl J Med.* April 12, 2012;366(15):1382-1392.

72. Despierre E, Vergote I, Anderson R, et al. Epidermal growth factor receptor (EGFR) pathway biomarkers in the randomized phase III trial of erlotinib versus observation in ovarian cancer patients with no evidence of disease progression after first-line platinum-based chemotherapy. *Target Oncol.* December 2015;10(4):583-596.

73. Pfisterer J, Plante M, Vergote I, et al. Gemcitabine plus carboplatin compared with carboplatin in patients with platinum-sensitive recurrent ovarian cancer: an intergroup trial of the AGO-OVAR, the NCIC CTG, and the EORTC GCG. *J Clin Oncol.* 2006;24(29):4699-4707.

74. Gordon AN, Tonda M, Sun S, et al. Long-term survival advantage for women treated with pegylated liposomal doxorubicin compared with topotecan in a phase 3 randomized study of recurrent and refractory epithelial ovarian cancer. *Gynecol Oncol.* 2004;95(1):1-8.

75. Aghajanian C, Blank SV, Goff BA, et al. OCEANS: a randomized, double-blind, placebo-controlled phase III trial of chemotherapy with or without bevacizumab in patients with platinum-sensitive recurrent epithelial ovarian, primary peritoneal, or fallopian tube cancer. *J Clin Oncol.* 2012;30(17):2039-2045.

76. Aghajanian C, Goff B, Nycum LR, et al. Overall survival and safety analysis of OCEANS, a phase 3 trial of chemotherapy with or without bevacizumab in patients with platinum-sensitive recurrent ovarian cancer. *Gynecol Oncol.* October 2015;139(1):10-16.

77. Pujade-Lauraine E, Wagner U, Aavall-Lundqvist E, et al. Pegylated liposomal doxorubicin and carboplatin compared with paclitaxel and carboplatin for patients with platinum-sensitive ovarian cancer in late relapse. *J Clin Oncol.* 2010;28(20):3323-3329.

78. Mahner S, Meier W, du Bois A, et al. Carboplatin and pegylated liposomal doxorubicin versus carboplatin and paclitaxel in very platinum-sensitive ovarian cancer patients: results from a subset analysis of the CALYPSO phase III trial. *Eur J Cancer.* February 2015;51(3):352-358.

79. Pujade-Lauraine E, Hilpert F, Weber B, et al. Bevacizumab combined with chemotherapy for platinum-resistant recurrent ovarian cancer: the AURELIA open-label randomized phase III trial. *J Clin Oncol.* May 1, 2014;32(13):1302-1308.

80. Poveda AM, Selle F, Hilpert F, et al. Bevacizumab combined with weekly paclitaxel, pegylated liposomal doxorubicin, or topotecan in platinum-resistant recurrent ovarian cancer: analysis by chemotherapy cohort of the randomized phase III AURELIA trial. *J Clin Oncol.* November 10, 2015;33(32):3836-3838.

81. Monk BJ, Poveda A, Vergote I, et al. Anti-angiopoietin therapy with trebananib for recurrent ovarian cancer (TRINOVA-1): a randomised, multicentre, double-blind, placebo-controlled phase 3 trial. *Lancet Oncol.* July 2014;15(8):799-808.

82. Monk BJ, Poveda A, Vergote I, et al. Final results of a phase 3 study of trebananib plus weekly paclitaxel in recurrent ovarian cancer (TRINOVA-1): Long-term survival, impact of ascites, and progression-free survival-2. *Gynecol Oncol.* October 2016;143(1):27-34.

83. Marth SN and Randall L. The European Society of Gynecology Oncology 19th biannual meeting: overview and summary of selected topics. *Gynecol Oncol.* 2016;140:377-380.

84. Raja F, Perren T, Embleton A, et al. Randomised double-blind phase III trial of cediranib (AZD 2171) in relapsed platinum sensitive ovarian cancer: results of the ICON6 trial. *Int J Gynecol Cancer.* 2013;23:47.

85. Mirza MR, Monk BJ, Herrstedt J, et al. Niraparib maintenance therapy in platinum-sensitive recurrent ovarian cancer. *N Engl J Med.* December 1, 2016;375:2154-2164.

86. Poveda A, Vergote I, Tjulandin S, et al. Trabectedin plus pegylated liposomal doxorubicin in relapsed ovarian cancer: outcomes in the partially platinum-sensitive (platinum-free interval 6-12 months) subpopulation of OVA-301 phase III randomized trial. *Ann Oncol.* January 2011;22(1):39-48.

87. Pignata S, Lorusso D, Scambia G, et al. Pazopanib plus weekly paclitaxel versus weekly paclitaxel alone for platinum-resistant or platinum-refractory advanced ovarian cancer (MITO 11): a randomised, open-label, phase 2 trial. *Lancet Oncol.* May 2015;16(5):561-568.

88. Thigpen JT, Blessing JA, Ball H, et al. Phase II trial of paclitaxel in patients with progressive ovarian carcinoma after platinum-based chemotherapy: a Gynecologic Oncology Group study. *J Clin Oncol.* 1994;12(9):1748-1753.

89. Monk BJ, Sill MW, Hanjani P, et al. Docetaxel plus trabectedin appears active in recurrent or persistent ovarian and primary peritoneal cancer after up to three prior regimens: a phase II study of the Gynecologic Oncology Group. *Gynecol Oncol.* March 2011;120(3):459-463.

90. Monk BJ, Sill M, Walker JL, et al. A randomized phase II evaluation of bevacizumab vs bevacizumab/fosbretabulin in recurrent ovarian, tubal, or peritoneal carcinoma: a Gynecologic Oncology Group Study. 15th Biennial Meeting of the International Gynecologic Cancer Society; November 2014; Melbourne, Australia.

91. Jackson AL, Davenport SM, Herzog TJ, et al. Targeting angiogenesis: vascular endothelial growth factor and related signalling pathways. *Transl Cancer Res.* 2015;491:70-83.

92. Coleman RL, Sill MW, Bell-McGuinn K, et al. A phase II evaluation of the potent, highly selective PARP inhibitor veliparib in the treatment of persistent or recurrent epithelial ovarian, fallopian tube, or primary peritoneal cancer in patients who carry a germline BRCA1 or BRCA2 mutation—an NRG Oncology/Gynecologic Oncology Group study. *Gynecol Oncol.* June 2015;137(3):386-391.

93. Kurzeder C, Bover I, Marme F, et al. Double-blind, placebo controlled randomized phase II trial evaluating pertuzumab combined with chemotherapy for low tumor human epidermal growth factor receptor 3 mRNA-expressing platinum resistant ovarian cancer (PENELOPE). *J Clin Oncol.* July 20, 2016;34(21):2516-2525.

94. Liu JF, Barry WT, Birrer M, et al. Combination cediranib and olaparib versus olaparib alone for women with recurrent platinum-sensitive ovarian cancer: a randomised phase 2 study. *Lancet Oncol.* October 2014;15(11):1207-1214.

95. Vergote I, Tropé CG, Amant F, et al. Neoadjuvant chemotherapy or primary surgery in stage IIIC or IV ovarian cancer. *N Engl J Med.* 2010;363(10):943-953.

96. Hirte H, Lheureux S, Fleming GF, et al. A phase 2 study of cediranib in recurrent or persistent ovarian, peritoneal or fallopian tube cancer: a trial of the Princess Margaret, Chicago and California Phase II Consortia. *Gynecol Oncol.* July 2015;138(1):55-61.

97. McNeish IA, Oza AM, Coleman RL, et al. Results of ARIEL2: a phase 2 trial to prospectively identify ovarian cancer patients likely to respond to rucaparib using tumor genetic analysis [abstract]. *J Clin Oncol.* 2015;33(suppl; abstract 5508).

98. Harter P, du Bois A, Hahmann M, et al. Surgery in recurrent ovarian cancer: the Arbeitsgemeinschaft Gynaekologische Onkologie (AGO) DESKTOP OVAR trial. *Ann Surg Oncol.* 2006;13(12):1702-1710.

99. Harter P, Sehouli J, Reuss A, et al. Prospective validation study of a predictive score for operability of recurrent ovarian cancer: the Multicenter Intergroup Study DESKTOP II. A project of the AGO Kommission OVAR, AGO Study Group, NOGGO, AGO-Austria, and MITO. *Int J Gynecol Cancer.* 2011;21(2):289-295.

100. Chan J, Brady WE, Brown J, et al. A phase II evaluation of sunitinib (SU11248) in the treatment of persistent or recurrent clear cell ovarian carcinoma: an NRG Oncology/Gynecologic Oncology Group (GOG) study. *Gynecol Oncol.* May 1, 2015;138(suppl 1):3.

101. Pujade-Lauraine E, Selle F, Weber B, et al. Volasertib versus chemotherapy in platinum-resistant or refractory ovarian cancer: a randomized phase II groupe des investigateurs nationaux pour l'etude des cancers de l'ovaire study. *J. Clin. Oncol.* March 1, 2016;34(7):706-713.

102. Senzer N, Barve M, Kuhn J, et al. Phase I trial of "bi-shRNAi(furin)/GMCSF DNA/autologous tumor cell" vaccine (FANG) in advanced cancer. *Mol Ther.* March 2012;20(3):679-686.

103. van der Burg ME, van Lent M, Buyse M, et al. The effect of debulking surgery after induction chemotherapy on the prognosis in advanced epithelial ovarian cancer. Gynecological Cancer Cooperative Group of the European Organization for Research and Treatment of Cancer. *N Engl J Med.* 1995;332(10):629-634.

104. Rose PG, Nerenstone S, Brady MF, et al. Secondary surgical cytoreduction for advanced ovarian carcinoma. *N Engl J Med.* 2004;351(24):2489-2497.

105. Coleman RL, Brady MF, Herzog TJ, et al. A phase III randomized controlled clinical trial of carboplatin and paclitaxel alone or in combination with bevacizumab followed by bevacizumab and secondary cytoreductive surgery in platinum sensitive recurrent ovarian peritoneal primary and fallopian tube cancer. Gynecologic Oncology Group 213. *Gynecol. Oncol.* 2015;137(suppl):3-4.

106. van de Laar R, Zusterzeel PL, Van Gorp T, et al. Cytoreductive surgery followed by chemotherapy versus chemotherapy alone for recurrent platinum-sensitive epithelial ovarian cancer (SOCceR trial): a multicenter randomised controlled study. *BMC Cancer.* January 14, 2014;14:22.

107. Soo Hoo S, Marriott N, Houlton A, et al. Patient-reported outcomes after extensive (ultraradical) surgery for ovarian cancer: results from a prospective longitudinal feasibility study. *Int J Gynecol Cancer.* November 2015;25(9):1599-1607.

108. Kehoe S, Hook J, Nankivell M, et al. Primary chemotherapy versus primary surgery for newly diagnosed advanced ovarian cancer (CHORUS): an open-label, randomised, controlled, non-inferiority trial. *Lancet.* July 18, 2015;386(9990):249-257.

109. van Meurs HS, Tajik P, Hof MH, et al. Which patients benefit most from primary surgery or neoadjuvant chemotherapy in stage IIIC or IV ovarian cancer? An exploratory analysis of the European Organisation for Research and Treatment of Cancer 55971 randomised trial. *Eur J Cancer.* October 2013;49(15):3191-3201.

110. Fagotti A, Vizzielli G, Fanfani F, et al. Phase III SCORPION trial in epithelial ovarian cancer patients with high tumor load receiving PDS versus NACT: an interim analysis on peri-operative outcomes. *Gynecol Oncol.* 2015;158(suppl 1):1-4.

111. Fagotti A, Vizzielli G, Delaco P, et al. A multicentric trial (Olympia-MITO 13) on the accuracy of laparoscopy to assess peritoneal spread in ovarian cancer. *Am J Obstet Gynecol.* November 2013;209(5):462.e1-462.e11.

112. Petrillo M, Vizzielli G, Fanfani F, et al. Definition of a dynamic laparoscopic model for the prediction of incomplete cytoreduction in advanced epithelial ovarian cancer: proof of a concept. *Gynecol Oncol.* October 2015;139(1):5-9.

113. Tozzi R, Giannice R, Cianci S, et al. Neo-adjuvant chemotherapy does not increase the rate of complete resection and does not significantly reduce the morbidity of Visceral-Peritoneal Debulking (VPD) in patients with stage IIIC-IV ovarian cancer. *Gynecol Oncol.* August 2015;138(2):252-258.

114. Rosen B, Laframboise S, Ferguson S, et al. The impacts of neoadjuvant chemotherapy and of debulking surgery on survival from advanced ovarian cancer. *Gynecol Oncol.* September 2014;134(3):462-467.

115. Chekerov R, Braicu I, Castillo-Tong DC, et al. Outcome and clinical management of 275 patients with advanced ovarian cancer International Federation of Obstetrics and Gynecology II to IV inside the European Ovarian Cancer Translational Research Consortium-OVCAD. *Int J Gynecol Cancer.* February 2013;23(2):268-275.

116. Winter WE III, Kucera PR, Rodgers W, et al. Surgical staging in patients with ovarian tumors of low malignant potential. *Obstet Gynecol.* 2002;100:671-676.

117. Gershenson DM, Silva EG, Tortolero-Luna G, et al. Serous borderline tumors of the ovary with noninvasive peritoneal implants. *Cancer.* 1998;83(10):2157-2163.

118. Crispens MA, Bodurka D, Deavers M, et al. Response and survival in patients with progressive or recurrent serous ovarian tumors of low malignant potential. *Obstet Gynecol.* 2002;99(1):3-10.

119. Stewart SL, Wike JM, Foster SL, et al. The incidence of primary fallopian tube cancer in the United States. *Gynecol Oncol.* 2007;107(3):392-397.

120. Hu CY, Taymour ML, Hertig AT. Primary carcinoma of the fallopian tube. *Am J Obstet Gynaecol.* 1950;59:58-67.

121. Sedlis A. Carcinoma of the fallopian tube. *Surg Clin North Am.* 1978;58:121-129.

122. Slayton RE, Park RC, Silverberg SG, et al. Vincristine, dactinomycin, and cyclophosphamide in the treatment of malignant germ cell tumors of the ovary. A Gynecologic Oncology Group study (a final report). *Cancer.* 1985;56(2):243-248.

123. Williams SD, Blessing JA, Moore DH. Cisplatin, vinblastine, and bleomycin in advanced and recurrent ovarian germ-cell tumors: a trial of the Gynecologic Oncology Group. *Ann Intern Med.* 1989;111(1):22-27.

124. Li J, Yang W, Wu X. Prognostic factors and role of salvage surgery in chemorefractory ovarian germ cell malignancies: a study in Chinese patients. *Gynecol Oncol.* 2007;105(3):769-775.

125. Williams S, Blessing JA, Liao SY, et al. Adjuvant therapy of ovarian germ cell tumors with cisplatin, etoposide, and bleomycin: a trial of the Gynecologic Oncology Group. *J Clin Oncol.* 1994;12(4):701-706.

126. Williams SD, Blessing JA, Hatch KD, et al. Chemotherapy of advanced dysgerminoma: trials of the Gynecologic Oncology Group. *J Clin Oncol.* 1991;9(11):1950-1955.

127. Williams SD, Kauderer J, Burnett AF, et al. Adjuvant therapy of completely resected dysgerminoma with carboplatin and etoposide: a trial of the Gynecologic Oncology Group. *Gynecol Oncol.* 2004;95(3):496-499.

128. Brown J, Sood AK, Deavers MT, et al. Patterns of metastasis in sex cord-stromal tumors of the ovary: can routine staging lymphadenectomy be omitted? *Gynecol Oncol.* 2009;113(1):86-90.

129. Tavassoeli FA, Devilee P, eds. *WHO Classification of Tumours, Pathology and Genetics: Tumours of the Breast and Female Genital Organs*. Lyon, France: IARC; 2003.

130. Wolf JK, Mullen J, Eifel PJ, et al. Radiation treatment of advanced or recurrent granulosa cell tumor of the ovary. *Gynecol Oncol* 1999;73(1):35-41.

131. Wilson MK, Fong P, Mesnage S, et al. Stage I granulosa cell tumours: a management conundrum? Results of long-term follow up. *Gynecol Oncol*. August 2015;138(2):285-291.

132. Homesley HD, Bundy BN, Hurteau JA, et al. Bleomycin, etoposide, and cisplatin combination therapy of ovarian granulosa cell malignancies and other stromal malignancies: a Gynecologic Oncology Group study. *Gynecol Oncol*. 1999;72(2):131-137.

133. Mangili G, Ottolina J, Cormio G, et al. Adjuvant chemotherapy does not improve disease-free survival in FIGO stage 1C ovarian granulosa cell tumors: the MITO-9 study. *Gynecol Oncol*. 2016;143:276-280.

134. Billmire DF, Cullen JW, Rescorla FJ, et al. Surveillance after initial surgery for pediatric and adolescent girls with stage I ovarian germ cell tumors: report from the Children's Oncology Group. *J Clin Oncol*. February 10, 2014;32(5):465-470.

135. Williams SD, Blessing JA, DiSaia PF, et al. Second-look laparotomy in ovarian germ cell tumors: the gynecologic oncology group experience. Gynecol Oncol 1994:52;287-91.

136. SGO Annual Meeting National Harbor Maryland March 2017.

Uterine Cancer

CHARACTERISTICS

- Uterine corpus cancer is the most common female gynecologic cancer in the United States with an estimated 61,380 cases and 10,920 deaths in the United States in 2017. Currently, endometrial adenocarcinoma is the most common malignancy of the female genital tract and ranks as the fourth most common cancer in females.
- **Risk factors** for endometrial cancer include the triad of obesity, diabetes, and hypertension. Other risk factors are a prolonged exposure to estrogens, nulliparity, early menarche, late menopause, and unopposed estrogen hormone therapy.
- Most women present with abnormal uterine bleeding. Of those postmenopausal women who do present with bleeding, 10% result in a diagnosis of uterine cancer.
- Other presenting signs and symptoms can be menorrhagia, intermenstrual bleeding, pain, pyometria, hematometria, and an abnormal Pap smear.
- Hyperplasia and cellular atypia, alone or combined, have known rates for progression to uterine cancer (Table 2.16) (1).
  - According to one collaborative study, a diagnosis of complex atypical hyperplasia was associated with a 43% chance of concurrent endometrial cancer. Of these specimens, 31% had myometrial invasion and 10% had greater than 50% myometrial invasion (2).

Table 2.16 Uterine Hyperplasia and Risk of Progression to Cancer

Type of hyperplasia	Total cases	Persisted (%)	Progressed (%)	Mean years follow-up
Simple	93	19	1	15.2
Complex	29	17	3	13.5
Atypical simple	23	23	8	11.4
Atypical complex	45	14	29	11.4

PROGNOSTIC FACTORS

Stage is the most important prognostic factor. Other factors include depth of myometrial invasion (DOI), LVSI, grade, histology, tumor size, patient age, and hormone receptor status.

PRE-TREATMENT WORKUP

- Workup for abnormal bleeding begins with a history and physical examination. Evaluation involves endometrial biopsy (EMB) with endocervical curettage or D&C. Pelvic ultrasound and Pap smear may also be performed, but are insufficient modalities used alone for persistent abnormal bleeding.
- An endometrial stripe thickness that is 5 mm or greater in a postmenopausal patient is abnormal and biopsy should be performed. The accuracy of EMB and D&C are relatively the same, between 91% and 99%, when compared with final pathology (2).
- Women with the following should be ruled out for cancer via endometrial biopsy: postmenopausal women with bleeding; postmenopausal patients with pyometria; asymptomatic postmenopausal women with endometrial cells on Pap smear (especially if atypical); perimenopausal patients with intermenstrual bleeding or increasingly heavy periods; and premenopausal patients with abnormal uterine bleeding, particularly if there is a history of anovulation.
- In women over the age of 35 years with abnormal bleeding, an EMB should be performed. 25% of cancers occur in premenopausal women and 5% occur in women less than 40 years of age.
- The pre-treatment workup for uterine cancer includes a CXR and abdominal-pelvic imaging. This can be with a pelvic ultrasound, CT, or MRI. Lab tests include a CBC, comprehensive metabolic panel (CMP), and CA-125 (which can predict LN metastasis) (Figure 2.8).

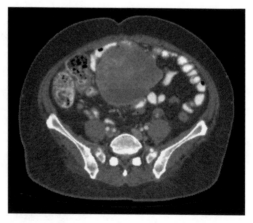

Figure 2.8 Uterine cancer on CT.

CATEGORICAL DIVISIONS

- **Histologic grouping:** epidemiological and clinical studies suggest that endometrial cancers be separated by histologic appearance and behavior into two groups: type I and II tumors. Genetic evaluation is moving toward categorizing tumors outside standard histological status into four separate categories.
  - ○ Type I tumors are the most common. The main risk factor in type I carcinomas is hyperestrogenism. These tend to be hormonally responsive and have an 83% all stage 5Y survival. These cancers typically have a favorable prognosis with appropriate therapy (Figure 2.9).
    - The most common type I cancer is endometrioid adenocarcinoma, which occurs in 75% of cases.
    - Adenosquamous carcinoma is diagnosed in 18% to 25% of uterine cancers. The behavior is similar to that of endometrioid cancer.
    - Villoglandular carcinoma occurs in 6% of uterine cancers. This subtype is distinguished by delicate fibrovascular cores. It is usually of low grade and is more differentiated than endometrioid adenocarcinoma.
    - Secretory carcinoma occurs in 2% of uterine cancers and appears as a well-differentiated glandular pattern with intracytoplasmic vacuoles containing glycogen, similar to secretory endometrium. It is usually grade 1.
    - Mucinous carcinoma is diagnosed in 5% of cases and mucin is present as the major cellular component. There are columnar cells that are basally oriented or pseudostratified. It is necessary to rule out other cancers such as colon, mucinous ovarian, and primary endocervical cancers. It has the same prognosis as endometrioid cancer.
    - Squamous carcinoma is associated with cervical stenosis, pyometria, and chronic inflammation. It is important to rule out a primary cervical cancer origin. It has a poorer prognosis.
    - IHC to differentiate type I tumors from type II includes: estrogen receptor (ER)/progesterone receptor (PR)+, p53–, and WT-1 negative.

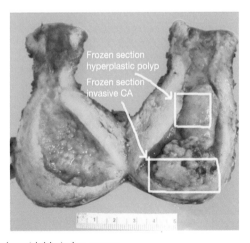

Figure 2.9 Endometrioid uterine cancer.

○ Type II cancers are poorly differentiated tumors, and are histologically represented by the serous, clear cell (CC) and malignant mixed Müllerian tumors (MMMT) histologies. Type II tumors are more biologically aggressive and have a 53% 5 YS for all stages. Type II tumors account for 15% of uterine carcinomas, but represent 50% of all relapses. These type II tumors are classified as high risk, high grade, and are unresponsive to hormonal therapy.

- **Serous** uterine carcinoma is diagnosed in 10% to 15% of endometrial cancers. If there is 10% or less serous component, it is called a mixed tumor. This subtype resembles serous carcinoma of the ovary. It is often found at an advanced stage. The depth of invasion is often not predictive of LN metastasis, and extrauterine disease is found in 60% of tumors. If the cancer is identified in a polyp without other evidence of uterine disease, 38% of patients will be found to have extrauterine spread. Intraperitoneal spread is common even when myometrial invasion is minimal. When comprehensively staged, 70% of patients are found to have advanced-stage disease: 25% of apparent stage I cancers (3) have omental metastasis and 25% of patients have upper abdominal disease (4). Microscopically, there are fibrous papillary fronds, picket fencing of the terminal cells, LVSI is common, and psammoma bodies are often present. It is high grade by definition. There is a 2% rate of *BRCA1* mutations in uterine serous cancer patients. Nine percent of women with a history of breast cancer followed by uterine serous cancer have a *BRCA 1/2* mutation (5).
- IHC for serous cancers: ER/PR variable, WT-1 negative, p53+.
- Clear cell carcinoma is diagnosed in 5% of uterine cancers. It also is an aggressive tumor. The cells contain a large amount of glycogen and when processed for histology, the glycogen in the cells gives an appearance of cellular clearing and nuclear hobnailing.
- Mixed Müllerian mesodermal tumors (MMMT; carcinosarcoma) are now thought to be metaplastic epithelial (or carcinomatous) cancers. These tumors tend to occur in older women with a median age of 65 to 75 years. Other characteristics include obesity, nulliparity, and diabetes. Tumor can be seen via speculum examination in 50% of women. Pathologically, there is a mixture of carcinomatous and sarcomatous tissues. The carcinomatous component is most commonly endometrioid, but can be of serous or CC histology. Prognosis is mainly dependent on the epithelioid histology. The sarcomatous/nonepithelial component is commonly an endometrial stromal sarcoma (ESS), but can be leiomyosarcoma (LMS), rhabdosarcoma, or chondrosarcoma. The presence or absence of heterologous elements is not predictive of outcome. Studies have shown similar allelic losses present in both the carcinomatous and sarcomatous areas of MMMTs in multiple patients. This suggests a late divergence in phenotype and a common abnormal clone for the entire cancer. Prior tamoxifen use has been implicated in this tumor's development. The median time of exposure to diagnosis of MMMT was 9 years and ranges to a relative risk (RR) of 15.9 (6). Prior pelvic XRT has also been noted to have a causal effect: in 23 patients with prior pelvic XRT,

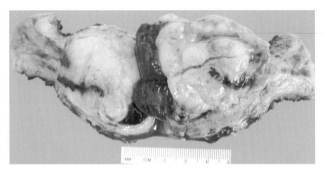

Figure 2.10 Mixed Müllerian mesodermal tumor (MMMT) uterine cancer.

35% had an MMMT uterine cancer. Surgical management is critical for staging and optimization of treatment. 20% of patients with clinical stage I and II are upstaged by LND. Cytoreduction in advanced stage disease (III and IV) with optimal resection was associated with improved survival of 52.3 months versus 8.6 months ($p < 0.0001$), with another study showing similar results in debulking to no residual versus optimal (less than 1 cm) and suboptimal disease with a PFS of 0.8 versus 8.6 versus 13 months and OS of 4.5 versus 12.7 versus 29.6 months, respectively (Figure 2.10) (7).

- **Genetic groupings:** adjuvant recommendations may be determined by genetic grouping in the future (8).
  ○ POL-E: ultramutated
  ○ Copy number high: serous/CC/some G3 adenocarcinomas
  ○ Copy number low: commonly G1/2 endometrioid adenocarcinomas
  ○ Microsatellite instability (MSI): genomic, somatic, and epigenetic (hypermethlyated)

STAGING
- Staging is **surgical**. In 1988, the staging was changed from clinical to surgical. Surgical staging was further revised in 2009 (Table 2.17A–D).
- **Grade** is specified as a three-tiered system: grade 1 tumors are highly differentiated, with less than 5% of the tumor containing solid areas; grade 2 tumors are moderately differentiated with 6% to 50% solid areas; grade 3 tumors are poorly differentiated carcinomas with greater than 50% of the tumor containing solid components. If nuclear atypia is present at a higher degree than the stated histological grade, the overall grade is increased by one grade.

TREATMENT
- Treatment is primarily surgical staging to include: pelvic washings, hysterectomy, bilateral salpingo-oophorectomy, LND, omentectomy and peritoneal biopsies (especially for the type II tumors), and surgical debulking of extrauterine/metastatic disease.

Table 2.17A AJCC 8th Edition: T Category		
T	**FIGO**	**T Criteria**
TX		Primary tumor cannot be assessed.
T0		No evidence of primary tumor.
T1	I	Tumor confined to the corpus uteri, including endocervical glandular involvement.
T1a	IA	Tumor limited to the endometrium or invading less than half the myometrium.
T1b	IB	Tumor invading one half or more of the myometrium.
T2	II	Tumor invading the stromal connective tissue of the cervix but not extending beyond the uterus.
T3	III	Tumor involving serosa, adnexa, vagina, or parametrium.
T3a	IIIA	Tumor involving the serosa and/or adnexa (direct extension or metastasis).
T3b	IIIB	Vaginal involvement (direct extension or metastasis) or parametrial involvement.
T4	IVA	Tumor invading the bladder mucosa and/or bowel mucosa (bullous edema is not sufficient to classify a tumor as T4).

Table 2.17B N Category		
N	**FIGO**	**N Criteria**
NX		Regional LNs cannot be assessed
N0		No regional LN metastasis
N0(i+)		Isolated tumor cells in regional LN(s) not >0.2 mm
N1	IIIC1	Regional LN metastasis to pelvic LNs
N1mi	IIIC1	Regional LN metastasis (>0.2 mm but not >2.0 mm in diameter) to the pelvic nodes
N1a	IIIC1	Regional LN metastasis (>2.0 mm in diameter) to pelvic LNs
N2	IIIC	Regional LN metastasis to para-aortic LNs, with or without positive pelvic LNs
N2mi	IIIC2	Regional LN metastasis (>0.2 mm but not >2.0 mm in diameter) to the para-aortic LNs, with or without positive pelvic LNs
N2a	IIIC2	Regional LN metastasis (>2.0 mm in diameter) to para-aortic LNs, with or without positive pelvic LNs
LN, lymph node.		

Table 2.17C M Category		
M	**FIGO**	**M Criteria**
M0		No distant metastasis
M1	IVB	Distant metastasis (includes metastasis to inguinal LNs, intraperitoneal disease, lung, liver, or bone)
LN, lymph node.		

Table 2.17D Stage Grouping			
When T is	**And N is**	**And M is**	**The stage group is**
T1	N0	M0	I
T1a	N0	M0	IA
T1b	N0	M0	IB
T2	N0	M0	II
T3	N0	M0	III
T3a	N0	M0	IIIA
T3b	N0	M0	IIIB
T1-T3	N1/N1mi/N1a	M0	IIIC1
T1-T3	N2/N2mi/N2a	M0	IIIC2
T4	Any N	M0	IVA
Any T	Any N	M1	IVB
Source: From Amin MB, Edge SB. (2017). *AJCC Cancer Staging Manual* 8th Edition. Chicago, IL: American Joint Committee on Cancer. With permission.			

- Treatment approaches:
  - Laparotomy
  - Minimally invasive (preferred)
    - Laparoscopic assisted vaginal
    - Robotic assisted
- Treatment modifications:
  - Conversion to laparotomy from laparoscopy: in one study this occurred in 17.5% of patients with body mass index (BMI) of 25, 26.5% with a BMI 34 to 35, and 57% of patients with BMI greater than 40. Port site metastasis occurred in 1% (9).
  - The ability of infrarenal/PA-LND was 81% in one study when the BMI was greater than 35 kg/m^2, compared to 95% when the BMI was less than 35 (10).

- Ovarian conservation in young women with uterine cancer: only 18% of women less than 45 years old have stage IAG1 disease. The risk of a synchronous ovarian malignancy can be as high as 19%–25% in younger women. Bilateral salpingo-oophorectomy (BSO) should be considered for all women with uterine cancer per Society of Gynecologic Oncology (SGO) guidelines. If ovarian conservation is desired, patients should be stage IA and G1-2. A retrospective review showed that conservation was not independently associated with survival (HR 0.94; 95% CI: 0.65–1.37) (11). Younger women have a higher risk of genetic mutations. The risk of hereditary nonpolyposis colorectal cancer (HNPCC) syndrome and ovarian malignancy is up to 10% if women harbor this genetic mutation. MRI is the best mode to evaluate for DOI and cervical involvement when considering preoperative radiologic staging for possible ovarian preservation (12).
- Morcellation: the risk of a fibroid harboring a LMS is 0.3% to 0.49%. Regardless, morcellation is not recommended for uterine cancer cases to avoid tumor spill and spread, or alter pathologic evaluation. Alternatives to morcellation for laparoscopic approaches to surgery are minilaparotomy or morcellation within an endoscopic bag after vaginal delivery of the specimen (13).
- Sentinel LND: this strategy remains under investigation (category 3) and careful consideration should be given to not performing this procedure with type II tumors. If it is considered, surgeon experience, adherence to an sentinel LND algorithm or clinical study, and the use of pathologic "ultrastaging" are key factors for successful SLN mapping. Serous/CC/MMMT histologies should not undergo this type of LN assessment.
- **Lymph node dissection**
  - The boundaries for pelvic LND (P-LND) are the following: the distal half of the common iliac vessels, the anterior and medial aspect of the external iliac vessels, the ureter or (superior vesicle artery below the common iliacs) medially, the circumflex iliac vein distally, and the obturator nerve inferiorly. The PA-LN boundaries are the following: the fat pads over and lateral to the great vessels, the inferior mesenteric artery superiorly, and the mid common iliac vessels inferiorly. For a high PA dissection, the LNs up to the renal vessels are removed medial to the ureters and anterior to the great vessels.
  - There is much controversy to the benefit and/or extent of an LND. LND has been shown not to increase the duration of surgery significantly. Some practitioners perform an LND based on tumor risk factors. Others recommend a comprehensive LND for all surgical candidates. Others have provided data that show that a LND is not therapeutic but can provide staging information to guide adjuvant therapies.
  - For those providers who choose a selective LND, the **Mayo criteria** is often employed to determine if a patient is low risk for LN metastasis. The Mayo criteria are: grade 1 or 2 disease; necessarily tumor size that is 2 cm or less; and ≤50% myometrial invasion. If all these criteria are met, patients have a less than 5% chance of positive LNs (14). Frozen section should be employed for this decision analysis. The accuracy of frozen section decreases with

grade: 87% accurate with grade 1, 65% with grade 2, only 31% with grade 3 (15). Doering et al correlated visual inspection for DOI with frozen section and found 91% accuracy (16), and Franchi et al supported this data with 85% accuracy and 72% sensitivity (17).

o For those who perform comprehensive LND, the following benefits are cited: there may be a therapeutic benefit with removal of micrometastasis; there is a 22% chance of extrauterine disease found with surgical staging; and 20% of tumors are upgraded at final pathology. Data have shown that removing nodes provides a survival benefit (18,19). An improvement in survival from 72% to 88% has been reported for patients undergoing lymphadenectomy with more than 11 LNs removed (20). Using Surveillance, Epidemiology, and End Results (SEER) data, Chan et al showed that in patients staged IB grade 3 and above, more than 20 LNs removed was found to provide the best OS (21). In low-risk patients, there was no association with LN count and survival. The PORTEC 1 trial subset of stage IC grade 3 (unstaged) patients who were treated with pelvic XRT had a 5 YS of only 58%. Most recurrences were distant (22). In contrast, stage IIIC patients staged and treated have a 5 YS of 57% to 72% (23,24).

o In some instances, LND is not performed. This can occur when cancer is found incidentally after hysterectomy. Postoperative pathological review can risk stratify patients for possible post hoc staging. There can be intraoperative complications that prevent full staging, or the patient may be medically intolerant of the procedure. Body habitus may also prohibit adequate staging: in the Lap-2 data, 50% of patients with a BMI greater than 40 were not able to have a para-aortic (PA-LND) performed (9). For those who support no LND, data from the following two randomized studies are commonly used.

▪ The Bendetti Panici study evaluated 514 eligible clinical stage I uterine cancer patients. Patients were randomly assigned to systematic P-LND versus no LND. Researchers found that early and late postoperative complications were higher in the systematic LND group. LND improved staging as more patients were found to have advanced stage disease with LN involvement. (13.3% vs. 3.2%). However, the 5 Y DFS and OS were similar (81% vs. 85.9% in the lymphadenectomy arm and 81.7% vs. 90% in the nonlymphadenectomy arm) (25).

▪ The ASTEC A Study in the Treatment of Endometrial Cancer, study (26, 27) evaluated 1,408 women with clinical stage I endometrial cancer and randomized them to standard surgery (hysterectomy, BSO, washings with PA LN palpation) or standard surgery plus lymphadenectomy. The primary outcome for this study was OS. The HR for death was higher in those who underwent comprehensive staging with LND, 1.16 ($p = 0.3$; 95% CI: 0.87–1.54). The absolute difference in 5Y OS was 1%.

▪ Based on a surgical/pathological review, in patients thought to have disease confined to the uterus, extrauterine disease has been found in 22% of patients, LN metastasis has been found to occur in 9% to 13% of patients, and isolated para-aortic LNs have been found in 2% of patients. The rate of positive PA LNs is approximately half the rate of positive pelvic LNs (Figure 2.11). For those who were identified with positive PA LNs, 47 of

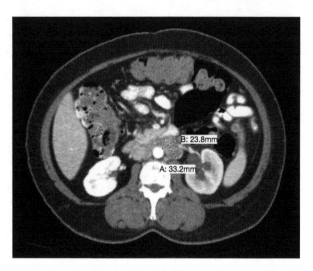

Figure 2.11 Uterine cancer on CT with para-aortic lymphadenopathy.

48 patients had one or more of the following: grossly positive pelvic LN; grossly positive adnexal metastasis; or outer one-third myometrial invasion (28). Omental metastasis has been found in up to 8% of patients (Table 2.18).

- If gross cervical involvement is seen at diagnosis: cervical biopsy and pelvic MRI should be performed for confirmation. If negative, TH-BSO and staging can be considered. If cervical biopsy is positive, a radical hysterectomy with BSO and surgical staging as primary treatment should be performed. Preoperative XRT consisting of external beam radiation therapy (EBXRT) and brachytherapy to a total dose of 75 to 80 Gy to point A can be alternative management. An adjuvant simple hysterectomy can then be considered. If not a surgical candidate, EBXRT and brachytherapy with consideration of systemic chemotherapy should be implemented. Reevaluation at a later date for surgical therapy should be performed. Systemic chemotherapy can also be an option alone for surgically inoperable patients.

- There are data to suggest that performing a radical hysterectomy, based on a positive endocervical curettage only, commonly shows no evidence of cancer on final pathology and may be overtreatment (29).

- If gross parametrial involvement is identified by physical examination or preoperative imaging, primary XRT with dosing analogous to that for cervical cancer (75–80 Gy) can be considered, followed by a simple hysterectomy, with or without chemotherapy.

- There are data to suggest that the incidence of omental metastasis is 6% to 8% and is associated with: grade of disease, extrauterine involvement, LN metastasis, deep myometrial invasion, and positive cytology.

- If there is **extrauterine disease** confirmed at presentation, neoadjuvant chemotherapy can be considered but most patients should proceed with

Table 2.18 GOG 33 Risk Factors for LN Metastasis

Risk factor	Pelvic*	Para-aortic
Grade		
1	3	2
2	9	5
3	18	11
Depth of myometrial invasion		
Superficial	5	3
Middle	6	1
Deep	25	17
Site of disease		
Fundus	8	4
Cervix	16	14
Lymphovascular space invasion		
Negative	7	9
Positive	27	19

*percentage who developed nodal metastasis

LN, lymph node.

total hysterectomy, BSO, and surgical staging and debulking. If tumor appears to be surgically unresectable at presentation, EBXRT with/without brachytherapy and consideration of chemotherapy should be offered. Systemic therapy alone is another option. If liver metastasis is present and biopsy confirmed, systemic therapy with or without EBXRT and/or hormonal therapy can be considered. Palliative TH-BSO can be considered.

- If cancer is found incidentally on post hysterectomy specimen and:
  - Stage IA G1-2, less than 50% DOI, no LVSI, and the tumor size is less than 2 cm, observation is recommended.
  - If stage IA G3, greater than 1/2 DOI, LVSI, or the tumor size is greater than 2 cm, stage 1B, or stage II, surgical staging should be considered. Imaging can also be considered and if negative, with other low risk features, protocols for adjuvant XRT can be considered.

- **Adjuvant treatment** is commonly recommended in patients with endometrial cancer. Treatment is based on stage and pathologic risk factors. Early stage disease is defined as stages I and II. Advanced stage is defined as stages III and IV.
  - High intermediate risk (HIR) early stage disease is often treated with adjuvant XRT. HIR is classified by two different studies.
    - PORTEC 1: stratified patients into an intermediate high-risk subgroup for which treatment was recommended: patient age older than 60 years, DOI greater than half myometrial thickness, or grade 2 or 3 tumor.
    - GOG 99 stratified patients by age and risk factors. If a patient fell into any of the following groups, they were considered HIR: patients age ≥70 years

with one risk factor, age 50 to 69 years with two risk factors, and any age with all three. The risk factors are: outer one-third myometrial invasion, grade 2 or 3 tumor, and LVSI.

- Absent RF:
  - □ Stage IA G1,2,3: can be observed or vaginal brachytherapy can be recommended
  - □ Stage IB G1,2,3: can be observed but more commonly vaginal brachytherapy with/without whole pelvic (WP) EBXRT (especially for G3) is recommended
- RF present:
  - □ Stage IA G1-2: observation or brachytherapy can be offered
  - □ Stage IAG3: brachytherapy, WP EBXRT, or observation can be offered
  - □ Stage IBG1-2: brachytherapy, WP EBXRT, or observation can be offered
  - □ Stage IBG3: brachytherapy with/without WP EBXRT with/without chemotherapy can be recommended

○ High-risk early stage disease is defined variably. Stage I serous, CC, MMMT, and variably grade 3 endometrioid cancers put patients into the high-risk early stage disease category. There are data to show that (FIGO 1988) stage 1CG3 type I tumors had a 58% 5 YS. Some clinicians recommend chemotherapy and XRT for these high-risk patients. Stage IA type II tumors are recommended to have adjuvant therapy: preferably a combination of XRT and chemotherapy (three cycles of chemotherapy with brachytherapy). Stage IB cancers are recommended to have chemotherapy (three to six cycles) with/without vaginal XRT and/or EBXRT.

○ Stage II disease: adjuvant XRT is recommended and cumulative data supports both WP EBXRT and brachytherapy treatment. Chemotherapy should be considered if a type II cancer is present and variably for G3 endometrioid cancer.

○ Advanced-stage endometrial cancer. For advanced-stage disease (stages III/IV) treatment is primarily surgical with comprehensive staging and cytoreduction to microscopic status if possible. Adjuvant therapy is commonly multimodal including both XRT and chemotherapy, and can include hormonal therapies.

  - Stage IIIA: chemotherapy, EBXRT and/or brachytherapy, or both is recommended.
  - Stage IIIB: chemotherapy and/or EBXRT, and brachytherapy.
  - Stage IIIC: chemotherapy and/or EBXRT and/or brachytherapy
  - Stage IV: chemotherapy with/without EBXRT and/or brachytherapy.
  - There is literature to support cytoreduction in advanced metastatic uterine cancer.
    - □ Greer treated 31 patients with stage IVB disease with whole abdominal XRT. Those with residual disease less than 2 cm had a corrected 5 YS of 80% and an absolute 5 YS of 63%, whereas there were no survivors in the group with residual greater than 2 cm (30).

- □ Goff evaluated patients with stage IV disease. Those who were cytoreduced had a longer median survival of 18 months compared to an 8-month survival in those who were not able to be cytoreduced (31).
- □ Bristow reviewed 65 patients with stage IVB endometrial cancer who underwent cytoreduction. Optimal cytoreduction (residual tumor ≤1 cm in maximal diameter) was accomplished in 55%. The median survival rate of patients who underwent optimal surgery was 34 months versus 11 months for patients with greater than 1 cm residual disease. Furthermore, patients with microscopic residual tumor survived significantly longer (median survival 46 months) compared to patients optimally cytoreduced but with macroscopic disease (32).
- □ Shih also suggested optimal cytoreduction for stage IV uterine cancer patients. Median survival: the median PFS was 40.3 months for patients with microscopic disease, 11 months for patients with any residual disease, and 2.2 months for patients who did not have attempted cytoreduction. The median OS was 42.2 months for patients with microscopic disease, 19 months for patients with any residual disease, and 2.2 months for patients that did not have attempted cytoreduction (33).
- □ There are data to support that most stage IIIA patients (adnexal spread of primary uterine disease) are clonally related metastatic tumors from one primary uterine tumor demonstrated on genetic analysis (34).
- ○ Type II cancers
  - ■ Early stage type II cancers (serous or CC histology): there are data to support platinum-based chemotherapy in addition to XRT for patients staged IA or above. Stage IA patients with no residual cancer in the hysterectomy specimen had no recurrences whether they received adjuvant therapy or not. 77% of stage IB patients not treated with adjuvant chemotherapy recurred versus no recurrences in the treated group; 20% of stage (FIGO 1988) IC patients who received chemotherapy recurred versus 80% who did not. Recurrences tended to occur at the vaginal cuff in patients not treated with brachytherapy, thus brachytherapy in combination with chemotherapy was recommended for all patients staged IA (with residual) or higher (35).
  - ■ Maximal cytoreduction for stage IV serous uterine cancer can offer an improvement in survival. Bristow showed that patients with optimal cytoreduction had a median survival of 26.2 months versus 9.6 months in patients with suboptimal surgery. Patients with microscopic residual tumor had a significantly longer median survival of 30.4 months versus those with 0.1 to 1 cm residual disease who had a median survival of 20.5 months. A 41-month versus a 34-month versus an 11-month OS was observed for those patients who were microscopically cytoreduced, optimally cytoreduced to less than 1 cm, or suboptimally cytoreduced, respectively (32).
  - ■ MMMT (carcinosarcoma) used to be classified as a uterine sarcoma. Recent data have suggested an improvement in survival with surgical cytoreduction (36). An adjuvant XRT trial from the EORTC eval-

uated a subset of carcinosarcoma patients and found a trend toward improvement in local control with whole-pelvic radiation therapy (WP-XRT), but there was no improvement in survival (37). Chemotherapy in combination with XRT has been shown to be effective in treatment of MMMTs. Ifosfamide and paclitaxel have been shown to produce a RR of 45% (38).

RECURRENCE

Recurrent disease can be broken into local recurrence or distant recurrence. Local recurrence is divided into vaginal and pelvic. A full metastatic workup should be performed with a physical examination; imaging of the chest, abdomen, and pelvis; lab tests for baseline organ function; and possibly PET imaging. Patients who were previously radiated in the pelvis tend to fail distantly at 70%, only 16% recur vaginally, and 14% recur in the pelvis. Patients without prior pelvic XRT tend to fail vaginally at 50%, 21% fail in the pelvis, and 30% distantly.

- If the recurrence is vaginal, XRT can be administered. Prior XRT does affect response. In the PORTEC 1 trial, data on relapsed patients showed a 5 YS of 65% if patients had no prior adjuvant XRT versus 19% if they had prior XRT. The treatment of recurrence is WP-XRT in combination with brachytherapy dosed to 75 to 80 Gy if no prior XRT. There are data to support surgical cytoreduction of vaginal lesions to less than 2 cm. This is associated with an improvement in OS to 43 months versus 10 months (39).
  - If no prior XRT to the site of recurrence, then surgical cytoreduction to <2 cm should occur if possible with/without intraoperative radiation therapy (IOXRT), or EBXRT and brachytherapy dosed at 75 to 80 Gy.
  - If prior XRT given:
    - And prior brachytherapy only, then EBXRT or surgical resection with/without IOXRT can be provided.
    - If prior EBXRT, surgical resection with/without IOXRT or hormonal therapy, or chemotherapy can be offered.
- For pelvic recurrence including pelvic LN involvement:
  - Surgical resection can be considered followed by tumor directed EBXRT with/without chemotherapy
  - EBXRT with/without chemotherapy
- For extrapelvic recurrences:
  - For isolated recurrence: surgical resection with/without XRT or ablative therapy can be considered.
  - If upper abdominal recurrence is resectable it should be surgically reduced, chemotherapy should follow, and consideration of EBXRT can be offered.
  - If not resectable and low grade, asymptomatic, or ER/PR positive, hormone therapy can be attempted and if progression, then systemic chemotherapy provided. If symptomatic, grade 2-3, or large volume disease, then chemotherapy with/without palliative XRT should be provided.
  - For widely metastatic disease: if low grade, asymptomatic, or ER/PR positive: hormone therapy can be attempted and if progression, then systemic

chemotherapy. If symptomatic, grade 2/3, or large volume disease, then chemotherapy with/without palliative XRT should be provided.

- Different chemotherapy regimens have been used. CAP: cyclophosphamide (500 mg/m^2), doxorubicin (40 mg/m^2), and cisplatin (70 mg/m^2), given every 4 weeks; single-agent paclitaxel at 250 mg/m^2 as 24-hr infusion (has shown a 36% response rate); or a combination of paclitaxel (175 mg/m^2), carboplatin AUC 6, and has shown a 40% response rate with an 8% complete response (40).
- Hormonal therapies, specifically progestins, have also been used. Medroxyprogesterone acetate (MPA) at a dose of 200 mg/day had a better response rate than 1,000 mg/day in the GOG 81 study. The overall response rate was 25%, and there was a higher response in ER and PR positive patients. Megace has also been used at a dose of 80 to 160 mg twice daily with an 18% to 34% response rate (41). For those patients who are ER positive on immunohistochemistry, tamoxifen or an aromatase inhibitor can be considered. If the patient is *Her-2/neu* positive, herceptin was found to have a 13% response rate in a phase II trial (GOG 181B) (42).
- Targeted therapies:
  - Cediranib monotherapy at 30 mg PO daily for a 28-day cycle was evaluated in 48 patients with recurrent or persistent endometrial cancer. The median age was 65.5 years, 52% had prior XRT and 73% had one prior chemotherapy regimen. A PR was seen in 12.5%. Median PFS was 2.65 months and median OS was 12.5 months and was well tolerated (43).
  - HNPCC/MSI confirmed patients: Pertulimuzab has been shown to be an actionable mutation medication.

FERTILITY SPARING OPTIONS (SEE ALSO CHAPTER 6)

- If the patient has fertility concerns, workup should include CT of the abdomen/pelvis; MRI of the pelvis, and pathology should be expertly reviewed.
- For consideration of fertility preservation: metastatic disease must be absent on workup, preferably no DOI seen on MRI, no contraindications (such as PE) should exist to medical therapy or desired pregnancy, grade must be well differentiated (G1), histology should be endometrioid subtype, and patients should undergo counseling with a reproductive endocrinologist as well as full informed consent that medical management is not the standard of care.
- Treatment: continuous progestin-based therapy with megace, medroxyprogesterone, or levonorgestrel intrauterine device (IUD). Resampling of the uterus should occur with D&C/EMB every 3 to 6 months. If there is a complete response by 6 months, conception can be encouraged. Completion hysterectomy should be offered at the end of desired fertility. If cancer is still present at 6 to 9 months, hysterectomy with BSO and staging is recommended.

POSTOPERATIVE HORMONAL REPLACEMENT THERAPY

Postoperative hormonal replacement therapy, namely estrogen, has been studied for quality of life and risk of recurrence. GOG 137 (44) evaluated estrogen HRT given to women with a history of uterine cancer. There was no increased risk of recurrence identified (RR was 1.27 80% CI: 0.916-1.77—the CI crossed 1.0, thus careful consideration of outcomes should be applied).

SYNCHRONOUS OVARIAN NEOPLASM

Five percent to 10% of women with a uterine cancer may have a **synchronous ovarian neoplasm.** Up to 25% of women under 40 years old can have this concurrent diagnosis. Concordant endometrioid histology in both the uterus and ovary are present 45% to 86% of the time. There is concordant grade in 69% of patients. Empirical criteria favoring metastatic uterine cancer over a synchronous ovarian tumor are: multinodular ovarian involvement, deep myometrial invasion, LVSI, bilateral ovarian involvement, and visualization of intratubal transit. Surgical staging or adjuvant recommendations are based on the worst-case scenario; that is, if the ovarian tumor is grade 3 and the uterine tumor is grade 1, chemotherapy would commonly be recommended.

SURVIVAL

Table 2.19A Endometrioid Uterine Cancer 5 YS by Stage	
Stage	**5 YS Endometrioid (%)**
1A	88
1B	75
II	69
IIIA	58
IIIB	50
IIIC	47
IVA	17
IVB	15
YS, year survival.	
Source: Ref. (45). Lewin SN, Herzog TJ, Barrena Medel NI, et al. Comparative performance of the 2009 International Federation of Gynecology and Obstetrics' staging system for uterine corpus cancer. Obstet Gynecol. 2010;116(5):1141-1149.	

Table 2.19B Serous Uterine Cancer 5 YS by Stage	
Stage	**5 YS Serous uterine cancer (%)**
I	50–80
II	50
III	20
IV	5–10
YS, year survival.	

Table 2.19C Carcinosarcoma Uterine Cancer 5 YS by Stage	
Stage	**5 YS Carcinosarcoma (%)**
I	70
II	45
III	30
IV	15
YS, year survival.	

FOLLOW-UP

- Every 3 months for the first 2 years
  Every 6 months for the next 3 years
  Then annual examinations thereafter
- Physical and pelvic examination should occur at each visit. Pap smears have not been found to increase the detection of recurrence, nor has annual chest x-ray. CA-125 can be drawn if it was initially elevated.

TAMOXIFEN AND UTERINE CANCER

Adjuvant treatment of pre- and postmenopausal women with hormone receptor positive **breast cancer** has been **tamoxifen**. There are known gynecologic side effects from this medication. Aromatase inhibitors have been evaluated as cross-over or primary therapy in some women, replacing tamoxifen treatment. Gynecologic side effects of tamoxifen can be vaginal bleeding, growth of uterine polyps in 8% to 36% of women, endometrial hyperplasia in 2% to 20%, and endometrial cancer ranging from 0% to 8%. The overall risk of subsequent uterine corpus cancer was increased more than twofold (observed-to-expected ratio [O/E] 2.17; 95% CI: 1.95–2.41) relative to the general SEER population in one study. The RR was substantially higher for malignant mixed Müllerian tumors (O/E 4.62; O 34; 95% CI: 3.20–6.46) than for endometrial adenocarcinomas (O/E 2.07, O 306; 95% CI: 1.85–2.32), although the excess absolute risk was smaller—an additional 1.4 versus 8.4 cancers per 10,000 women per year, respectively.

Ultrasound diagnoses an endometrial stripe that is greater than 5 mm in 50% of patients on tamoxifen; but endometrial stripes up to 8 mm can be considered normal in these patients. A routine annual EMB is not recommended unless these women are symptomatic with abnormal or postmenopausal bleeding of significant atypical vaginal discharge (46).

NOTABLE STUDIES IN UTERINE CANCER

High-Risk Early Stage Disease Adjuvant Therapy Studies

- Aalders studied 540 patients with stage I endometrial cancer status post TAH BSO, but who were not surgically staged. All received brachytherapy and were randomized to WP-XRT or no further treatment (NFT). There was no improvement in OS. The 5 YS was 89% in the EBXRT arm versus 91% in the NFT (NS).

Vaginal and pelvic recurrences were 6.9% in the NFT arm versus 1.9% if given pelvic XRT. Distant metastasis occurred more often in the XRT arm. In the subset of patients with stage IC grade 3 disease, there were fewer recurrences in the EBXRT arm, 18% versus 7% (47).

- PORTEC 1: 715 eligible patients underwent TAH and BSO without surgical staging or lymphadenectomy. Patients were included if they had either: grade 1 disease with greater than 50% invasion, grade 2 with any invasion, or grade 3 with less than 50% invasion. Less than 2% of histologies were other than endometrioid. Patients were randomized to no additional therapy versus WP-XRT to 46 Gy. The 5Y recurrence rate was 4% versus 14%, favoring XRT ($p < 0.001$) and the 5 YS was 81% versus 85% (NS). Distant metastasis was similar at 7% and 8%. The 8 Y RFS was 68% for both groups. The 8Y OS was 71% in the XRT group and 77% in the control group (NS) due to salvage of relapse in the NFT arm (85% of vaginal recurrences were salvageable). An HIR subgroup was identified: patient age older than 60 years, depth of invasion greater than half myometrial thickness, or grade 2 or 3 tumor. In this HIR group, the recurrence rate was 23% versus 5%, favoring XRT. 73% of recurrences were in the vagina. Survival after recurrence was better for the control group rather than XRT group. For the pelvic recurrence patients, 51% were salvaged if they had not received XRT versus 19% if they had received adjuvant XRT. Stage IB grade 3 patients had higher rates of distant metastasis (15%). A subgroup of patients staged IC grade 3 were not randomized but all received WP-XRT. These patients all had a 5 YS of 58%. A 15-year follow-up report yielded a median follow-up of 13.3 years, with a 5.8% locoregional recurrence in the XRT arm versus 15.5% in the NFT arm. 74% of these recurrences were isolated vaginal recurrences (48-50).
- Systemic pelvic lymphadenectomy randomized trial ILIADE II study: 514 eligible patients underwent hysterectomy with BSO and were randomized to systemic P-LND or no LND. LND improved surgical staging with 13.3% versus 3.2% of patients identified with LN metastasis. At 49 months of follow-up, the 5Y DFS and OS were 81% and 85.9% in the LND arm and 81.7% and 90% in the no LND arm. There was no improvement in DFS or OS with LND. Researchers found the rate of recurrence in LN beds was 1.5% in each arm; therefore, LN basins were not where patients recurred (26).
- GOG 99: 392 eligible patients with type I cancers staged IB, IC, IIA, and occult IIB were evaluated. All were surgically staged with TAH, BSO, pelvic and para-aortic LND. Of patients, 75% had endometrioid histology, 80% had grade 1 or 2 tumors, 25% had LVSI, and 10% were stage II. Patients were randomized to WP-XRT to 50.4 Gy without brachytherapy, or no further therapy (NFT). Median follow-up was 68 months. The overall recurrence rate was 12% in the NFT group and decreased to 3% with XRT. The OS was 86% in the NFT group versus 92% in the XRT arm (NS). A HIR group was identified, which accounted for 132 patients (one third of those enrolled) and two thirds of the study-related deaths. This HIR group included patients of age ≥70 years with one risk factor, age 50 to 69 years with two risk factors, and any age with all three. The risk factors were: outer one-third myometrial

invasion, grade 2 or 3 tumor, and LVSI. For this subgroup, the recurrence rate was reduced with adjuvant XRT from 26% to 6%. The major difference was the vaginal vault recurrences: 13 recurred vaginally in the NFT versus two that recurred in the XRT arm, and of these two, both had refused XRT. Five percent in each group had distant metastasis (51).

- PORTEC 2: this study evaluated 427 patients with stage I or stage IIA endometrial carcinoma with HIR factors. Patients were randomized to pelvic XRT (46 Gy) or vaginal brachytherapy (21 Gy high-dose rate or 30 Gy low-dose rate). The 5-year vaginal recurrence rate was 1.8% for vaginal brachytherapy versus 1.6% for pelvic XRT. The 5-year rates of locoregional relapse were 5.1% for vaginal brachytherapy and 2.1% for pelvic XRT. There were no differences in overall or disease-free survival. At 126 months, LVSI and unfavorable molecular alterations (TP53-mutation or > 10% L1CAM expression) (HR 8.53, 95% CI: 2.7-27.3) and EBXRT (HR 0.16 95%, CI: 0.04-0.70) were independent prognostic factors for pelvic recurrence and locoregional recurrence (HR 0.37, 95% CI: 0.14-0.95 and HR 6.7, 95% CI: 2.5-17.9, respectively), but not for vaginal recurrence. EBXRT should be considered for patients with HIR cancers and tumor with LVSI (52).

- PORTEC3: a multicenter trial of high-risk endometrial cancer patients randomly allocated (1:1) 686 patients to XRT alone (48.6 Gy) in 1.8 Gy fractions five times a week or chemoradiotherapy consisting of two cycles of concurrent cisplatin 50 mg/m^2 followed by four adjuvant cycles of carboplatin AUC 5 and paclitaxel 175 mg/m^2. Inclusion criteria were: surgical staging with TH-BSO and LND, histologically confirmed endometrial carcinoma, with one of the following postoperative FIGO 2009 stages and grade: stage IA with invasion, grade 3 with documented LVSI; stage IB grade 3; stage II; stage IIIA or IIIC; or IIIB if parametrial invasion only; stage IA (with invasion), IB, II, or III with serous or CC histology. The primary endpoints were OS and PFS analyzed in the intention-to-treat population. Median follow-up was 42.3 months. At 12 and 24 months, no significant differences in grade 3 or worse adverse events were found between groups; only grade 2 or higher sensory neuropathy adverse events persisted at 24 months (25 [10%] of 240 patients in the chemoradiotherapy group vs. one [<1%] of 247 patients in the XRT alone group; $p < 0.0001$). OS and PFS results are still pending. (53).

- PORTEC-4: this is a three-arm study that will evaluate approximately 500 patients in a 2:1 fashion with HIR endometrial cancer. Patients are randomized to receive vaginal brachytherapy (either 21 Gy in three fractions vs. 15 Gy in three fractions to 5 mm depth vaginal cuff) versus no additional therapy NAT (third arm). Eligible patients had histologically confirmed endometrioid type endometrial carcinoma, via hysterectomy BSO, FIGO 2009 stage I, with one of the following combinations of substage, age, and grade: stage IA, any age and grade 3 without LVSI; stage IB, age 60 years or above and grade 1 or 2; stage IB, any age, grade 1 and 2 with documented LVSI. NTR3263. Results pending (54).

- RTOG-9708: this was a phase II study in 46 patients with high-risk uterine cancer stages I to III cancer who underwent TAH, BSO, +/- LND. High-risk pathologic features were: grade 2/3, DOI greater than 1/2, and cervical stromal involvement, or pelvic confined extrauterine disease. Patients were given adjuvant pelvic XRT to 45 Gy with concurrent cisplatin 50 mg/m^2 on days 1 and 28. Vaginal brachytherapy was given after EBXRT. Four additional cycles of cisplatin 50 mg/m^2 and paclitaxel 175 mg/m^2 were given every 28 days after completion of XRT. The median follow-up was 4.3 years. At 4 years, the locoregional recurrence rate was 4% and distant recurrence rates 19%. OS and DFS rates at 4 years were 85% and 81%, respectively. 4Y rates for survival and DFS for stage III patients were 77% and 72%, respectively. There were no recurrences for patients with stage IC, IIA, or IIB (55).

- Japanese Gynecologic Oncology Group-2033: this study evaluated 385 patients with stage IC to stage IIIC endometrial carcinoma who were randomized to WP-XRT versus cyclophosphamide (333 mg/m^2), doxorubicin (40 mg/m^2), and cisplatin (50 mg/m^2) (CAP chemotherapy) every 4 weeks for three or more courses. The 5Y PFS was nearly the same at 83.5% in the pelvic XRT group and 81.8% in the CAP group. The 5Y OS was 85% in the XRT group versus 87% in the chemotherapy group (NS). A subgroup of HIR patients—who were defined as having (a) stage IC disease in patients over 70 years of age or having grade 3 tumor or (b) stage II or stage IIIA (positive cytology) with greater than 50% myometrial invasion—were found to have significantly better outcomes with chemotherapy: the PFS for the XRT arm was 66% versus 84% for the chemotherapy arm, and the OS was 74% in the XRT group versus 90% in the chemotherapy group (56).

- SEPAL study: Survival Effect of Para-Aortic Lymphadenectomy in endometrial cancer: cohorts from two different Japanese gynecologic oncology teams totaling 671 patients were retrospectively analyzed with respect to the use of PA-LND. Routine PA-LND was practiced standardly at one facility and not at the other. Both facilities offered systemic pelvic lymph node dissection (P-LND). A median P-LND count was 34 in the P-LND group versus 59 in the combined PA and P-LND group. Patients at intermediate or high risk of recurrence were offered adjuvant chemotherapy and XRT. The OS was longer in the combination PA and P-LND group with a HR of 0.53. The risk of death was reduced independent of adjuvant therapies so it was recommended that a combined PA and P-LND be performed for all intermediate and high-risk patients (57).

- GOG 249: 601 patients were randomized after TH BSO in a phase III trial of WP-XRT versus vaginal cuff brachytherapy followed by paclitaxel/carboplatin chemotherapy (VCB/C) in patients with high risk, early stage endometrial cancer. All patients were required to undergo hysterectomy. Staging was encouraged, but not required. All patients had stage I endometrioid disease with GOG 99 based high risk criteria (based on age, tumor grade, depth of invasion, and presence of LVSI), stage II, or stage I and II serous or clear cell tumors. Patients assigned to WP-XRT were treated with standard four-field or intensity-modulated radiation therapy (IMXRT) techniques. Additional VCB was optional for patients with serous or clear cell tumors or stage II disease. Patients assigned to VCB/C received high dose rate (HDR) or low dose rate (LDR) brachytherapy followed by paclitaxel 175 mg/m^2 (3 hours) plus carboplatin AUC 6 q21 days for a total of three cycles. Of the 601 patients, 289 received WP-XRT and 291 received VCB/C. The median age was 63 years, 74% had stage I disease, and 89% underwent lymphadenectomy; 71% had endometrioid histology, 15% had serous, and 5% had clear cell. Of patients, 91% completed WP-XRT and 87% completed VCB/C. Recurrence sites totaled 5 versus 3 vaginal, 2 versus 19 pelvic, and 32 versus 24 distant failures with WP-XRT versus VCB/C. With a median follow-up of 24 months, the 24-month RFS was 82% versus 84% for WP-XRT and VCB/C and treatment hazard ratio (HR) was 0.97 (95% CI: 0.635–1.43) (VCB/C relative to WP-XRT). The 24-month survival was 93% versus 92% for WP-XRT and VCB/C and treatment HR was 1.28 (95% CI: 0.689–2.36) (VCB/C relative to WP-XRT). There was no statistically significant treatment effect heterogeneity with respect to RFS among clinical–pathologic variables evaluated. There was higher toxicity in the chemotherapy arm (58).

- MaNGO ILIADE-III NSGO-EC-9501/EORTC-55991: This was a pooled study from two randomized trials evaluating 534 patients with FIGO 1988 staged I-IIIC (pelvic LN only involvement) endometrial cancer. The primary endpoint was PFS. Patients were randomly assigned to adjuvant XRT with or without sequential chemotherapy. Comprehensive surgical staging with LND was not mandatory and 30% did not have LND. Inclusion criteria were serous clear cell or anaplastic tumors by definition. Serous and clear cell tumors were included in the NSGO/EORTC trial only. Optional vaginal brachytherapy was decided before randomization. Pelvic XRT was given before chemotherapy in the combination arm. Chemotherapy consisted of either: 4 courses of doxorubicin/epirubicin 50 mg/m^2 and cisplatin 50 mg/m^2 every 4 weeks; paclitaxel 175 mg/m^2 and epirubicin 60 mg/m^2/doxorubicin 40 mg/m^2 and carboplatin AUC 5; or paclitaxel 175 mg/m^2 and carboplatin AUC 5-6 every 21 days. The PFS difference in the NSGO/EORTC trial favored combination XRT and chemotherapy with HR 0.64 (95% CI: 0.41-99; $p = 0.04$.) In the MaNGO trial the HR was 0.61 but was NS. When the data was pooled, the HR was 0.63 (95% CI: 0.41-0.99; $p = 0.009$) favoring combination therapy. The pooled trial data showed significant differences in cancer specific survival with a HR of 0.55 (95% CI: 0.35-0.88; $p = 0.01$). This trial then showed the sequential use of chemotherapy after XRT was associated with a 36% decrease in the rate of relapse or death and a 49% decrease in the rate in the risk of death from endometrial cancer.
- GOG 258: randomized phase III trial of cisplatin and tumor volume directed irradiation followed by carboplatin and paclitaxel versus carboplatin and paclitaxel. Results pending.
- RTOG-0921: this was a phase II study of postoperative IMRT with concurrent cisplatin and bevacizumab followed by carboplatin and paclitaxel for patients with endometrial cancer. 30 eligible patients with TH-BSO LND and had ≥1 of the following high-risk factors: grade 3 carcinoma with greater than 50% myometrial invasion, grade 2 or 3 disease with any cervical stromal invasion, or known extrauterine extension confined to the pelvis. Treatment consisted of pelvic IMRT and concurrent 50 mg/m^2 cisplatin on days 1 and 29 of XRT and bevacizumab (at a dose of 5 mg/kg on days 1, 15, and 29 of XRT) followed

by adjuvant carboplatin AUC 5 and paclitaxel 135 mg/m^2 for four cycles. 23.3% patients developed grade ≥3 treatment-related non-hematologic toxicities within 90 days; an additional six patients experienced grade ≥3 toxicities between 90 and 365 days after treatment. The 2Y OS rate was 96.7% and the disease-free survival rate was 79.1%. No patient developed a within-field pelvic failure and no stage IIIA and lower had recurrent disease with a median follow-up of 26 months (59).

Surgical-pathological findings in type 1 and 2 endometrial cancer: This NRG Oncology/Gynecologic Oncology Group study was a surgical pathological study of uterine adeno carcinoma or carcino-sarcoma cancer patients enrolled in GOG 210. 5,866 patients with extra-uterine disease were evaluated and all uterine histologies were included, with 1,630 of the total being type II tumors. Molecular analysis using data from The Cancer Genome Analysis identified certain predictive proteins: 16% of patients were found to have somatic *BRCA* mutations. Tumors with mutations of either *PTEN* and *BRCA2* were associated with improved survival (96).

Advanced and Recurrent Endometrial Cancer Studies

- GOG 28: this study evaluated melphalan, 5-fluorouracil (FU), and Megace versus doxorubicin, 5-FU and cyclophosphamide in 358 patients with FIGO stages III and IV or recurrent endometrial cancer. The overall response rate (ORR) in those with measurable disease was 38% in both groups; 36% of each group had stable disease, and only 26.4% progressed on treatment. The OS was 10.6 versus 10.1 months, respectively (both NS) (60).
- GOG 48: this study evaluated 356 eligible patients and compared doxorubicin to the doublet of doxorubicin and cyclophosphamide. All patients had received prior therapy with progestins subsequent to progression of disease. A response rate of 22% versus 32% was found and an OS of 6.8 versus 7.6 months was identified with a 17% reduction in the rate of death (61).
- GOG 94: this trial evaluated 77 stage III/IV type I and 103 type II endometrial cancers. A subgroup (phase II study) of patients with stage I/II serous and CC uterine cancer patients were also evaluated. Treatment was whole abdominal radiotherapy (WAR). The 3Y RFS was 29% and 27% for the type I and type II cancers, respectively. The OS were 31% and 35%, respectively. The 5Y PFS was 54%. The OS was 34%. This led to the development of GOG 122 (62,63).
- GOG 107: this study evaluated doxorubicin 60 mg/m^2 versus doxorubicin 60 mg/m^2 and cisplatin 50 mg/m^2 every 3 weeks in 281 eligible patients with stage III/IV or recurrent endometrial cancer. The ORR was 25% versus 42%. The median PFS was 3.8 versus 5.7 months, and the median OS was 9.2 versus 9 months for doxorubicin alone versus the doublet, respectively. The doublet improved RR and PFS with little impact on OS (64).
- GOG 122: this trial randomized 400 patients with stage III, IV, and recurrent disease to WAR versus doxorubicin 60 mg/m^2 and cisplatin 50 mg/m^2 (AP) for seven cycles plus an additional eighth cycle of cisplatin alone every 3 weeks. Of patients, 85% had a P-LND and 75% had a PA-LND. XRT was dosed at 45 Gy total (30 Gy WAR + 15 Gy boost to the PA LN and to the pelvis). 85% had

microscopic residual disease, 25% were stage IV, and 50% were stage IIIC. The PFS HR was 0.71 favoring AP demonstrating a 12% decrease in recurrence at 5 years with chemotherapy. The OS HR was 0.68 favoring chemotherapy. A 13% increase in OS was seen at 5 years in the chemotherapy arm. The 5 YS was 53% with chemotherapy versus 42% with XRT (65).

- GOG 139: this trial evaluated a possible circadian difference in the administration of doxorubicin and cisplatin in 342 patients with stages III, IV, and recurrent disease. No benefit was found to timing the administration of chemotherapy based on increased glutathione levels early in the morning. The RR was 46% versus 49%. The PFS was 6.5 months for the standard timed therapy and 5.9 months for the circadian timed therapy. The OS was 11.2 for standard versus 13.2 months for the circadian therapy (both NS) (66).

- GOG 163: this trial evaluated 328 chemotherapy-naïve uterine cancer patients FIGO staged III or IV or recurrent (prior XRT and hormone therapy not excluded), were randomly assigned to doxorubicin 60 mg/m^2 followed by cisplatin 50 mg/m^2 (arm 1, n = 157) or doxorubicin 50 mg/m^2 followed 4 h later by paclitaxel 150 mg/m^2 over 24 h plus filgrastim 5 mcg/kg on days 3-12 (arm 2, n = 160). Both regimens were repeated every 3 weeks for a maximum of seven cycles. There was no significant difference in response rate, PFS, or OS. The odds of response ratio in arm 2 relative to arm 1 stratified by PS was 1.12 [95% CI: 0.69–1.79; p = 0.36, one-tailed]. The median PFS was 7.2 months on arm 1 and 6 months on arm 2. The HR relative to arm 1 was 1.01 (95% CI: 0.80– 1.28; p = 0.46, one-tailed). The median OS was 12.6 months on arm 1 and 13.6 months on arm 2. The death HR relative to arm 1 was 1.00 (95% CI: 0.78–1.27; p = 0.49, one-tailed) Toxicities were primarily hematological, with 54% (arm 1) and 50% (arm 2) of patients experiencing grade 4 granulocytopenia. There was no difference in PFS or OS in either group. The response rate was 40% versus 43%; the PFS was 7.2 versus 6 months; and the OS was 12.6 versus 13.6 months (NS) (67).

- GOG 177: this study looked at the combination of paclitaxel 160 mg/m^2, doxorubicin 45 mg/m^2, and cisplatin 50 mg/m^2 (TAP) with G-CSF support versus the doublet of doxorubicin 60 mg/m^2 and cisplatin 50 mg/m^2 (AP): 273 patients with stage III, IV, or recurrent disease were treated every 3 weeks for seven cycles or until progression; 50% of patients on both arms received all cycles of therapy. There was a 22% complete response (CR) in the TAP arm versus a 7% CR on the AP arm and a PR of 36% versus 27%. The overall response rates were 57% versus 34%, the PFS was 8.3 versus 5.3 months, and the median OS was 15.3 versus 12.1 months, all favoring TAP (68).

- GOG 184: in this study, 552 eligible patients with stages III and IV disease were randomized to receive chemotherapy consisting of the triplet of cisplatin 50 mg/m^2, doxorubicin 45 mg/m^2, and paclitaxel 160 mg/m^2 (TAP) versus the doublet of cisplatin and doxorubicin (AP) at the same dosing for six cycles after volume directed XRT. 80% completed six cycles of chemotherapy. No difference in OS was found. The PFS was 64% for the TAP versus 62% for the AP arm HR 0.9 95% CI: 0.69-1.17 p = 0.21, one-tail). A subgroup analysis found that TAP was associated with a 50% reduction in recurrence or death if there was gross residual disease (69).

- GOG 209: this noninferiority trial compared carboplatin AUC 6 and paclitaxel 175 mg/m^2 given every 3 weeks for seven cycles to paclitaxel 160 mg/m^2, doxorubicin 45 mg/m^2, and cisplatin 50 mg/m^2 (TAP) with G-CSF support every 3 weeks for seven cycles in 1,312 patients with metastatic or recurrent endometrial cancer. Patients were allowed to receive volume directed XRT. A 14-month RFS was found in each arm (HR: 1.03), with an OS of 32 months versus 38 months, respectively (HR: 1.01). The neurotoxicity was 26% versus 19% favoring carboplatin and paclitaxel, thus this regimen is not inferior to TAP (70).

- GOG 238: this was a randomized trial of pelvic XRT with or without concurrent weekly cisplatin in patients with pelvic only recurrence of carcinoma of the uterine corpus. The two arms were: a) WP-XRT dosed at 4500 cGy in 25 fractions with interstitial or intracavitary brachytherapy or an external beam boost versus b) WP-XRT 4500 cGy in 25 fractions with weekly cisplatin at 40 mg/m^2 with interstitial or intracavitary brachytherapy or an external beam boost. Results pending.

- XRT salvage for vaginal recurrent disease: whole pelvic and HDR brachytherapy were used: 45 Gy of WP-XRT was delivered in 25 fractions and VB was given to a median dose of 23.75 Gy in five fractions. Complete clinical response (CCR) was seen in 95% of patients. 5Y local control, distant control, RFS, and OS were 95%, 61%, 68%, and 67%, respectively (71).

- Mundt et al found evidence to support the continued use of locoregional XRT in combination with chemotherapy for high-risk stage III/IV patients. 43 patients were reviewed retrospectively. Patients treated with doxorubicin and platinum chemotherapy alone were found to have a 67% incidence of recurrence; 31% relapsed in the pelvis, vagina, or both, making the case for adding radiation therapy for multimodality therapy (72).

- GOG 129F: single-agent paclitaxel was evaluated in a phase II trial for patients with persistent or recurrent endometrial cancer. Paclitaxel was dosed at 200 mg/m^2, and 175 mg/m^2 for patients with prior WP-XRT, every 3 weeks. A 27.3% overall RR was seen in 44 patients (73).

- GOG 139S: this study evaluated histology among different uterine cancer studies totaling 1,203 patients from four randomized trials. The response with different combinations of doxorubicin, cisplatin, and paclitaxel was not associated with histology except for the CC subtype (ORR for type I was 44%; type II serous, 44%; type II CC, 32%). A main predictor of OS was histology with the type II tumors having a HR of 1.2 for serous and 1.5 for CC carcinoma. The breakdown of histology by GOG study is: GOG 122 had 50% endometrioid, 20% serous, 5% CC, and 10% mixed histologies, 80% were grade 2, 3; GOG 177 had 15% and 19% serous in each arm; GOG 184 had 13% serous in each arm; GOG 99 had none (74).

- MITO-END2: this trial included 108 patients with advanced or recurrent endometrial cancer who had received 0 to 1 prior lines of chemotherapy. Bevacizumab was added to six to eight cycles of carboplatin and paclitaxel and then continued as maintenance therapy. This approach resulted in a significant improvement in median PFS (13 vs. 8.7 months, $p = 0.036$) and a numerical increase in median OS (23.5 vs. 18 months, $p = 0.24$), although these OS data are not yet mature (75).

- GOG 229H: phase II study of cediranib, a multitargeted tyrosine kinase inhibitor (VEGF/PDGF/FGF) in endometrial cancer. 48 evaluable patients were administered single-agent cediranib 30 mg PO daily for a 28-day cycle. The median age was 65.5 years, 52% of patients had received prior XRT, and 73% of patients received only one prior chemotherapy regimen. PR was seen in 12.5%, 29% had a 6-month event free survival (EFS). The median PFS was 3.65 months and median OS was 12.5 months (43).
- Lenvatinib: a phase II trial of 133 patients with recurrent disease found a RR of 22%, with 44% having SD and a median duration of response of 9 months (76).

MMMT-Carcinosarcoma Trials

- GOG 108: 194 patients with stages III/IV and recurrent disease were randomized between ifosfamide versus ifosfamide and cisplatin. The response rate was 36% versus 54%. The PFS was 4 months versus 6 months with a RR of response 0.73 ($p = 0.02$). PFS and survival data suggest that the combination offers a slight prolongation of PFS (RR, 0.73; 95% upper CI: 0.94; $p = 0.02$, one-tailed test), but not significant for OS (RR, 0.80, 95% CI: 1.03; $p = 0.071$, one-tailed test) (77).
- GOG 150: this trial evaluated 206 patients with stage I to IV optimally debulked carcinosarcoma, and randomized them to WAR with a pelvic boost versus ifosfamide with mesna and cisplatin. The recurrence rate was 58% in the WAR arm versus 52% in chemotherapy arm (NS). There was a significant survival benefit to chemotherapy (HR 0.67) with a 5 YS of 47% versus 37%. Recurrence was vaginal in 3.8% of patients who received WAR compared to 9.9% in the chemotherapy arm. The final recommendation was that chemotherapy and vaginal brachytherapy may be the best combination for carcinosarcoma (38).
- GOG 161: this trial evaluated 179 patients with stage III/IV, persistent, or recurrent disease. Ifosfamide/mesna dosed at 1.6 g/m^2 IV daily for 3 days plus paclitaxel 135 mg/m^2 every 3 weeks was compared to ifosfamide/mesna 2 g/m^2 IV daily for 3 days every 3 weeks up to eight cycles. A higher RR of 45% was seen with the doublet compared to 29% with the single agent. The PFS was found to be significant at 5.8 versus 3.6 months (a 31% decrease in the HR of death 0.69; 95% CI: 0.49-0.97, $p = 0.3$), as was the OS of 13.5 versus 8.4 months (HR 0.71; 95% CI: 0.51-0.97, $p = 0.3$), both favoring the doublet (78).
- GOG 261: stages I-IV and recurrent uterine MMMT (also including TOC and peritoneal MMMT), chemotherapy naïve patients are randomized in a phase III noninferiority trial to ifosphamide 1.6 g/m^2 days 1,2,3 and paclitaxel 135 mg/m^2 versus carboplatin AUC 6 and paclitaxel 135 mg/m^2. Cycles are every 3 weeks for 6 to 10 cycles. Results pending.
- SEER study: 1,891 patients with stages I and II MMMT demonstrated that pelvic XRT was associated with a 21% reduction in cancer specific mortality. For

patients who did not have an LND, radiation therapy was associated with a 25% reduction in mortality (7).

- EORTC 55874: this was a phase III randomized trial for 224 patients of adjuvant pelvic XRT versus observation for all early stage sarcomas. There were 103 LMS, 91 MMMT, and 28 ESS. All patients underwent TAH and BSO and washings (166 patients): nodal sampling was not required and 25% had an LND. Patients were randomized to either observation or pelvic XRT, 51 Gy in 28 fractions over 5 weeks. 112 patients were in each arm. A reduction in local relapse (14 vs. 24, $p = 0.004$) was seen but no effect on either OS or PFS was seen. The MMMT patients trended toward better local control versus LMS patients, but they had a higher rate of distant metastasis and there was no change in OS with additional XRT (79).
- TOTEM: Trial Of Two follow up regimens in EndoMetrial cancer: this is a study evaluating two follow-up regimens with different test intensity in endometrial cancer-treated patients: does a more intensive routine investigation lead to a survival advantage. Results pending.
- FIGURE: follow-up In Gynecological Care Units: addressing whether a routine compared with patient-initiated follow-up strategy is superior. Results pending.
- ENDAT: endometrial cancer telephone follow-up trial: assessing whether a nurse-led telephone follow-up is as beneficial as standard follow-up care. Results pending.

UTERINE SARCOMAS

I. Characteristics
  - Sarcomas arise from the mesodermal tissues of the body. In gynecology, they most commonly originate in the uterus.
  - Sarcomas are estimated to comprise 5%-6% of the total 61,380 uterine cancers in 2017 in the United States. There is a 3% risk of adnexal metastasis (80).
  - Clinically patients can present with postcoital bleeding, intermenstrual bleeding, an enlarged uterus, or the cancer can mimic a prolapsed fibroid on examination.
  - The main risk factor is a history of prior pelvic XRT.
  - The route of spread can be lymphatic, peritoneal, or hematogenous.
II. Pre-treatment workup includes an EMB or D&C, a CXR, CT of the abdomen and pelvis, and consideration of a chest CT if there is a confirmed diagnosis of sarcoma. 19% of patients with LMS have lung metastasis. Routine preoperative lab tests are important.
III. Staging is surgical. This includes hysterectomy, BSO, exploration of the abdomen and pelvis, possible LND, biopsy of any suspicious extrauterine lesions, and omentectomy. Histology was updated in 2014. It differentiates **LMS**, low-grade and high-grade **ESS**, and undifferentiated sarcoma from adenosarcomas (ASs) (81).

- Staging for LMS and ESS was last amended by FIGO in 2009 (Table 2.20A–D).

Stage I: tumor limited to uterus
  - IA: < 5 cm
  - IB: > 5 cm

Stage II: tumor extends to the pelvis
  - IIA: adnexal involvement
  - IIB: extrauterine pelvic tissue

Stage III: abdominal involvement
- o IIIA: invades the abdomen 1 site
- o IIIB: invades the abdomen > 1 site
- o IIIC: involvement of pelvic and/or para-aortic LN

Stage IV:
- o IVA: involves bladder or rectum
- o IVB: distant metastasis (Table 2.21A–D)

Table 2.20A AJCC Staging 8th Edition for ESS and LMS: T Category		
T	**FIGO**	**T criteria**
TX		Primary tumor cannot be assessed
T0		No evidence of primary tumor
T1	I	Tumor limited to the uterus
T1a	IA	Tumor 5 cm or less in greatest dimension
T1b	IB	Tumor more than 5 cm
T2	II	Tumor extends beyond the uterus, within the pelvis
T2a	IIA	Tumor involves adnexa
T2b	IIB	Tumor involves other pelvic tissues
T3	III	Tumor infiltrates abdominal tissues
T3a	IIIA	One site
T3b	IIIB	More than one site
T4	IVA	Tumor invades bladder or rectum

ESS, endometrial stromal sarcoma; LMS, leiomyosarcoma.

Table 2.20B N Category		
N	**FIGO**	**N criteria**
NX		Regional LNs cannot be assessed
N0		No reginal LN metastasis
N0(i+)		Isolated tumor cells in regional LN(s) no greater than 0.2 mm
N1	IIIC	Reginal LN metastasis

LN, lymph node.

Table 2.20C M Category		
M	**FIGO**	**M criteria**
M0		No distant metastasis
M1	IVB	Distant mestasis

Table 2.20D Stage Grouping

When T is	And N is	And M is	The stage group is
T1	N0	M0	I
T1a	N0	M0	IA
T1b	N0	M0	IB
T1c	N0	M0	IC
T2	N0	M0	II
T3a	N0	M0	IIIA
T3b	N0	M0	IIIB
T1-T3	N1	M0	IIC
T4	Any N	M0	IVA
Any T	Any N	M1	IVB

Source: From Amin MB, Edge SB. (2017). *AJCC Cancer Staging Manual* 8th Edition. Chicago, IL: American Joint Committee on Cancer. With permission.

- FIGO staging for adenosarcoma (AS) Table 2.21A

Table 2.21A AJCC Staging 8th Edition for AS: T Category

T	FIGO	T criteria
TX		Primary tumor cannot be assessed
T0		No evidence of primary tumor
T1	I	Tumor limited to the uterus
T1a	IA	Tumor limited to the endometrium/endocervix
T1b	IB	Tumor invades less than half of the myometrium
T1c	IC	Tumor invades more than half of the myometrium
T2	II	Tumor extends beyond the uterus, within the pelvis
T2a	IIA	Tumor involves adnexa
T2b	IIB	Tumor involves other pelvic tissues
T3	III	Tumor infiltrates abdominal tissues
T3a	IIIA	One site
T3b	IIIB	More than one site
T4	IVA	Tumor invades bladder or rectum

AS, adenosarcoma.

Table 2.21B N Category

N	FIGO	N criteria
NX		Regional LNs cannot be assessed
N0		No regional lymph node metastasis
N0(i+)		Isolated tumor cells in regional LN(s) no greater than 0.2 mm
N1	IIIC	Regional LN metastasis

LN, lymph node.

Table 2.21C M Category

M	FIGO	M criteria
M0		No distant metastasis
M1	IVB	Distant metastasis

Table 2.21D Stage Grouping

When T is	And N is	And M is	The stage group is
T1	N0	M0	I
T1a	N0	M0	IA
T1b	N0	M0	IB
T2	N0	M0	II
T3a	N0	M0	IIIA
T3b	N0	M0	IIIB
T1–T3	N1	M0	IIIC
T4	Any N	M0	IVA
Any T	Any N	M1	IVB

Source: From Amin MB, Edge SB. (2017). *AJCC Cancer Staging Manual* 8th Edition. Chicago, IL: American Joint Committee on Cancer. With permission.

IV. There are four main histologic types of uterine sarcoma: LMS, low-grade and high-grade ESS, and undifferentiated sarcoma. More uncommon uterine sarcoma subtypes are AS, PEComa, and rhabdomyosarcoma.

o LMS is the most common uterine sarcoma. It originates from the uterine smooth muscle. It represents 40% of uterine sarcomas. It can present at any age but most commonly arises in women aged 45 to 55 years old. Only 15% are diagnosed preoperatively with an EMB or D&C. For diagnosis, it is necessary to demonstrate coagulative necrosis. One or both of the following are also necessary: cellular atypia, or more than 10 mitosis/HPF. The rate of ovarian metastasis is 3% (82) and the rate of LN metastasis is 6.6% to 11% (83,84). LND has not shown to be of benefit for staging as up to 70% of women with positive LN already have extrauterine disease (85). Ten percent have pulmonary metastasis at presentation so a baseline CXR or chest CT at diagnosis is indicated. BSO has not been shown to reflect on outcome. Adjuvant pelvic XRT reduces local recurrence but does not change OS.

- If an LMS is found incidentally after hysterectomy, a second staging surgery should be considered if there was morcellation of the uterus; a supracervical hysterectomy was performed initially (in these cases, the cervix should be removed on reoperation), or there was no evaluation of the abdomen or pelvis. A second staging surgery for an LND or BSO has not been found to be beneficial (86).
- Adjuvant therapy is considered based on stage. Chemotherapy can consist of single-agent doxorubicin with a RR of 25%, single-agent ifosfamide with an RR of 17%, combination ifosfamide and doxorubicin with an RR of 30%, or combination gemcitabine and docetaxel with an RR of 53%. Aromatase inhibitors can be considered if the tumor is ER positive.
  □ **Stage I:** observe or consider chemotherapy
  □ **Stage II, III:** consider chemotherapy and/or tumor directed EBXRT
  □ **Stage IVA:** chemotherapy and/or EBXRT
  □ **Stage IVB:** chemotherapy with/without palliative EBXRT
- For isolated lung recurrences, thoracotomy with resection can yield a survival benefit. The 5 YS was 43% in one series (87).

o **Low-grade ESS:** it is commonly diagnosed in women aged 42 to 53 years. This tumor represents about 8% of uterine sarcomas and arises from the stromal cells between the endometrial glandular cells. LGESS are characterized by small cells with low-grade cytology and features resembling stromal cells in proliferative endometrium. Mitotic activity is usually low (<5 MF/10 HPF). It cannot be diagnosed by D&C. Final pathology needs to document LVSI and invasion. If one of these two components is absent, then the diagnosis is an endometrial stromal nodule. There is a 20% risk of pelvic LN metastasis, so consideration for a LND should be entertained. Removal of the ovaries is recommended as these are hormone-dependent cancers and can respond to endogenous estrogen. Reoperation for BSO and LND, if ESS was an incidental finding should be performed if the ovaries were not initially resected. Stage is the most important prognostic factor. Adjuvant therapy is considered based on stage.

- For stage I, consider observation versus hormonal therapy.
- For stages II, III, and IVA: hormone therapy with/without tumor directed XRT. 20% of recurrences have been documented in the pelvis.

- For stage IVB, consider hormonal therapy with or without palliative XRT.
- Hormonal therapy can include: Megace (40–160 mg daily); an 88% RR with a 50% CR has been seen (88). Aromatase inhibitors and gonadotropin-releasing hormone (GnRH) agonists may also be considered. Estrogen replacement therapy may increase the chance of recurrence. For recurrent disease, a 33% response rate was seen with ifosfamide and doxorubicin. Aromatase inhibitors can also be considered in these tumors.
- **Radiation:** there are data to show that 33.3% of recurrences are pelvic only, if no adjuvant XRT was given—so pelvic XRT can be considered.
- **High-grade ESS:** it is characterized by small cells with high-grade cytology, frequent necrosis, and brisk mitotic activity (>10 MF/10 HPF). HGESS can contain areas of conventional LGESS. Adjuvant therapy is based on stage:
  - Stage 1: observe or consider chemotherapy.
  - Stage II, III: consider chemotherapy and/or EBXRT.
  - Stage IVA: chemotherapy and/or EBXRT.
  - Stage IVB: chemotherapy with/without palliative EBXRT.
- **Undifferentiated uterine sarcomas (UUS)** are characterized by cells with high-grade cytologic features lacking any resemblance to the stromal cells in proliferative endometrium or any other specific type of determination. Adjuvant therapy is based on stage: chemotherapy should be considered with a single agent or combination agents to include: doxorubicin, ifosfamide, cisplatin, gemcitabine, and docetaxel. Responses to chemotherapy can occur but at low rates.
  - Stage I: observe or consider chemotherapy.
  - Stage II, III: consider chemotherapy and/or tumor directed EBXRT.
  - Stage IVA: chemotherapy and/or EBXRT.
  - Stage IVB: chemotherapy with/without palliative EBXRT.
- WHO 2003 uterine sarcoma classifies ESS as a category into itself, removing LG and HG. HG is termed undifferentiated endometrial sarcoma. This is slightly different from NCCN terminology (97).
- **Adenosarcoma:** represents 1% of uterine sarcomas. The median age of diagnosis is 50 years old. Abnormal bleeding is common and speculum examination can visualize tumor in 50% of cases. These are mixed tumors with sarcomatous stroma and benign epithelium with a favorable prognosis unless sarcomatous overgrowth or stromal invasion is present. They stain for CD10 and express ER/PR. Extrauterine disease occurs in 20% of cases, staging is appropriate, and BSO should be considered. These are low-grade malignancies, and if recur do so locally. Those with sarcomatous overgrowth may have distant metastasis. 20% can recur more than 5 years after surgery. There is an increased risk of recurrence if deep myometrial invasion is present. Adjuvant XRT and chemotherapy for the subsets of sarcomatous overgrowth or deep stromal invasion can be considered. Ifosfamide, plus doxorubicin, and/or cisplatin or gemcitabine plus docetaxel have produced a few responses for metastatic or recurrent disease. Consider XRT and chemotherapy for sarcomatous overgrowth, heterologous elements, or deep stromal invasion.
  - **Prognostic factors:** stage is the most important prognostic factor; the depth of myometrial invasion, LVSI, grade, histology, tumor size, patient age, and hormone receptor status can all affect outcome (Tables 2.22–2.24).

5Y SURVIVAL

Table 2.22 Uterine LMS 5 YS	
Stage	5Y LMS survival (%)
Localized	63
Regional	36
Distant	14
LMS, leiomyosarcoma; YS, year survival.	

Table 2.23 Uterine ESS 5 YS	
Stage	5Y ESS survival (%)
Localized	99
Regional	94
Distant	69
ESS, endometrial stromal sarcoma; YS, year survival.	

Table 2.24 Uterine Undifferentiated Sarcoma 5 YS	
Stage	5Y undifferentiated survival (%)
Localized	70
Regional	43
Distant	23

FOLLOW-UP
- Every 3 months for the first 2 years
  - Every 6 months for the next 3 years
  - Annual examinations thereafter
- Physical and pelvic examination should occur at each visit. Pap smears have not been found to increase the detection of recurrence. CT imaging of the chest/abdomen/pelvis can occur every 3 to 6 months for 2 to 3 years, then every 6 months for the next 2 years, then annually for high-grade sarcomas.

RECURRENT DISEASE
- Local recurrence in the vagina or pelvis with negative CT of the chest/abdomen/pelvic:
  - If prior XRT:
    - Surgical exploration and resection with/without IOXRT with/without systemic therapy *or*
    - Systemic therapy *or*
    - Tumor directed re-irradiation

○ If no prior XRT:
  ▪ Surgical exploration with resection and/or IOXRT
  ▪ Tumor directed XRT with/without systemic therapy can also be offered
- Isolated distant metastasis:
  ○ If resectable: consider resection or ablative therapy and consider postoperative systemic therapy with/without EBXRT
  ○ If unresectable: consider systemic therapy and/or tumor directed EBXRT or local ablative therapy. If there is a response, surgical resection can be considered
- If disseminated disease:
  ○ Systemic therapy with/without palliative radiation therapy *or*
  ○ Best supportive care

NOTABLE STUDIES IN SARCOMA

- ESS: in a retrospective review, overall there was a 64% recurrence. The 10Y PFS was 43%, with an OS of 85%. Those who received HRT had ORR of 27% and 53% had stable disease with a median TTP of 24 months. 89% of those without BSO had recurrence, 55% who had a BSO did not recur; 32% had LVSI so LND may be beneficial (89).
- Another retrospective study evaluated ESS stage I and II. There were no relapses in those who received adjuvant XRT, 13 of 30 relapsed if no XRT was administered. Thus pelvic EBXRT may improve local control but may not affect OS (90).
- GOG 277: this was a phase III, double-blind, placebo-controlled trial in patients with chemotherapy-naive, metastatic, unresectable uterine leiomyosarcomas. 107 patients were enrolled, 54 were randomized to gemcitabine–docetaxel plus placebo and 53 to gemcitabine–docetaxel plus bevacizumab. Accrual was stopped early for futility. The gemcitabine–docetaxel—placebo group compared to the gemcitabine–docetaxel—bevacizumab group had median PFS of 6.2 months and 4.2 months, respectively (HR 1.12; $p = 0.58$). Objective responses were seen in 31.5% in the gemcitabine–docetaxel—placebo group and 35.8% in the gemcitabine–docetaxel—bevacizumab group. The mean response duration was 8.6 months vs 8.8 months. The median OS was 26.9 months vs 23.3 months (HR 1.07; $p = 0.81$).
- PALETTE: patients with metastatic soft tissue sarcoma (STS) (all sites) in a multicenter, international, double-blind, placebo-controlled phase III trial that were angiogenesis inhibitor-naïve, and had failed at least one anthracycline containing regimen, were eligible. A total of 369 patients were randomized (246 pazopanib, 123 placebo), 2:1 to receive either pazopanib 800 mg once daily or placebo until tumor progression, unacceptable toxicity, death, or patient's request. The median age was 56. Median duration of follow-up at clinical cut-off date was 15 months. The primary endpoint was PFS. PFS was significantly prolonged with pazopanib (median 20 versus 7 weeks; HR 0.31; 95% CI: 0.24–0.40; $p < 0.0001$). The interim analysis for OS showed a not statistically significant (NS) improvement of pazopanib versus placebo (median: 11.9 vs. 10.4 months; HR 0.83; 95% CI: 0.62–1.09). Main grade 3

to 4 toxicities in the pazopanib versus placebo arm were respectively: fatigue (13%, 6%), hypertension (7%, nil), anorexia (6%, nil), diarrhea (5%, 1%), thromboembolic events (grades 3–5) (3%, 2%), left ventricular ejection fraction (LVEF) decrease of greater than 15% (8% and 3%). Thus, pazopanib is an active drug in anthracycline pre-treated metastatic STS patients with an increase in median PFS of 13 weeks (92).

- SAR-3007: a subgroup analysis of recurrent uterine LMS patients after prior chemotherapy evaluating trabectedin versus dacarbazine (DTIC). This phase III study randomized in a 2:1 fashion 577 LMS and liposarcoma patients; 140 uterine LMS patients were in the trabectedin arm versus 81 uterine LMS in the DTIC group. Dosing was 1.5 mg/m^2 as a 24-hour infusion for every 3 weeks versus DTIC 1 g/m^2 IV every 3 weeks. The PFS was 4.2 months versus 1.5 months with the OS was 13.4 versus 12.9 for trabectedin versus DTIC, respectively (93).

- Study 309: this trial randomized 452 sarcoma patients to eribulin 1.4 mg/m^2 IV days 1 and 8 q21 days or DTIC 850–1200 mg/m^2 IV day 1 q21 days until progression. 228 patients were randomized to eribulin and 224 patients were given DTIC. OS in the DTIC group was a median of 13.5 months compared to 11.5 months in the eribulin group (95% CI: 10.9–15.6; HR 0.77; 95% CI: 0.62–0.95; $p = 0.0169$). Adverse effects were seen in 97% of those in the DTIC group and 99% in the eribulin group (94).

- From the PALETTE and EORTC 62043 trials: 44 uterine sarcoma patients who were treated with pazopanib were reviewed; 61.3% were heavily pretreated with greater than two lines of chemotherapy; 11% had a partial response. Median PFS was 3 months, median OS was 17.5 months. Response to pazopanib was similar for uterine sarcoma compared to nonuterine STS (95).

REFERENCES

1. Kurman RJ, Kaminski PF, Norris HJ. The behavior of endometrial hyperplasia. A long-term study of "untreated" hyperplasia in 170 patients. *Cancer.* 1985;56(2):403-412.
2. Trimble CL, Kauderer J, Zaino R, et al. Concurrent endometrial carcinoma in women with a biopsy diagnosis of atypical endometrial hyperplasia: a Gynecologic Oncology Group Study. *Cancer.* 2006;106(4):812-819.
3. Chan JK, Loizzi V, Youssef M, et al. Significance of comprehensive surgical staging in noninvasive papillary serous carcinoma of the endometrium. *Gynecol Oncol.* 2003;90(1): 181-185.
4. Geisler JP, Geisler HE, Melton ME, et al. What staging surgery should be performed on patients with uterine papillary serous carcinoma? *Gynecol Oncol.* 1999;74(3): 465-467.
5. Pennington KP, Walsh T, Lee M, et al. BRCA1, TP53, and CHEK2 germline mutations in uterine serous carcinoma. *Cancer.* January 15, 2013;119(2):332-338.
6. Brinton LA, Felix AS, McMeekin DS, et al. Etiologic heterogeneity in endometrial cancer: evidence from a Gynecologic Oncology Group trial. *Gynecol Oncol.* May 2013;129(2): 277-284.
7. Cantrell LA, Blank SV, Duska LR. Uterine carcinosarcoma: a review of the literature. *Gynecol Oncol.* June 2015;137(3):581-588.
8. Talhouk A, McConechy MK, Leung S, et al. A clinically applicable molecular-based classification for endometrial cancers. *Br J Cancer.* July 14, 2015;113(2):299-310.

9. Walker JL, Piedmonte MR, Spirtos NM. Laparoscopy compared with laparotomy for comprehensive surgical staging of uterine cancer: Gynecologic Oncology Group Study LAP2. *J Clin Oncol.* November 10, 2009;27(32):5331-5336.

10. James JA, Rakowski JA, Jeppson CN. Robotic transperitoneal infra-renal aortic lymphadenectomy in early-stage endometrial cancer. *Gynecol Oncol.* February 2015;136(2): 285-292.

11. Wright JD, Jorge S, Tergas AI. Utilization and outcomes of ovarian conservation in premenopausal women with endometrial cancer. *Obstet Gynecol.* January 2016;127(1): 101-108.

12. SGO Clinical Practice Endometrial Cancer Working Group, Burke WM, Orr J, Leitao M. Endometrial cancer: a review and current management strategies: part I. *Gynecol Oncol.* August 2014;134(2):385-392.

13. Kho KA, Anderson TL, Nezhat CH. Intracorporeal electromechanical tissue morcellation: a critical review and recommendations for clinical practice. *Obstet Gynecol.* October 2014;124(4):787-793.

14. Mariani A, Webb MJ, Keeney GL, et al. Low-risk corpus cancer: is lymphadenectomy or radiotherapy necessary? *Am J Obstet Gynecol.* 2000;182(6):1506-1519.

15. Goff BA, Rice LW. Assessment of depth of myometrial invasion in endometrial adenocarcinoma. *Gynecol Oncol.* 1990;38(1):46-48.

16. Doering DL, Barnhill DR, Weiser EB, et al. Intraoperative evaluation of depth of myometrial invasion in stage I endometrial adenocarcinoma. *Obstet Gynecol.* 1989;74(6):930-933.

17. Franchi M, Ghezzi F, Melpignano M, et al. Clinical value of intraoperative gross examination in endometrial cancer. *Gynecol Oncol.* 2000;76(3):357-361.

18. Cragun JM, Havrilesky LJ, Calingaert B, et al. Retrospective analysis of selective lymphadenectomy in apparent early-stage endometrial cancer. *J Clin Oncol.* 2005;23:3668-3675.

19. Chan JK, Cheung MK, Huh WK, et al. Therapeutic role of lymph node resection in endometrioid corpus cancer: a study of 12,333 patients. *Cancer.* 2006;107(8):1823-1830.

20. Kilgore LC, Partridge EE, Alvarez RD, et al. Adenocarcinoma of the endometrium: survival comparisons of patients with and without pelvic node sampling. *Gynecol Oncol.* 1995;56:29-33.

21. Chan JK, Kapp DS, Cheung MK, et al. The impact of the absolute number and ratio of positive lymph nodes on survival of endometrioid uterine cancer patients. *Br J Cancer.* 2007;97(5):605-611.

22. Creutzberg CL, van Putten WL, Wárlám-Rodenhuis CC, et al. Outcome of high-risk stage IC, grade 3, compared with stage I endometrial carcinoma patients: the Postoperative Radiation Therapy in Endometrial Carcinoma Trial. *J Clin Oncol.* 2004;22(7):1234-1241.

23. Nelson G, Randall M, Sutton G, et al. FIGO stage IIIC endometrial carcinoma with metastases confined to pelvic lymph nodes: analysis of treatment outcomes, prognostic variables, and failure patterns following adjuvant radiation therapy. *Gynecol Oncol.* 1999;75(2):211-214.

24. Ayhan A, Taskiran C, Celik C, et al. Surgical stage III endometrial cancer: analysis of treatment outcomes, prognostic factors and failure patterns. *Eur J Gynaecol Oncol.* 2002;23(6):553-556.

25. Benedetti Panici P, Basile S, Maneschi F, et al. Systematic pelvic lymphadenectomy vs. no lymphadenectomy in early-stage endometrial carcinoma: randomized clinical trial. *J Natl Cancer Inst.* 2008;100(23):1707-1716.

26. Blake P, Swart AM, Orton J, et al. Adjuvant external beam radiotherapy in the treatment of endometrial cancer (MRC ASTEC and NCIC CTG EN.5 randomised trials): pooled trial results, systematic review, and meta-analysis. *Lancet.* 2009;373(9658):137-148.

27. Kitchener H, Swart AM, Qian Q, et al. Efficacy of systemic pelvic lymphadenectomy in endometrial cancer (MRC ASTEC trail): a randomised study. *Lancet.* 2009;373(9658): 125-136.

28. Morrow CP, Bundy BN, Kurman RJ, et al. Relationship between surgical-pathological risk factors and outcome in clinical stage I and II carcinoma of the endometrium: a Gynecologic Oncology Group Study. *Gynecol Oncol.* 1991;40(1):55-65.

29. Disaia PJ. Predicting parametrial involvement in endometrial cancer: is this the end for radical hysterectomies in stage II endometrial cancers? *Obstet Gynecol.* 2011;116(5): 1016-1017.

30. Greer BE, Hamberger AD. Treatment of intraperitoneal metastatic adenocarcinoma of the endometrium by the whole-abdomen moving-strip technique and pelvic boost irradiation. *Gynecol Oncol.* 1983;16(3):365-373.

31. Goff BA, Kato D, Schmidt RA, et al. Uterine papillary serous carcinoma: patterns of metastatic spread. *Gynecol Oncol.* 1994;54(3):264-268.

32. Bristow RE, Duska LR, Montz FJ. The role of cytoreductive surgery in the management of stage IV uterine papillary serous carcinoma. *Gynecol Oncol.* 2001;81(1):92-99.

33. Shih KK, Yun E, Gardner GJ, et al. Surgical cytoreduction in stage IV endometrioid endometrial carcinoma. *Gynecol Oncol.* 2011;122(3):608-611.

34. Chao A, Wu RC, Jung SM, et al. Implication of genomic characterization in synchronous endometrial and ovarian cancers of endometrioid histology. *Gynecol Oncol.* 2016;143(1):60-67.

35. Kelly MG, O'Malley DM, Hui P, et al. Improved survival in surgical stage I patients with uterine papillary serous carcinoma (UPSC) treated with adjuvant platinum-based chemotherapy. *Gynecol Oncol.* 2005;98(3):353-359.

36. Tanner EJ, Leitao MM Jr, Garg K, et al. The role of cytoreductive surgery for newly diagnosed advanced-stage uterine carcinosarcoma. *Gynecol Oncol.* 2011;123(3):548-552.

37. Reed NS, Mangioni C, Malmstrom H, et al. First results of a randomized trial comparing radiotherapy versus observation postoperatively in patients with uterine sarcomas. An EORTC-GCG study. *Int J Gynecol Cancer.* 2003;13:4.

38. Homesley HD, Filiaci V, Markman M. Phase III trial of ifosfamide with or without paclitaxel in advanced uterine carcinosarcoma: a Gynecologic Oncology Group Study. *J Clin Oncol.* 2007;25(5):526-531.

39. Awtrey CS, Cadungog MG, Leitao MM, et al. Surgical resection of recurrent endometrial carcinoma. *Gynecol Oncol.* 2006;102(3):480-488.

40. Scudder SA, Liu PY, Wilczynski SP, et al. Paclitaxel and carboplatin with amifostine in advanced, recurrent, or refractory endometrial adenocarcinoma: a phase II study of the Southwest Oncology Group. *Gynecol Oncol.* 2005;96(3):610-615.

41. Thigpen JT, Brady MF, Alvarez RD, et al. Oral medroxyprogesterone acetate in the treatment of advanced or recurrent endometrial carcinoma: a dose-response study by the Gynecologic Oncology Group. *J Clin Oncol.* 1999;17(6):1736-1744.

42. Fleming GF, Sill MW, Darcy KM, et al. Phase II trial of trastuzumab in women with advanced or recurrent, HER2-positive endometrial carcinoma: a Gynecologic Oncology Group Study. *Gynecol Oncol.* 2010;116(1):15-20.

43. Bender D, Sill MW, Lankes HA, et al. A phase II evaluation of cediranib in the treatment of recurrent or persistent endometrial cancer: An NRG Oncology/Gynecologic Oncology Group Study. *Gynecol Oncol.* September 2015;138(3):507-512.

44. Barakat RR, Bundy BN, Spirtos NM, et al. Randomized double-blind trial of estrogen replacement therapy versus placebo in stage I or II endometrial cancer: a Gynecologic Oncology Group Study. *J Clin Oncol.* 2006;24:587-592.

45. Lewin SN, Herzog TJ, Barrena Medel NI, et al. Comparative performance of the 2009 International Federation of Gynecology and Obstetrics' staging system for uterine corpus cancer. *Obstet Gynecol.* 2010;116(5):1141-1149.

46. Curtis RE, Freedman DM, Sherman ME, Fraumeni JF, Jr. Risk of malignant mixed mullerian tumors after tamoxifen therapy for breast cancer. *J Nat Cancer Instit.* 2004;96(1):70-74.

47. Aalders J, Abeler V, Kolstad P, et al. Postoperative external irradiation and prognostic parameters in stage I endometrial carcinoma: clinical and histopathologic study of 540 patients. *Obstet Gynecol.* 1980;56(4):419-427.
48. Creutzberg CL, van Putten WL, Koper PC, et al. Surgery and postoperative radiotherapy versus surgery alone for patients with stage-1 endometrial carcinoma: multicentre randomised trial. PORTEC Study Group. Postoperative radiation therapy in endometrial carcinoma. *Lancet.* 2000;355(9213):1404-1411.
49. Creutzberg CL, Nout RA, Lybeert ML, et al. Fifteen-year radiotherapy outcomes of the randomized PORTEC-1 trial for endometrial carcinoma. *Int J Radiat Oncol Biol Phys.* 2011;81(4):e631-e638.
50. Nout RA, van de Poll-Franse LV, Lybeert ML. Long-term outcome and quality of life of patients with endometrial carcinoma treated with or without pelvic radiotherapy in the post-operative radiation therapy in endometrial carcinoma 1 (PORTEC-1) trial. *J Clin Oncol.* May 1, 2011;29(13):1692-1700.
51. Keys HM, Roberts JA, Brunetto VL, et al. A phase III trial of surgery with or without adjunctive external pelvic radiation therapy in intermediate risk endometrial adenocarcinoma: a Gynecologic Oncology Group Study. *Gynecol Oncol.* 2004;92(3):744-751.
52. Nout RA, Smit VT, Putter H, et al. Vaginal brachytherapy versus pelvic external beam radiotherapy for patients with endometrial cancer of high-intermediate risk (PORTEC-2): an open-label, non-inferiority, randomised trial. *Lancet.* 2010;375(9717):816-823.
53. De Boer SM, Powell ME, Mileshkin L, et al. Toxicity and quality of life after adjuvant chemoradiotherapy versus radiotherapy alone for women with high-risk endometrial cancer (PORTEC-3): an open label, multicenter randomized, phase 3 trial. *Lancet Oncol.* August 2016;17(8):1114-1126.
54. PORTEC-4: Randomised phase III trial comparing vaginal brachytherapy (two doses schedules: 21 or 15 Gy HDR in 3 fractions) and observation after surgery in patients with endometrial carcinoma with high-intermediate risk features.
55. Greven K, Winter K, Underhill K. Final analysis of RTOG 9708: adjuvant postoperative irradiation combined with cisplatin/paclitaxel chemotherapy following surgery for patients with high-risk endometrial cancer. Gynecol Oncol. October 2006;103(1):155-159.
56. Susumu N, Sagae S, Udagawa Y, et al. Randomized phase III trial of pelvic radiotherapy versus cisplatin-based combined chemotherapy in patients with intermediate- and high-risk endometrial cancer: a Japanese Gynecologic Oncology Group Study. *Gynecol Oncol.* 2008;108(1):226-233.
57. Todo Y, Kato H, Kaneuchi M, et al. Survival effect of para-aortic lymphadenectomy in endometrial cancer (SEPAL study): a retrospective cohort analysis. *Lancet.* 2010;375(9721):1165-1172.
58. McMeekin DS, Filiaci VL, Aghajanian C, et al. GOG-0249/Endorsed study: a randomized phase III trial of pelvic radiation therapy (PXRT) versus vaginal cuff brachytherapy followed by paclitaxel/carboplatin chemotherapy (VCB/C) in patients with high risk (HR), early stage endometrial cancer (EC): a Gynecologic Oncology Group trial. *Gynecol Oncol.* 2014;134:438.
59. Viswanathan AN, Moughan J, Miller BE, et al. NRG Oncology/RTOG 0921: a phase 2 study of postoperative intensity modulated radiotherapy with concurrent cisplatin and bevacizumab followed by carboplatin and paclitaxel for patietns with endometrial cancer. *Cancer.* July 1, 2015;121(13):2156-2163.
60. Cohen CJ, Bruckner HW, Deppe G, et al. Multidrug treatment of advanced and recurrent endometrial carcinoma: a Gynecologic Oncology Group Study. *Obstet Gynecol.* 1984;63(5):719-726.

61. Thigpen JT, Blessing JA, DiSaia PJ, et al. A randomized comparison of doxorubicin alone versus doxorubicin plus cyclophosphamide in the management of advanced or recurrent endometrial carcinoma: a Gynecologic Oncology Group Study. *J Clin Oncol.* 1994;12(7):1408-1414.

62. Sutton G, Axelrod JH, Bundy BN, et al. Adjuvant whole abdominal irradiation in clinical stages I and II papillary serous or clear cell carcinoma of the endometrium: a phase II study of the Gynecologic Oncology Group. *Gynecol Oncol.* 2006;100(2):349-354.

63. Sutton G, Axelrod JH, Bundy BN, et al. Whole abdominal radiotherapy in the adjuvant treatment of patients with stage III and IV endometrial cancer: a Gynecologic Oncology Group Study. *Gynecol Oncol.* 2005;97:755-763.

64. Thigpen JT, Brady MF, Homesley HD, et al. Phase III trial of doxorubicin with or without cisplatin in advanced endometrial carcinoma: a Gynecologic Oncology Group Study. *J Clin Oncol.* 2004;22(19):3902-3908.

65. Randall ME, Filiaci VL, Muss H, et al. Randomized phase III trial of whole-abdominal irradiation versus doxorubicin and cisplatin chemotherapy in advanced endometrial carcinoma: a Gynecologic Oncology Group Study. *J Clin Oncol.* 2006;24(1):36-44.

66. Gallion HH, Brunetto VL, Cibull M, et al. Randomized phase III trial of standard timed doxorubicin plus cisplatin versus circadian timed doxorubicin plus cisplatin in stage III and IV or recurrent endometrial carcinoma: a Gynecologic Oncology Group Study. *J Clin Oncol.* 2003;21(20):3808-3813.

67. Fleming GF, Filiaci VL, Bentley RC, et al. Phase III randomized trial of doxorubicin 1 cisplatin versus doxorubicin 1 24-h paclitaxel 1 filgrastim in endometrial carcinoma: a Gynecologic Oncology Group Study. *Ann Oncol.* 2004;15(8):1173-1178.

68. Fleming GF, Brunetto VL, Cella D, et al. Phase III trial of doxorubicin plus cisplatin with or without paclitaxel plus filgrastim in advanced endometrial carcinoma: a Gynecologic Oncology Group Study. *J Clin Oncol.* 2004;22(11):2159-2166.

69. Homesley HD, Filiaci V, Gibbons SK, et al. A randomized phase III trial in advanced endometrial carcinoma of surgery and volume directed radiation followed by cisplatin and doxorubicin with or without paclitaxel: a Gynecologic Oncology Group Study. *Gynecol Oncol.* 2009;112:543-552.

70. Miller D, Filiaci V, Fleming G, et al. Randomized phase III noninferiority trial of first line chemotherapy for metastatic or recurrent endometrial carcinoma: a Gynecology Oncology Group Study. *Gynecol Oncol.* 2012;125:771-773.

71. Vargo JA, Kim H, Houser CJ, et al. Definitive salvage for vaginal recurrence of endometrial cancer: the impact of modern intensity-modulated-radiotherapy with image-based HDR brachytherapy and the interplay of the PORTEC 1 risk stratification. *Radiother Oncol.* October 2014;113(1):126-131.

72. Mundt AJ, McBride R, Rotmensch J, et al. Significant pelvic recurrence in high-risk pathologic stage I–IV endometrial carcinoma patients after adjuvant chemotherapy alone: implications for adjuvant radiation therapy. *Int J Radiat Oncol Biol Phys.* 2001;50(5): 1145-1153.

73. Lincoln S, Blessing JA, Lee RB, et al. Activity of paclitaxel as second-line chemotherapy in endometrial carcinoma: a Gynecologic Oncology Group Study. *Gynecol Oncol.* 2003;88(3):277-281.

74. McMeekin DS, Filiaci VL, Thigpen JT, et al. The relationship between histology and outcome in advanced and recurrent endometrial cancer patients participating in first-line chemotherapy trials: a Gynecologic Oncology Group Study. *Gynecol Oncol.* 2007;106(1):16-22.

75. Lorusso D, Ferrandina G, Colombo N, et al. Randomized phase II trial of carboplatin-paclitaxel (CP) compared to carboplatin-paclitaxel-bevacizumab (CP-B) in advanced (stage III–IV) or recurrent endometrial cancer: The MITO END-2 trial. *J Clin Oncol.* 2015;33(suppl; abstract 5502).

76. Vergote I, Teneriello M, Powell MA, et al. A phase 2 trial of lenvatinib in patients with advanced or recurrent endometrial cancer: angiopoietin-2 as a predictive marker for clinical outcomes. *J Clin Oncol.* 2013;31 (suppl; abstract 5520)

77. Sutton G, Brunetto VL, Kilgore L. A phase III trial of ifosfamide with or without cisplatin in carcinosarcoma of the uterus: a Gynecologic Oncology Group Study. *Gynecol Oncol.* November 2000;79(2):147-153.

78. Wolfson AH, Brady MF, Rocereto T, et al. A gynecologic oncology group randomized phase III trial of whole abdominal irradiation (WAI) vs. cisplatin-ifosfamide and mesna (CIM) as post-surgical therapy in stage I-IV carcinosarcoma (CS) of the uterus. *Gynecol Oncol.* 2007;107(2):177-185.

79. Reed NS, Mangioni C, Malmström H, et al. Phase III randomised study to evaluate the role of adjuvant pelvic radiotherapy in the treatment of uterine sarcomas stages I and II: an European Organisation for Research and Treatment of Cancer Gynaecological Cancer Group Study (protocol 55874). *Eur J Cancer.* April 2008;44(6):808-818.

80. Sutton G. Uterine sarcomas 2013. *Gynecol Oncol.* July 2013;130(1):3-5.

81. Kurman RJ, Carcangiu ML, Herrington CS, Young RH. *WHO Classification of Tumours,* Vol 6, IARC WHO Classification of Tumours, No 6. ISBN-10 9283224353. Available at: cancer.org. Accessed April 17, 2017.

82. Leitao MM, Sonoda Y, Brennan MF, et al. Incidence of lymph node and ovarian metastasis in leiomyosarcoma of the uterus. *Gynecol Oncol.* 2003;91(1):209-212.

83. Giuntoli RL II, Metzinger DS, DiMarco CS, et al. Retrospective review of 208 patients with leiomyosarcoma of the uterus: prognostic indicators, surgical management, and adjuvant therapy. *Gynecol Oncol.* 2003;89(3):460-469.

84. Kapp DS, Shin JY, Chan JK. Prognostic factors and survival in 1396 patients with uterine leiomyosarcoma: emphasis on impact of lymphadenectomy and oophorectomy. *Cancer.* 2008;112(4):820-830.

85. Goff BA, Rice LW, Fleischhaker D, et al. Uterine leiomyosarcoma and endometrial stromal sarcoma: lymph node metastases and sites of recurrence. *Gynecol Oncol.* 1993;50(1): 105-109.

86. O'Cearbhaill R, Hensley ML. Optimal management of uterine leiomyosarcoma. *Expert Rev Anticancer Ther.* 2010;10(2):153-169.

87. Levenback C, Rubin SC, McCormack PM, et al. Resection of pulmonary metastases from uterine sarcomas. *Gynecol Oncol.* 1992;45(2):202-205.

88. Chu MC, Mor G, Lim C, et al. Low-grade endometrial stromal sarcoma: hormonal aspects. *Gynecol Oncol.* 2003;90(1):170-176.

89. Cheng X, Yang G, Schmeler KM. Recurrence patterns and prognosis of endometrial stromal sarcoma and the potential of tyrosine kinase-inhibiting therapy. *Gynecol Oncol.* May 1, 2011;121(2):323-327.

90. Malouf GG, Duclos J, Rey A. Impact of adjuvant treatment modalities on the management of patients with stages I-II endometrial stromal sarcoma. *Ann Oncol.* October 2010;21(10):2102-2106.

91. Hensley ML, Miller A, O'Malley DM, et al. Randomized phase III trial of gemcitabine plus docetaxel plus bevacizumab or placebo as first-line treatment for metastatic uterine leiomyosarcoma: an NRG Oncology/Gynecologic Oncology Group Study. *J Clin Oncol.* April 1, 2015;33(10):1180-1185.

92. van der Graaf WT, Blay JY, Chawla SP, et al. Pazopanib for metastatic soft-tissue sarcoma (PALETTE): a randomised, double-blind, placebo-controlled phase 3 trial. *Lancet.* May 19, 2012;379(9829):1879-1886.

93. Demetri GD, von Mehren M, Jones RL et al. Efficacy and safety of trabectedin or dacarbazine for metastatic liposarcoma or leiomyosarcoma after failure of conventional chemotherapy: results of a phase III randomized multicenter clinical trial. *J. Clin Oncol.* March, 2016;34(8): 786-793.

94. Schoffski P, Chawla S, Maki RG et al. Eribulin versus dacarbazine in previously treated patients with advanced liposarcoma or leiomyosarcoma; a randomised open-label, multicentre, phase 3 trial. *Lancet.* April 16, 2016;387(10028):1629-1637.

95. Benson C, Ray-Coquard I, Sleijer S, et al. Outcome of uterine sarcoma patients treated with pazopanib: a retrospective analysis based on two European organisation for research and treatment of cancer (EORTC) soft tissue and bone sarcoma group (STBSG) clinical trial 62043 and 62072. *Gynecol Oncol.* 2016;142:89-94.

96. Creasman WT, Ali S, Mutch DG, et al. Surgical-pathological findings in type 1 and 2 endometrial cancer: an NRG Oncology/Gynecologic Oncology Group study on GOG-210 protocol. *Gynecol Oncol.* 2017. doi:10.1016/j.ygyno.2017.03.017

97. Tavassoli FA, Devilee P. WHO Classification of Pathology and genetics of tumours of the breast and female genital organs. In: Tavassoli FA, Devilee P, editors. Lyon, France: IARC Press; 2003. pp. 233–236.

Vulvar Cancer

CHARACTERISTICS

- Vulvar cancer represents 3% to 5% of all female genital cancers and 1% of all malignancies in women. In 2017, there are 6,020 new cases and 1,150 deaths predicted to occur. The average age at diagnosis is 65 years, although it is trending toward a younger age.
- Clinical features include pruritus, ulceration, or a mass. The most common location of lesions is the labia majora (40%), the labia minora (20%), periclitoral region (10%), and perineal area (15%). The route of spread is either by direct extension, lymphatic embolization to the groin nodes, or lymphatic or hematogenous spread to distant sites.
- Risk factors are multifactorial: age greater than 70 years, lower socioeconomic status, hypertension, diabetes, prior lower genital tract dysplasia or cancer, immunosuppression, and human papillomavirus (HPV) infection are known to increase the risk of vulvar cancer. Vulvar SIL/dysplasia is the precancerous state and 76% of patients with vulvar HSIL are HPV positive. There is a 22% rate of subclinical invasive disease in vulvar HSIL, usually less than 1 mm DOI (31).
- Groin lymph node (LN) metastasis: subclinical LN metastasis can occur in 10% to 36% of normally palpated groins (1). Clinical staging clearly under-stages patients. On the contrary, 20% of palpably enlarged LNs are pathologically negative; 28% of patients with positive groin LNs will have positive pelvic LNs.
- The risk for nodal metastasis is related to both depth of invasion and tumor size. The risk of positive LNs with 1 mm DOI is minimal at less than 1%. For a DOI of 2 mm, the risk is 7% to 8%. For a DOI of 3 mm, the risk is 12% to 17%. For a DOI of 5 mm, there is a 15% to 17% risk of LN metastasis. The risk of LN metastasis by lesion size is significant: for a size of 0 to 1 cm, there is a 7.7% risk of positive LNs; for a 2-cm lesion, the risk is 22%; for a 3-cm lesion, the risk is 27%; and for a 5-cm lesion, the risk is 35% to 40% (2).

HISTOLOGY

- Squamous cell carcinoma represents 85% of all vulvar cancers. Other histologic types are basal cell carcinoma, adenocarcinoma, sarcoma, and verrucous carcinoma and melanoma.
- Malignant melanoma represents 5% of vulvar cancers. There are four histologic subtypes of melanoma: superficial spreading, lentigo, acral, and nodular.
- Vulvar Paget's disease has cutaneous and noncutaneous (bladder/colorectal) subtypes. Underlying invasive adenocarcinoma is present in 4% to 17% of cases; 30% to 42% of patients may have, or will later develop, an adenocarcinoma at another nonvulvar location such as the breast, rectum, colon, or uterus.

- Grading: FIGO grading is the most commonly used grading system and is as follows:
  - G1: Well differentiated
  - G2: Moderately differentiated
  - G3: Poorly or undifferentiated.

  GOG grading in vulvar cancer is slightly different than for other tumors. G1 tumors are well differentiated, G2 tumors are composed of less than one third of G3 cells. G3 tumors are composed of greater than one third yet less than one half of G3 cells. G4 tumors have greater than one half of the tumor composed of G3 cells.
- The depth of invasion is measured from the epithelial–stromal junction of the adjacent most superficial dermal papilla to the deepest point of invasion.

PRE-TREATMENT WORKUP

- Pre-treatment workup includes a physical exam with careful evaluation of the vagina and cervix. Five percent of invasive lesions are multifocal. Biopsy for diagnosis should occur at the center of any suspicious area.
- Imaging with CT, MRI, or PET can be obtained if positive groin or pelvic LNs are suspected. Chest x-ray should be obtained, as well as standard lab tests. EUA with cystoscopy can assist in determination of the extent of an anterior lesion's involvement of the urethra. Proctoscopy can be helpful in determination of anorectal involvement if there is a large lesion impinging on the posterior perineal triangle.
- Single-photon emission computed tomography with CT (SPECT/CT) for sentinel lymph node detection (SLND) has been shown to improve SLN dissection by preoperative three-dimensional anatomical localization. In preoperative imaging, SPECT/CT was shown to identify more SLNs (mean 8.7 LN per patient) versus lymphoscintigraphy (mean 5.9) and led to high spatial resolution and anatomical localization. It also identified aberrant lymphatic drainage in 17.5% of patients. Aberrant sentinel lymph nodes were found in the following locations: 31.7% pelvic, 2% paravesical, 7.5% para-aortic, 2% gluteal. Sensitivity for all who underwent complete groin LND was 100%, NPV 100%, the FN rate was 0%. For dissection, distances were calculated from the ASIS or symphysis based on SPECT/CT (3).
- If the groin LNs appear positive, FNA can be considered before a groin LND. If cytology from the FNA is positive, then aggressive surgical removal of bulky LNs should be considered because the usual doses of EBXRT are not adequate to control large volume disease. There is no need to perform a complete LND in light of bulky LNs; instead, remove the bulky disease and mark the area with hemoclips before XRT. If the LNs are fixed and unresectable, consider neoadjuvant chemotherapy and XRT.
- The workup for melanoma is CT of the chest/abdomen/pelvis, MRI of the brain, LDH, and baseline PET. *BRAFV600E* gene mutation information should be obtained via IHC on the tumor.

STAGING

- Vulvar cancer is staged **surgically** and last updated by FIGO in 2009. FIGO modifies the staging systems and the TNM categories have been defined to correspond to the FIGO stages; however there are notable differences between FIGO staging and AJCC staging for positive lymph node status (Table 2.25) (Table 2.26A–D).

Table 2.25 2009 FIGO Staging: Carcinoma of the Vulva

FIGO stage	Description
Stage I	Tumor confined to the vulva and/or perineum. Multifocal lesions should be designated as such.
• IA	Lesions 2 cm or less, confined to the vulva and/or perineum, and with stromal invasion of 1.0 mm or less
• IB	Lesions more than 2 cm, or any size with stromal invasion of more than 1.0 mm, confined to the vulva and/or perineum
Stage II	Tumor of any size with extension to adjacent perineal structures (lower/distal third of the urethra, lower/distal third of the vagina, anal involvement) with negative nodes
Stage III	Tumor of any size with or without extension to adjacent perineal structures (lower/distal third of the urethra, lower/distal third of the vagina, anal involvement) with positive inguino-femoral lymph nodes
• IIIA(i) • IIIA(ii) • IIIB(i) • IIIB(ii) • IIIC	One LN metastasis ≥ 5 mm One or two LN metastases each < 5 mm Two or more LN metastasis ≥ 5 mm Three or more LN metastasis < 5 mm LN(s) with extranodal extension
Stage IV	Tumor of any size with extension to any of the following or distant structures:
• IVA(i)	Tumor invading upper/proximal two thirds of the urethra, upper/proximal two thirds of the vagina, bladder mucosa, or rectal mucosa, or fixed to the pelvic bone
• IVA(ii)	Fixed or ulcerated regional LN metastasis
• IVB	Distant metastasis (including pelvic LN metastasis)

Source: International Federation of Gynecology and Obstetrics.

Table 2.26A AJCC 8th Edition: T Category

T	FIGO stage	T criteria
Tx		Primary tumor cannot be assessed
T0	I	Tumor confined to the vulva and/or perineum. Multifocal lesions should be designated as such. The largest lesion or the lesion with the greatest depth of invasion will be the target lesion identified to address the highest pT stage. Depth of invasion is defined as the measurement of the tumor from the epithelial-stromal junction of the adjacent most superficial dermal papilla to the deepest point of invasion
T1a	IA	Lesions 2 cm or less, confined to the vulva and/or perineum, and with stromal invasion of 1.0 mm or less

(continued)

Table 2.26A AJCC 8th Edition: T Category (*continued*)

T	FIGO stage	T criteria
T1b	IB	Lesions more than 2 cm, or any size with stromal invasion of more than 1.0 mm, confined to the vulva and/or perineum
T2	II	Tumor of any size with extension to adjacent perineal structures (lower/distal third of the urethra, lower/distal third of the vagina, anal involvement)
T3	IVA(i)	Tumor of any size with extension to any of the following: upper/proximal two thirds of the urethra, upper/proximal two thirds of the vagina, bladder mucosa, or rectal mucosa, or fixed to the pelvic bone

Table 2.26B AJCC 8th Edition: N Category

N	FIGO stage	N criteria
NX		Regional LNs cannot be assessed
N0		No regional LN metastasis
N0(i+)		Isolated tumor cells in regional LN(s) no greater than 0.2 mm
N1	III	Regional LN metastasis with one or two LN metastasis each <5 mm, or one LN metastasis ≥5 mm
N1a	IIIA	One or two LN metastases each <5 mm
N1b	IIIA	One LN metastasis ≥5 mm
N2		Regional LN metastasis with three or more LN metastases, each <5 mm, or two or more LN metastases ≥5 mm, or LN(s) with extranodal extension
N2a*	IIIB	Three or more LN metastases each <5 mm
N2b	IIIB	Two or more LN metastases each ≥5 mm
N2c	IIIC	LN(s) with extranodal extension
N3	IVA(ii)	Fixed or ulcerationed regional LN metastasis

LN, lymph node.
*Includes micrometastasis N1mi and N2mi.

Table 2.26C AJCC 8th Edition: M Category

M	FIGO stage	M criteria
M0		No distant metastasis (no pathological M0; use clinical M to complete stage group)
M1	IVB	Distant metastasis (including pelvic LN metastasis)

LN, lymph node.

Table 2.26D AJCC 8th Edition: Stage Grouping			
When T is	**And N is**	**And M is**	**The stage group is**
T1	N0	M0	I
T1a	N0	M0	IA
T1b	N0	M0	IB
T2	N0	M0	II
T1–2	N1–2c	M0	III
T1–2	N1a, N1b	M0	IIIA
T1–2	N2a, N2b	M0	IIIB
T1–2	N2c	M0	IIIC
T1–3	N3	M0–M1	IV
T1–2	N3	M0	IVA(ii)
T3	Any N	M0	IVA(i)
Any T	Any N	M1	IVB

Source: From Amin MB, Edge SB. (2017). *AJCC Cancer Staging Manual* 8th Edition. Chicago, IL: American Joint Committee on Cancer. With permission.

- Melanoma is surgically staged in a similar fashion. There are a few different methods of staging. Stage is the most important prognostic factor. Breslow's staging is used by the AJCC because it is more reproducible and better for ulcerated lesions.
  ○ Stage:

Stage	Clark's level	Chung's level	Breslow's level/depth
I	Intraepithelial	Intraepithelial	<0.76 mm
II	Papillary dermis	<1 mm from granular layer	0.76–1.5 mm
III	Fills dermal papillae	1.1–2 mm from granular layer	1.51–2.25 mm
IV	Reticular layer	>2 mm from granular layer	2.26–3 mm
V	Subcutaneous fat	Subcutaneous fat	>3 mm

  ○ Chung's staging has replaced Clark's staging because it did not take into account that vulvar skin is non–hair-bearing and contains less subcutaneous tissue.
    ■ **Stage Grouping** Table 2.27D
    ■ **Mitotic rate** assessment: a higher mitotic rate is porportional to growth and spread (Tables 2.27A-E and 2.28).

Table 2.27A AJCC 8th Edition Staging: Melanoma T Category

T	Thickness	Ulceration status
TX: primary tumor thickness cannot be assessed (diagnosis was by curettage)	NA	NA
T0: no evidence of primary tumor (unknown primary or completely regressed)	NA	NA
Tis: (melanoma in situ)	NA	NA
T1	≤1.0 mm	Unknown or unspecified
T1a	<0.8 mm	Without ulceration
T1b	<0.8 mm 0.8–1.0 mm	With ulceration Without ulceration
T2	>1.0–2.0 mm	Unknown or unspecified
T2a	>1.0–2.0 mm	Without ulceration
T2b	>1.0–2.0 mm	With ulceration
T3	>2.0–4.0 mm	Unknown or unspecified
T3a	>2.0–4.0 mm	Without ulceration
T3b	>2.0–4.0 mm	With ulceration
T4	>4.0 mm	Unknown or unspecified
T4a	>4.0 mm	Without ulceration
T4b	>4.0 mm	With ulceration

Table 2.27B AJCC 8th Edition Staging: N Category

N	Number of tumor-involved regional LN (s)	Presence of in-transit, satellite, and/or microsatellite metastases
NX	Regional nodes not assessed (SLND not performed, regional nodes previously removed for unrelated reason. Exception: pathological N category is not required for T1 melanomas, use cN	No
N0	No regional metastases	No
N1	One tumor-involved node or in-transit, satellite, and/or microsatellite metastases with no tumor-involved nodes	No
N1a	One clinically occult LN (i.e., detected by SLND)	No

(continued)

Table 2.27B AJCC 8th Edition Staging: N Category (*continued*)

N	Number of tumor-involved regional LN (s)	Presence of in-transit, satellite, and/or microsatellite metastases
N1b	One clinically detected LN	No
N1c	No regional LN disease	Yes
N2	Two or three tumor-involved nodes or in-transit, satellite, and/or microsatellite metastases with one tumor-involved node	
N2a	Two or three clinically occult (i.e., detected by SLND)	No
N2b	Two or three, at least one of which was clinically detected	No
N2c	One clinically occult or clinically detected	Yes
N3	Four or more tumor-involved nodes or in-transit, satellite, and/or microsatellite metastases with two or more tumor-involved nodes, or any number of matted nodes without or with in-transit satellite, and/or microsatellite metastases	
N3a	Four or more clinically occult (i.e., detected by SLND)	No
N3b	Four or more, at least one of which was clinically detected, or presence of any number of matted nodes	No
N3c	Two or more clinically occult or clinically detected and/or presence of any number of matted nodes	Yes

LN, lymph node; SLND, sentinel lymph node dissection.

Table 2.27C AJCC 8th Edition Staging: M Category

M	M criteria/anatomic site	LDH level
M0	No evidence of distant metastasis	NA
M1	Evidence of distant metastasis	See the following
M1a	Distant metastasis to skin, soft tissue including muscle, and/or nonregional LN	Not recorded or unspecified
M1a (0)		Not elevated
M1a (1)		Elevated

(*continued*)

Table 2.27C AJCC 8th Edition Staging: M Category (*continued*)

M1b	Distant metastasis to lung with or without M1a sites of disease	Not recorded or unspecified
M1b (0)		Not elevated
M1b (1)		Elevated
M1c	Distant metastasis to non-CNS visceral sites with or without M1a or M1b sites of disease	Not recorded or unspecified
M1c (0)		Not elevated
M1c (1)		Elevated
M1d	Distant metastasis to CNS with or without M1a, M1b, or M1c sites of disease	Not recorded or unspecified
M1d (0)		Normal
M1d (1)		Elevated

Suffixes for M category: (0) LDH not elevated, (1) LDH elevated. No suffix is used if LDH is not recorded or is unspecified.

Table 2.27D AJCC 8th Edition Staging: Clinical Stage Grouping (cTMN)

When T is	And N is	And M is	Then the clinical stage group is
Tis	N0	M0	0
T1a	N0	M0	IA
T1b	N0	M0	IB
T2a	N0	M0	Ib
T2b	N0	M0	IIA
T3a	N0	M0	IIA
T3b	N0	M0	IIB
T4a	N0	M0	IIB
T4b	N0	M0	IIC
Any T, Tis	≥N1	M0	III
Any T	Any N	M1	IV
Tis	N0	M0	0
T1a	N0	M0	IA

Table 2.27E AJCC 8th Edition Staging: Pathological Stage Grouping (pTNM)

When T is	And N is	And M is	Then the pathological stage group is
T1b	N0	M0	IA
T2a	N0	M0	Ib
T2b	N0	M0	IIA
T3a	N0	M0	IIA

(*continued*)

Table 2.27E AJCC 8th Edition Staging: Pathological Stage Grouping (pTNM) (*continued*)

When T is	And N is	And M is	Then the pathological stage group is
T3b	N0	M0	IIB
T4a	N0	M0	IIB
T4b	N0	M0	IIC
T0	N1b, N1c	M0	IIIB
T0	N2b, N2c, N3b, or N3c	M0	IIIC
T1a/b–T2a	N1a or N2a	M0	IIIA
T1a/b–T2a	N1 b/c or N2b	M0	IIIB
T2b/T3a	N1a–N2b	M0	IIIB
T1a–T3a	N2c or N3a/b/c	M0	IIIC
T3b/T4a	Any N ≥ N1	M0	IIIC
T4b	N1a–N2c	M0	IIIC
T4b	N3a/b/c	M0	IIID
Any T, Tis	Any N	M1	IV

Source: From Amin MB, Edge SB. (2017). *AJCC Cancer Staging Manual* 8th Edition. Chicago, IL: American Joint Committee on Cancer. With permission.

Table 2.28 5Y Survival (YS) for Melanoma

Stage	5 YS for Melanoma
IA	5 YS rate of 95%
IB	5 YS rate of approximately 91%
IIA	5 YS rate of 77%–79%
IIB	5 YS rate of 63%–67%
IIC	5 YS rate of 45%
IIIA	(T1-4aN1aM0) have a 5 YS rate of 70% ; (T1-4aN2aM0) 5 YS of 63%
IIIB	(T1-4bN1aM0) or (T1-4bN2aM0) have a 5 YS rate of 50%–53%; (T1-4aN1bM0) or (T1-4aN2bM0) have a 5 YS rate of 46%–59%
IIIC	(T1-4bN1bM0); (T1-4bN2bM0); or ≥4 metastatic LNs, matted LNs, or in-transit met(s)/satellite(s) have a 5 YS rate of 24%–29%
IV	(M1a) has a 5 YS rate of 19%; (M1b) has a 5 YS rate of 7%; (M1c) has a 5 YS rate of 10%

TREATMENT

• Management of squamous cell and adenocarcinomas has been wide radical excision (radical hemi/vulvectomy) with a 1-cm to 2-cm gross margin with groin (S)LND. For lesions that invade less than a depth of 1 mm, the groin LND can be omitted. If the lesion is lateral (more than 2 cm from the midline), dissection of the contralateral groin can be omitted. If the lesion is midline, or within 2 cm of a midline structure, a bilateral groin SLND should be performed.

○ Early stage T1 and ≤ 4 cm T2 lesions:
  ▪ Less than 1 mm DOI: wide local resection
  ▪ Greater than 1 mm DOI: radical local resection or modified radical vulvectomy with groin SLND
○ Larger T2 and T3 lesions: obtain radiology imaging to evaluate LN status.
  ▪ If radiologically negative:
    □ Can offer EBXRT to primary tumor/groins/pelvis with concurrent platinum-based chemotherapy *or*
    □ Perform complete groin LND:
      – If positive LN: EBXRT to primary tumor/groins/pelvis with concurrent platinum-based chemotherapy
      – If negative: EBXRT to primary tumor and selective EBXRT to groin LN with concurrent platinum-based chemotherapy.
      After completion of neoadjuvant chemoradiation: biopsy of the tumor bed to confirm complete pathologic response is indicated, or resection of residual tumor with wide surgical margins is appropriate. If pathologic margins are still positive, consider re-resection, additional EBXRT, and/or chemotherapy. If unresectable, additional EBXRT can be considered, and/or systemic therapy, or best supportive care.
    □ If bulky inguinofemoral LN are present with an unresectable T3 lesion:
      – Resection of the bulky LN before commencement of chemoradiation can be performed *or*
      – Chemoradiation alone can be performed.
    □ For T4a lesions:
      – Radical vulvectomy with bilateral groin LND or a pelvic exenteration can be considered.
      – Neoadjuvant combination chemotherapy and XRT ± LND.
    □ Metastatic disease beyond the pelvis: any T, any N, M1
      – EBXRT for locoregional control and/or chemotherapy for control and symptom palliation, or best supportive care.
    □ Management of a positive SLN:
      – EBXRT with concurrent cisplatin chemotherapy to the bilateral groins and whole pelvis (WP)
      – Complete bilateral inguinofemoral LND:
    □ Management of positive LN from complete inguinofemoral LND: adjuvant XRT and cisplatin chemotherapy if:
      – Greater than 2 LN are positive
      – Greater than 1 LN is positive with greater than 2-mm sized metastasis *or*
      – Extracapsular LN involvement is present.
    □ Neoadjuvant combination chemotherapy and XRT is considered as upfront therapy in larger T2 lesions, as well as T3 and T4 lesions. These patients can be treated with 50.4 Gy groin and WP-XRT with concurrent cisplatin at 40 to 50 mg/m^2 weekly. A groin LND/SLND can be performed before XRT, and if negative WP XRT can be omitted and XRT fields tailored to the primary tumor including potential en face therapy. Posttreatment surgical evalu-

ation with resection of residual tumor and/or groin LND should be performed.

□ Fixed or ulcerated LN can be surgically resected with XRT to follow; or if unresectable, preoperative chemoradiation with postoperative resection of any macroscopic residual disease.

- The femoral triangle is anatomically bordered by the inguinal ligament superiorly, the sartorius muscle laterally, and the adductor longus muscle medially. The incision site for the groin LND starts 2 cm below a line drawn between the ASIS and the pubic tubercle. The skin flap is preserved. The upper flap is dissected toward the inguinal ligament. The LN-bearing tissue, which is attached to the inguinal ligament, is removed, and the superficial epigastric and superficial circumflex vessels should be ligated. The lower flap is then dissected. The saphenous vein, which runs through the medial aspect of the triangle, should be conserved, and its tributaries ligated.

- If an **ipsilateral groin LN** is found to be positive at final pathology for a unilateral tumor, management of the contralateral groin should be considered. Options include dissection of the contralateral groin, adjuvant bilateral groin and pelvic XRT, or a combination of contralateral groin LND and if negative, unilateral groin/pelvic XRT.

- The risk of contralateral positive LN with a negative ipsilateral groin LND is between 0.4% and 2.6%. GOG 74 demonstrated a 2.4% risk of isolated contralateral positive LNs in tumors 2 cm or less in size. If the DOI was less than 5 mm, contralateral LN metastasis occurred in 1.2% (4). Contralateral positive LNs have been found in 0.9% of patients if the tumor was less than 2-cm wide (5). In another study, a 1.8% rate of positive contralateral LNs was demonstrated if the ipsilateral groin LNs were found to be negative. In no patients were contralateral positive groin LNs found if the tumor was less than 2-cm wide and invasion was less than 5 mm (6).

- Sentinel groin LND can potentially decrease the extent and complication rate of the groin LND. The combined sequenced injection of Technetium-99m (^{99m}Tc) radiolabeled albumin and blue dye to the primary tumor, followed by intraoperative scintillation, has proven sensitive and specific enough for sentinel node identification. If frozen section is positive for LN metastasis, a complete bilateral groin LND should be performed. Radiation without completion LND is under investigation. Indications for performing a SLND are:
  ○ Negative clinical groin examination and imaging
  ○ Primary unifocal tumor
  ○ Tumor size less than 4 cm
  ○ No prior vulvar surgery to have altered lymphatic flow

- There is a relationship between margin status and recurrence. Heaps et al (7) reported on margin status: if there is less than 8 mm of fixed tumor-free tissue at resection, 13 of 23 patients recurred locally, whereas if the margins were greater than 8 mm, only 8 of 112 patients recurred. Thus, for positive or close margins, re-excision, and/or adjuvant XRT to the vulva can decrease the local recurrence rate. Those treated with adjuvant XRT had a 44% recurrence rate versus those observed who had a 75% recurrent rate (8). Tumor thickness greater than 5 mm, tumor >4 cm in size or LVSI, may also be indications for adjuvant local XRT.

- Adjuvant groin and WP-XRT is indicated for FIGO stages 3B, 3C, and 4A. Concurrent radiosensitizing cisplatin chemotherapy should be considered.

- There are complications of a radical vulvectomy and groin LND. The wound infection rate is 29%. The wound breakdown rate is 38% for triple incision surgery versus 68% for en bloc resection. Lymphedema occurs at a rate of 7% to 19%. Lymphocytes occur at a rate of 7% to 28%. Cellulitis or lymphangitis can occur due to *beta Streptococcus*. Prophylactic antibiotics are warranted in patients with chronic lymphedema and if prone to cellulitis. Nerve injuries or paresthesias can also occur.
- Basal cell carcinomas are rarely metastatic. Treatment is with excisional biopsy to include a minimum margin of 1 cm and no LND.
- Verrucous carcinoma is a low grade tumor that is locally invasive and rarely metastasizes. Treatment is wide radical excision. Radiation therapy is commonly avoided due to concerns about aggressive transformation and metastasis.
- Vulvar sarcomas are also treated with wide radical excision. Combination chemotherapy and XRT may assist in disease management.
- Vulvar melanoma patients should undergo a wide radical excision with bilateral groin SLND.
  - There are data to suggest that radical surgery versus wide local excision yields no difference in overall survival (OS) (9).
  - LND in vulvar melanoma is of prognostic indication only; it is not therapeutic. Removal of enlarged nodes is adequate treatment.
  - Margins: the surgically desired margin for in situ disease is 0.5 mm; for a 1-mm thick tumor, a 1-cm margin; for 1.01- to 2-mm thick lesions, a 1- to 2-cm margin; for 2.01- to 4-mm thick lesions, a 2-cm margin; and for a lesion greater than 4-mm thick, a 2-cm margin.
  - Most failures are distant.
  - AJCC stage is the most important prognostic factor.
  - Adjuvant therapy for vulvar melanoma can be single-agent chemotherapy including dacarbazine, temozolomide, cisplatin, vinblastine, or paclitaxel. Combination chemotherapy can consist of cisplatin and paclitaxel.
  - Biological agents can be used with standard cytotoxic drugs or alone. Biologicals include ipilimumab, alpha-interferon, and vemurafenib.
- Paget's disease:
  - For noncutaneous vulvar Paget's disease, there is no benefit to an extensive resection or deep vulvectomy.
  - Treatment: for cutaneous vulvar Paget's, surgical resection is the mainstay. Other treatments are:
    - Surgery: a simple wide resection is recommended, with a 1-cm clinically negative margin. Response rates range from 33% to 70%. The risk of recurrence is high at 58% overall. If margins are negative the risk is 18% to 38% and if positive range between 45% and 61%. Frozen section of the margins has not been found to be better than visual inspection (false-negative rate 35%–38%). Permanent section margin status also did not predict recurrence: with 33% recurrence if negative margins versus 40% recurrence if positive margins (10).
    - Radiation therapy: response rate of 62% to 100% with a recurrence rate of 0% to 35%.
    - **Topical** chemotherapy with bleomycin or 5FU: response rate of 57% to 100%, with a recurrence rate of 25%. Adverse events: pain, moist desquamation, allergic reactions.

- Photodynamic therapy: 5-aminolevulinic acid with light wavelengths. Response rate of 14% to 50%, with a recurrence rate of 38% to 56%.
- Laser therapy: response rate of 53% to 75% with a recurrence rate of 67%.
- Imiquimod: response rate 52% to 80%, recurrence rate 19%.

RECURRENCE

- The risk for local recurrence is close surgical margins. There are data to support that an 8-mm fixed margin (a 1-cm fresh margin) is adequate to diminish local recurrence from 50% if margins were less than 8 mm, to 0% if margins were greater than 8 mm. Surgical margins of 2 cm are still recommended, but if anatomy does not permit (urethral, anal, or vaginal margins that would significantly compromise function), a 1-cm margin can be adequate (7). Farias-Eisner et al (11) looked at radical local excision and LND for stages I and II vulvar cancers, and found that radical local excision had the same survival as those treated more radically with vulvectomy, and LN status had the largest impact on survival (98% OS if negative nodes were identified vs. 45% if positive nodes were found).
- For local recurrence, a radical excision should be performed with complete bilateral groin LND if not done previously. If groin LN were previously irradiated and clinically negative at the time of recurrence, resection of vulvar recurrence alone is recommended. If margins are negative, observation or additional XRT can be considered. If margins are positive and LN is negative, re-excision or EBXRT with or without brachytherapy XRT ± chemotherapy can be considered. If margins are negative and LN is positive, then concurrent chemoradiation should be offered, and if margins are positive and LN is positive, EBXRT with/without brachytherapy and concurrent chemotherapy ± re-excision should be considered. If radical re-excision is contraindicated or declined, EBXRT with or without brachytherapy and concurrent chemotherapy is recommended. This can be followed by surgical resection of residual tumor if present.
- Isolated perineal recurrences can be cured 75% of the time with salvage surgery. If the recurrence is central and regional, a pelvic exenteration can be considered.
- If groin nodal recurrence is detected: resection of the involved LN or a complete LND can be performed, followed by concurrent chemoradiation, if not previously performed. If the groin recurrence is fixed or large, then concurrent chemoradiation should be offered.
- If there is an isolated pelvic nodal recurrence: resection can be considered, and/or concurrent chemoradiation should be offered to follow.
- If distant metastases are identified on comprehensive workup, palliative chemotherapy and/or EBXRT should be considered.
- For LN recurrence in melanoma, pathology should be confirmed via biopsy, and imaging should also be obtained with PET/CT or CT of the chest/abdomen/pelvis. If the LN recurrence is in the groin, the entire LN basin should be dissected if not previously performed, and the enlarged LN should be resected. If a prior LND was performed, removal of the node itself is adequate. If the disease is completely resected, XRT, alpha interferon, and/or a clinical trial can be offered. If the disease is unresectable, systemic therapy, XRT, or a clinical trial can be offered. If there are clinically positive superficial LNs or there are three or greater positive LNs, iliac and obturator LND should be considered.

SURVIVAL

The 2Y survival (YS) for nonmelanoma vulvar cancer patients with positive groin LN is 68%, and for those with positive pelvic LN is 23% (Table 2.29).

FOLLOW-UP

- Every 3 months for the first 2 years
- Every 6 months for the next 3 years
- Annual visits thereafter

NOTABLE TRIALS

- GOG 36: this surgical pathology study evaluated 637 patients with vulvar cancer, all of whom had tumors of less than 5 mm DOI. Risk factors for local recurrence and LN metastasis were studied. Multivariate risk factors that were predictive of groin LN metastasis were: tumor size less than 2 cm (18.9% + LN); greater than 2 cm (41.6% + LN). Independent predictors of groin LN metastasis were: tumor grade, LVSI, depth of invasion, age, and fixed or ulcerated LN. A clinically negative groin examination had a false-negative rate of 23.9%. Those patients in GOG 36 who were identified with positive groin LNs were randomized to GOG 37 (12,13).
- GOG 37: this study identified 114 patients with positive groin LNs after a radical vulvectomy and bilateral groin LND, and randomized them to an ipsilateral pelvic LND or to groin and pelvic XRT. The XRT was dosed at 45 to 50 Gy. 5% recurred in the XRT group, and 24% recurred in the pelvic LND group. The 2 YS was 68% for those treated with groin and pelvic XRT versus 54% for those who received the pelvic LND. The number of positive LNs influenced survival: one positive LN yielded an 80% OS, whereas 4 or more positive LNs had a 27% OS. The incidence of positive pelvic LNs if groin LNs were positive was 28%. There was a 9% incidence of local vulvar recurrence in both arms. A follow-up analysis was performed (15): the 6 YS for patients who received XRT was 61% versus 41% for those who received the pelvic LND. The 6 YS for cancer-related deaths was 51% versus 29% for the pelvic XRT versus pelvic LND groups, respectively (HR, 50.49). Poor prognostic factors were: clinically suspicious or fixed LNs, or greater than two positive groin LNs. A ratio of 20% positive LNs to total LNs was associated with contralateral metastasis, relapse, and cancer-related death, thus the cutoff for recommending XRT. 44% of patients in the XRT arm died secondary to other causes. The actual 3Y disease specific death rate was 25% (14).

Table 2.29 Vulvar Cancer 5 YS by Stage	
Stage	5 YS (%)
I	95
II	75–85
III	55
IVA	20
IVB	5

- GOG 74: this study surgically evaluated the outcomes of 143 patients with early stage vulvar tumors who underwent a superficial groin LND with a modified radical vulvectomy. Overall, 7% developed isolated groin recurrences, and of those with a groin recurrence, 91.7% died. The median time to recurrence in the vulva was 35.9 months, and 7 months for recurrence in the groin. The median survival time after recurrence was 52.4 months for vulvar recurrence and 9.4 months for groin recurrence. This study is criticized for a high number of grade 3 tumors (28%) and that of the nine groin recurrences, three were in an undissected groin (patients who refused groin dissection) (4,16).

- GOG 88: because patients in GOG 37 with positive groin LNs had favorable outcomes with XRT the question as to whether a groin LND was necessary if prophylactic XRT was administered was investigated. This study evaluated 50 patients after a radical vulvectomy and randomized them to prophylactic groin XRT or to groin LND. In this study, 0 out of 25 patients recurred if a LND was performed, followed by XRT for positive LN (of which 20% were indeed positive), versus an 18.5% recurrence if prophylactic groin XRT was administered to an undissected groin with, therefore, an unknown LN status. Criticisms of this study were: underdosing of the groins as the dose prescription point was to 3 cm and on review, the average vessel depth was 6.1 cm (range 2–18.6 cm) with an average BMI of 25.6 (17,18).

- GOG 101: this phase II study evaluated 73 patients with T3 or T4 disease treated with neoadjuvant chemotherapy and XRT. The XRT total dose was 47.6 Gy administered in 1.7 Gy fractions as a hyper-fractionated split dose regimen of 23.8 Gy BID for 4 days and daily for 6 days with a 2-week break, with two concurrent cycles of cisplatin 50 mg/m^2 day 1 and 5-FU 1,000 mg/m^2 days 1 to 4 given week 1 of each course of XRT. 69 of 71 women were converted to a resectable status, with 68 patients keeping urinary and fecal capacity. 47% (33 of 71) had a CCR and 70% of these were CPR. 2.8% remained unresectable. There was a 55% OS. A companion study to GOG 101 was done for patients with unresectable positive groin LNs (N2/3 nodes); 38 of 40 patients became resectable, with 15 of 37 patients having a CPR. Overall, 29 of 38 patients had local control of their disease. 19 patients recurred: 9 locally and 8 distant (19,20).

- GOG 205: this phase II study evaluated 58 patients with T3 or T4 disease treated with neoadjuvant chemotherapy and XRT. XRT was dosed at 57.6 Gy with concurrent weekly cisplatin dosed at 40 mg/m^2. Surgical resection followed for residual tumor (or biopsy to confirm CCR). 64% of patients had a CCR (37 of 58) and 78% of these had a CPR. In this study, there was no hyper-fractionation, no mid-treatment break, and no 5-FU. Management of the groin LNs in these studies was standardized. Clinically negative or resectable groin LNs underwent groin LND before neoadjuvant therapy. If there were unresectable groin LNs, the groin dissection was performed after neoadjuvant therapy (21).

- GOG 173: in this study, 452 eligible patients with a tumor size ≥2 cm, ≤6 cm, and with at least 1-mm invasion underwent radical vulvectomy with groin lymphatic mapping. 772 groin dissections were performed. A sentinel LN (SLN) was identified in 418 of 452 patients. LN metastases were found in 132 of 418 patients (31.6%). The SLN was positive in 121 of 418 patients. 11 (8.3%) patients with a negative SLN were found to have positive LNs identified on final complete dissection pathology (thus 132 total SLN positive patients). 23% of the true-positive patients were detected by immunohistochemistry (IHC) analysis of the SLN. The sensitivity of SLN dissection was 91.7% and the FNPV was 3.7% (90% upper confidence bound = 6.1%). In patients with tumors less than 4 cm, the false-negative rate was 2% (22).

- GOG 195: 137 patients were evaluable for analysis of lymphedema after randomization to receive sutured closure versus fibrin sealant applied in the wound followed by sutured closure. The incidence of grade 2/3 lymphedema was 67% in the sutured closure arm and 60% in the fibrin sealant arm; thus no benefit to fibrin sealant was found. The incidence of lymphedema was correlated strongly with inguinal infection and not increased in those who received adjuvant XRT (23).

- DiSaia et al recommended omitting the deep LND to decrease morbidity without compromising survival. 50 stage I patients with negative superficial nodes were retrospectively reviewed. No deep LND was performed. There were no recurrences after 12 months (24).

- GROINSS-V-1/GOG 270 **GRO**ningen **IN**ternational **S**tudy on **S**entinel nodes in **V**ulvar cancer: this study evaluated 403 patients. 623 groin dissections were performed. All tumors were greater than 1 mm DOI, unifocal, squamous, and less than 4 cm in size with clinically negative groin LN. A radical vulvectomy and sentinel groin LND were performed in all patients. Follow-up was 35 months. A combination of radioactive tracer and blue dye was used. 67% had negative SLN, 32.9% had a positive SLN. Of 259 patients with unifocal vulvar disease and a negative sentinel node (median follow-up time, 35 months), 6 had groin recurrences diagnosed, for a false-negative rate of 2.3%. The 3 YS rate was 97%. The 3Y DSS rate for patients with SLN metastasis greater than 2 mm was 69.5%, the 3Y DSS of the SLN metastasis less than 2 mm was 94.4%. The short-term morbidity was decreased in the SLN patients compared with those patients with a positive sentinel node who underwent a complete inguinofemoral lymphadenectomy. Wound breakdown in the groin was 11.7% versus 34.0%, and cellulitis occurred at 4.5% versus 21.3%. The long-term morbidity was also less with recurrent erysipelas occurring at a rate of 0.4% versus 16.2%, and lymphedema of the legs seen in 1.9% versus 25.2% of patients. GROINSS-V-I 10Y follow-up: the median follow-up was 105 months. The overall recurrence rate was 37.2% at 5 years, at a median time of 27 months. The local recurrence rate was 27.2% at 5Y and 39.5% at 10Y after primary treatment. The primary isolated groin recurrence rate was 4.1% and distant recurrence was 2%. In SLN– patients, the isolated groin recurrence was 2.5%. The local recurrence rate for SLN– patients was 24.6% at 5Y and 36.4% at 10Y. In SLN+ patients, the groin recurrence was 8% and distant recurrence 6.8% at 5 and 10Y. Local recurrence was 33.2% at 5Y and 46.4% at 10Y. SLN– patients had 5 and 10Y DSS of 93.5% and 90.8% compared to SLN+ patients of 75.5% and 64.5%. For all patients, 10Y DSS decreased from 90.4% to 68.7% for local recurrence. For SLN– patients, 10Y DSS decreased from 96.1% to 80.8%, and SLN+ patients, 10Y DSS decreased from 77.7% to 44.6% for local recurrence (25,26).

- **GRO**ningen **IN**ternational **S**tudy on **S**entinel nodes in **V**ulvar cancer (GROINSS-V) **II** NCT01500512: eligible patients undergo planned radical vulvectomy and sentinel LND. These are patients with unifocal tumors less than 4 cm in size and less than

N3 disease. Patients without pathologic LN involvement undergo observation. Patients with less than 2 mm LN involvement undergo XRT. Patients with significant LN involvement undergo inguinofemoral lymphadenectomy and XRT with or without chemotherapy according to institutional guidelines. Results pending.

- AGO-CaRE-1 (Chemo **a**nd **R**adiotherapy in **E**pithelial Vulvar Cancer): this was a retrospective multicenter cohort study in Germany, from 1998 to 2008 reviewing 1,618 documented patients with primary squamous-cell vulvar cancer stage IB and higher. Of the patients, 1,249 had surgical groin staging and known LN status and were further analyzed. Of the 1,249 patients, 447 (35.8%) had LN metastases (N+). The majority of N+ patients had one (172 [38.5%]) or two (102 [22.8%]) positive nodes. The 3Y PFS of N+ patients was 35.2%, and the OS was 56.2% compared with 75.2% and 90.2% in node-negative patients (N−). 244 (54.6%) N+ patients had adjuvant therapy, of which 183 (40.9%) had XRT directed at the groins (± other fields). 3Y PFS and OS rates in these patients were better compared with N+ patients without adjuvant treatment (PFS: 39.6% vs. 25.9%, hazard ratio [HR] 0.67; 95% confidence interval [CI]: 0.51–0.88; $p = 0.004$; OS: 57.7% vs. 51.4%; HR 0.79; 95% CI: 0.56 to 1.11; $p = 0.17$). This effect was statistically significant in multivariable analysis adjusted for age, ECOG PS, FIGO stage, grade, invasion depth, and number of positive nodes (PFS: HR 0.58; 95% CI: 0.43–0.78; $p < 0.001$; OS: HR 0.63; 95% CI: 0.43–0.91; $p = 0.01$). Thus, adjuvant XRT was associated with improved prognosis in node-positive patients; however, outcomes after adjuvant XRT remains poor compared with node-negative patients. Adjuvant chemoradiation should improve therapy beyond XRT alone (27).
- Impact of adjuvant chemotherapy in addition to XRT for node-positive vulvar cancer: a National Cancer Data Base (NCDB) analysis. A total of 1,792 patients were reviewed: 26.3% received adjuvant chemotherapy in addition to XRT, and 76.6% had one to three involved LN. The median unadjusted survival with and without adjuvant chemotherapy was 29.7 and 44 months, $p = 0.001$. Delivery of adjuvant chemotherapy resulted in a 38% reduction in the risk of death (HR 0.62; 95% CI: 0.48–0.79; $p < 0.001$) for node positive vulvar cancer patients in the NCDB. A propensity adjusted analysis was performed and able to show a significant improvement in 3Y OS of 53.9% versus 46.9% in patients receiving chemoradiation (28).
- GOG 279: this is a phase II trial of approximately 52 patients evaluating cisplatin and gemcitabine concurrent with IMRT for the treatment of locally advanced squamous cell carcinoma of the vulva. Eligible patients are T2 to T3, N0 to N3 squamous cell cancers not amenable to primary surgical resection. Pre-treatment SLND or groin dissection is performed. Patients will be treated with 64 Gy IMRT total dose to the vulva and 50 Gy to the nonmalignant groin or 60 Gy to involved LN (>3 +LN, extracapsular involvement, or close margins), concordant with gemcitabine 50 mg/m^2 and cisplatin 40 mg/m^2 weekly during XRT. Surgical resection of residual disease is scheduled at 6 to 8 weeks post-therapy. Results are pending.
- Debulking of clinically involved LN followed by XRT (compared to complete groin LND or SLND followed by XRT for node positive disease) had fewer complications. There was no increase in groin recurrences or changes in OS in 68 patients (29).

- Vemurafenib is an antibody against the *BRAF* receptor. The V600E mutation occurs in some melanomas and constitutively activates the *BRAF* gene. In a randomized trial of 675 untreated metastatic melanoma patients stage IIIc or IV who were *BRAF* V600E positive, vemurafenib was compared to dacarbazine. Vemurafenib was dosed at 960 mg orally twice daily and dacarbazine at 1,000 mg/m^2 IV every 3 weeks. The 6-month OS was 84% in the vemurafenib group and 64% in the dacarbazine group. Response rates were 48% for vemurafenib and 5% for dacarbazine (30).
- RTM-0905: a phase II trial of dasatinib 70 mg PO BID in c-KIT-positive patients with unresectable locally advanced or stage IV mucosal, sacral, and vulvovaginal melanoma. Results pending.

REFERENCES

1. Iversen T, Aalders JG, Christensen A, et al. Squamous cell carcinoma of the vulva: a review of 424 patients, 1956-1974. *Gynecol Oncol.* 1980;9(3):271-279.
2. Gonzalez Bosquet J, Kinney WK, Russell AH, et al. Risk of occult inguinofemoral lymph node metastasis from squamous carcinoma of the vulva. *Int J Radiat Oncol Biol Phys.* 2003;57(2):419-424.
3. Klapdor R, Länger F, Gratz KF. SPECT/CT for SLN dissection in vulvar cancer: improved SLN detection and dissection by preoperative three-dimensional anatomical localisation. *Gynecol Oncol.* September 2015;138(3):590-596.
4. Stehman FB, Bundy BN, Dvoretsky PM, et al. Early stage I carcinoma of the vulva treated with ipsilateral superficial inguinal lymphadenectomy and modified radical hemivulvectomy: a prospective study of the Gynecologic Oncology Group. *Obstet Gynecol.* 1992;79(4):490-497.
5. de Hullu JA, van der Zee AG. Surgery and radiotherapy in vulvar cancer. *Crit Rev Oncol Hematol.* 2006;60(1):38-58.
6. Gonzalez Bosquet J, Magrina JF, Magtibay PM, et al. Patterns of inguinal groin metastases in squamous cell carcinoma of the vulva. *Gynecol Oncol.* 2007;105(3):742-746.
7. Heaps JM, Fu YS, Montz FJ, et al. Surgical-pathologic variables predictive of local recurrence in squamous cell carcinoma of the vulva. *Gynecol Oncol.* 1990;38(3):309-314.
8. Faul CM, Mirmow D, Huang Q, et al. Adjuvant radiation for vulvar carcinoma: improved local control. *Int J Radiat Oncol Biol Phys.* 1997;38(2):381-389.
9. Trimble EL, Lewis JL Jr, Williams LL, et al. Management of vulvar melanoma. *Gynecol Oncol.* 1992;45(3):254-258.
10. Fishman DA, Chambers SK, Schwartz PE, et al. Extramammary Paget's disease of the vulva. *Gynecol Oncol.* 1995;56(2):266-270.
11. Farias-Eisner R, Cirisano FD, Grouse D, et al. Conservative and individualized surgery for early squamous carcinoma of the vulva: the treatment of choice for stage I and II (T1-2N0-1M0) disease. *Gynecol Oncol.* 1994;53(1):55-58.
12. Homesley HD, Bundy BN, Sedlis A, et al. Assessment of current International Federation of Gynecology and Obstetrics staging of vulvar carcinoma relative to prognostic factors for survival (a Gynecologic Oncology Group study). *Am J Obstet Gynecol.* 1991;164(4):997-1003; discussion 1003-1004.
13. Homesley HD, Bundy BN, Sedlis A, et al. Prognostic factors for groin node metastasis in squamous cell carcinoma of the vulva (a Gynecologic Oncology Group study). *Gynecol Oncol.* 1993;49(3):279-283.
14. Homesley HD, Bundy BN, Sedlis A, et al. Radiation therapy versus pelvic node resection for carcinoma of the vulva with positive groin nodes. *Obstet Gynecol.* 1986;68(6):733-740.

15. Kunos C, Simpkins F, Gibbons H, et al. Radiation therapy compared with pelvic node resection for node-positive vulvar cancer: a randomized controlled trial. *Obstet Gynecol.* 2009;114(3):537-546.
16. Stehman FB, Bundy BN, Ball H, et al. Sites of failure and times to failure in carcinoma of the vulva treated conservatively: a Gynecologic Oncology Group study. *Am J Obstet Gynecol.* 1996;174(4):1128-1132; discussion 1132-1133.
17. Stehman FB, Bundy BN, Thomas G, et al. Groin dissection versus groin radiation in carcinoma of the vulva: a Gynecologic Oncology Group study. *Int J Radiat Oncol Biol Phys.* 1992;24(2):389-396.
18. Koh WJ, Chiu M, Stelzer KJ, et al. Femoral vessel depth and the implications for groin node radiation. *Int J Radiat Oncol Biol Phys.* 1993;27(4):969-974.
19. Moore DH, Thomas GM, Montana GS, et al. Preoperative chemoradiation for advanced vulvar cancer: a phase II study of the Gynecologic Oncology Group. *Int J Radiat Oncol Biol Phys.* 1998;42(1):79-85.
20. Montana GS, Thomas GM, Moore DH, et al. Preoperative chemo-radiation for carcinoma of the vulva with N2/N3 nodes: a Gynecologic Oncology Group study. *Int J Radiat Oncol Biol Phys.* 2000;48(4):1007-1013.
21. Moore DH, Ali S, Koh WJ, et al. A phase II trial of radiation therapy and weekly cisplatin chemotherapy for the treatment of locally-advanced squamous cell carcinoma of the vulva: a Gynecologic Oncology Group study. *Gynecol Oncol.* 2012;124(3):529-533.
22. Levenback CF, Ali S, Coleman RL, et al. Lymphatic mapping and sentinel lymph node biopsy in women with squamous cell carcinoma of the vulva: a Gynecologic Oncology Group study. *J Clin Oncol.* November 1, 2012;30(31):3786-3791.
23. Carlson JW, Kauderer J, Walker JL, et al. A randomized phase III trial of VH fibrin sealant to reduce lymphedema after inguinal lymph node dissection: a Gynecologic Oncology Group study. *Gynecol Oncol.* July 2008;110(1):76-82.
24. DiSaia PJ, Creasman WT, Rich WM. An alternate approach to early cancer of the vulva. *Am J Obstet Gynecol.* 1979;133(7):825-832.
25. van der Zee AG, Oonk MH, de Hullu JA, et al. Sentinel node dissection is safe in the treatment of early-stage vulvar cancer. *J Clin Oncol.* 2008;26(6):884-889.
26. Te Grootenhuis NC, van der Zee AG, van Doorn HC, et al. Sentinel nodes in vulvar cancer: long-term follow-up of the GROningen International Study on Sentinel nodes in Vulvar cancer (GROINSS-V) I. *Gynecol Oncol.* January 2016;140(1):8-14.
27. Mahner S, Jueckstock J, Hilpert F, et al. Adjuvant therapy in lymph node-positive vulvar cancer: the AGO-CaRE-1 study. *J Natl Cancer Inst.* January 24, 2015;107(3):dju426. doi:10.1093/jnci/dju426
28. Gill BS, Bernard ME, Lin JF, et al. Impact of adjuvant chemotherapy with radiation for node-positive vulvar cancer: a National Cancer Data Base (NCDB) analysis. *Gynecol Oncol.* June 2015;137(3):365-372.
29. Nooij LS, Ongkiehong PJ, van Zwet EW, et al. Groin surgery and risk of recurrence in lymph node positive patients with vulvar squamous cell carcinoma. *Gynecol Oncol.* December 2015;139(3):458-464.
30. Chapman PB, Hauschild A, Robert C, et al. Improved survival with vemurafenib in melanoma with BRAF V600E mutation. *N Engl J Med.* 2011;364(26):2507-2516.
31. Modesitt SC, Waters AB, Walton L, et al. Vulvar intraepithelial neoplasia III: occult cancer and the impact of margin status on recurrence. *Obstet Gynecol.* 1998;92(6):962-966.

Vaginal Cancer

CHARACTERISTICS

- Vaginal cancer represents 1% to 2% of all female genital tract malignancies. The median age at diagnosis is 60 years. Most vaginal cancers are metastatic lesions from other sites, including the cervix, uterus, breast, gestational trophoblastic disease, and the gastrointestinal (GI) tract. Primary vaginal cancers are commonly found in the upper one third of the vagina, often in the posterior fornix. There are 4,810 new cases with 1,240 deaths estimated for 2017.
- Symptoms include vaginal discharge, vaginal bleeding, tenesmus, pelvic pain, bladder irritation, and pelvic fullness.
- If the patient has a history of uterine, cervical, or vulvar cancer, the vaginal lesion is considered a recurrent cancer unless proven otherwise by discriminating pathology or greater than 5 years have intervally passed since prior diagnosis.
- Risk factors for vaginal cancer include human papillomavirus (HPV) infection, chronic vaginal irritation, prior treatment for cervical cancer, prior CIN, and a history of in-utero exposure to DES.
- DES was used from 1940 to 1971. Vaginal adenosis and vaginal adenocarcinoma are characteristics of exposure. Other physical representations are a cockscomb cervix. The risk of clear cell carcinoma is 1:1,000 with a history of DES. The peak age at diagnosis was 19 years. Surveillance for women who were exposed to DES in utero includes at least yearly gynecologic exams with cervicovaginal cytology (and colposcopy as indicated) to occur indefinitely.
- The route of spread is direct, lymphatic, or hematogenous. The route of lymphatic spread depends on the location of the lesion. If the lesion is in the upper two thirds of the vagina, metastasis is often directly to the pelvic lymph nodes (LNs). If the lesion is in the lower one third of the vagina, metastasis can often be to the inguinal-femoral LNs, and/or pelvic lymph nodes. Hematogenous spread often occurs late in the disease process.
- The most important prognostic factor is stage of disease. Age is also an important factor. Melanomas and sarcomas have the worst prognosis. Lesions of the distal vagina tend to have a worse prognosis than proximal lesions. Size less than 3 cm has a better prognosis than if larger than 5 cm. LN status also confers prognosis, with a 5-year survival (YS) of 33% for positive LNs compared to 56% for negative LNs.

PRE-TREATMENT WORKUP

The pre-treatment workup is colposcopy of the entire genital tract and physical examination. Diagnosis is via biopsy often guided with colposcopy. It may be necessary to perform an examination under anesthesia with cystoscopy and proctoscopy. These procedures may also help with initial staging. Chest x-ray, intravenous pyelography (IVP), cystoscopy, proctoscopy, and barium enema are FIGO-approved diagnostic studies. CT, MRI, and PET imaging may assist in evaluating extent of disease and aid in treatment planning.

HISTOLOGY

- 80% of vaginal cancers are of squamous cell histology.
- 5% to 9% are adenocarcinomas.
- Malignant melanoma represents 2.8% to 5% of vaginal neoplasms. Vaginal melanomas are more often found in the lower one third of the vagina.
- Rhabdomyosarcoma is usually found as the botryoid variant of embryonal rhabdomyosarcoma and is the most common malignant tumor of the vagina in infants and children; 90% of patients are younger than 5 years. On clinical examination, grape-like edematous masses may protrude from the vagina. The histologic pearl is the presence of a cambium layer beneath an intact vaginal epithelium.
- Leiomyosarcoma can also be found, and this can occur in women with a prior history of radiation therapy (XRT).

STAGING

Staging continues to be clinical, closely following cervical cancer parameters (Tables 2.30A–D).

Table 2.30A AJCC 8th Edition: T Category		
T	FIGO stage	T criteria
TX		Primary tumor cannot be assessed
T0		No evidence of primary tumor
T1	I	Tumor confined to the vagina
T1a	I	Tumor confined to the vagina, measuring ≤2.0 cm
T1b	I	Tumor confined to the vagina, measuring >2.0 cm
T2	II	Tumor invading paravaginal tissues but not to pelvic sidewall
T2a	II	Tumor invading paravaginal tissues but not to pelvic wall, measuring ≤2.0 cm
T2b	II	Tumor invading paravaginal tissues but not to pelvic wall, measuring >2.0 cm
T3	III	Tumor extending to the pelvic sidewall and/or involving the lower third of the vagina and/or causing hydronephrosis or nonfunctioning kidney
T4	IVA	Tumor invading the mucosa of the bladder or rectum and/or extending beyond the true pelvis (bullous edema is not sufficient evidence to classify a tumor as T4)

Table 2.30B AJCC 8th Edition: N Category		
N	**FIGO stage**	**N criteria**
NX		Regional LNs cannot be assessed
N0		No regional LN metastasis
N0(i+)		Isolated tumor cells in regional LN(s) not greater than 0.2 mm
N1	III	Pelvic or inguinal LN metastasis
LN, lymph node.		

Table 2.30C AJCC 8th Edition: M Category		
M	**FIGO stage**	**M criteria**
M0		No distant metastasis
M1	IVB	Distant metastasis

Table 2.30D AJCC 8th Edition: Stage Grouping			
When T is	**And N is**	**And M is**	**Then the stage group is**
T1a	N0	M0	IA
T1b	N0	M0	IB
T2a	N0	M0	IIA
T2b	N0	M0	IIB
T1–3	N1	M0	III
T3	N0	M0	III
T4	Any N	M0	IVA
Any T	Any N	M1	IVB
Source: From Amin MB, Edge SB. (2017). *AJCC Cancer Staging Manual* 8th Edition. Chicago, IL: American Joint Committee on Cancer. With permission.			

If there is clinical involvement of the cervix or the vulva, the tumor should be classified as a primary cervical or vulvar cancer, respectively; tumors limited to the urethra should be classified as urethral cancers.

TREATMENT

Treatment depends on the location and depth of the lesion, the stage of the cancer, and medical comorbidities.

- Treatment for stage I squamous cell or adenocarcinomas that involve the upper two thirds of the vagina can include a radical hysterectomy with upper vaginectomy and LND, or an upper vaginectomy and parametrectomy with LND if the uterus has previously been removed. XRT without surgery has equivalent outcomes. Concurrent platinum-based chemotherapy has been adopted to follow cervical cancer guidelines. If the lower one third of the vagina is involved, external beam radiation therapy (EBXRT) fields should include the groins. Dosing is 50.4 Gy EBXRT to a total of 80 to 85 Gy with interstitial or Fletcher-Suit brachytherapy.
- Treatment for stages II, III, and IV is definitive XRT with concurrent platinum-based chemotherapy. If the lesion size is 2 cm or greater, surgical resection can be considered to potentially optimize XRT. XRT usually includes EBXRT and intracavitary or interstitial therapy to a total dose of 85 to 90 Gy. If the lower one third of the vagina is involved, the groins should also be irradiated.
- Treatment for melanoma is radical surgical resection if possible. Exenterative surgery has not been found to provide additional survival benefit. Chemotherapy with biologic therapy may provide adjuvant benefits.
- The treatment of rhabdomyosarcoma is usually multimodal with therapy consisting of surgical resection, XRT, and systemic chemotherapy. Commonly used agents are vincristine, actinomycin, and cyclophosphamide. Another regimen is cyclophosphamide, doxorubicin, and dacarbazine.
- Leiomyosarcoma is treated with radical surgical resection and the consideration of adjuvant XRT and/or chemotherapy.

RECURRENT DISEASE

If recurrent disease is identified, a full metastatic workup should be employed. If only local disease is confirmed, a wide local excision or a partial (radical) vaginectomy can be performed. If central disease is identified, a pelvic exenteration can be considered. If there is distant metastasis, chemotherapy with or without XRT can be considered (Table 2.31).

SURVIVAL

Table 2.31 Vaginal Cancer 5Y Survival by Stage	
Stage	5 YS (%)
I	84
II	75
III	57
IV	10

FOLLOW-UP

- Physical and pelvic examinations are recommended: a Pap smear may help with detection of recurrence but at most annually.
  - Every 3 months for the first 2 years
  - Every 6 months for the next 3 years
  - Annual examinations thereafter

Gestational Trophoblastic Disease

CHARACTERISTICS

- Gestational trophoblastic disease (GTD) describes a group of tumors that arise from trophoblastic cells. This is usually the result of an abnormal fertilization event and includes molar pregnancy, choriocarcinoma, placental site trophoblastic tumor (PSTT) and epitheliod trophobblastic tumor (ETT).
- Hydatidiform molar pregnancy occurs in approximately 1 out of 1,000 pregnancies in North America. Clinical features of a mole are vaginal bleeding in the first trimester or early second trimester; uterine size large for dates; ovarian theca-lutein cysts (seen in 46% of patients, 2% of which may torse); early preeclampsia less than 20 weeks (12%–17%); hyperthyroidism due to the similarity between the alpha subunit of both human chorionic gonadotropin (hCG) and thyroid-stimulating hormone (TSH) hormones; hyperemesis gravidarum (20%); passage of vesicles per vagina; and respiratory complaints due to tumor emboli or increased progesterone (27%).
- Risk factors for a molar pregnancy include age (<20 years or >40 years of age), history of a prior mole, and Asian ethnicity.
- WHO has classified GTD into two states: premalignant and malignant. The premalignant tumors are the complete and the partial moles. The malignant tumors are the invasive mole, gestational choriocarcinoma, ETT and PSTT. Within the malignant tumors are the categories of nonmetastatic and metastatic. Within the metastatic category are low-risk metastatic and high-risk metastatic disease.
- There is an increased risk for a second mole after a first molar pregnancy. This is usually paternally related. The risk of another molar pregnancy increases from 1 out of 1,000 to 1 out of 100. There is a familial recurrent hydatidiform mole syndrome (FRHM). This is an autosomal recessive disorder with mutations in NLRP7 (in 70% of cases) or KHDC3L (5% of cases) that results in a diploid complete mole of biparental origin.
- A mole and fetus have been diagnosed at a rate of 1 out of 100,000 pregnancies. There are data to suggest a 40% chance of a live birth. Persistent GTD is diagnosed in 55% of these patients, and 22.7% are found to have metastatic disease. There is an increased risk for hemorrhage, preeclampsia, and metastatic disease. The pregnancy should be terminated if these life-threatening complications occur.
- Tumors from other primary sites can produce hCG. Genetic studies should be performed on patient's tumors who are refractory to common first line and salvage therapies to rule out nongestational choriocarcinoma.

HISTOLOGY

- Complete and partial moles are usually diagnosed at the time of uterine evacuation. Histopathology is the main diagnostic method. Other abnormal pregnancies/fetuses can be mistaken for a partial mole. These include Turner's, Beckwith-Wiedemann, and Edward's syndromes.
- A complete mole has no fetal components. Furthermore, the placental villi are hydropic (or edematous) with no identifiable vasculature. The origin of this mole is considered to arise from fertilization of an anuclear oocyte with either two sperm or one sperm that duplicates itself, thus all nuclear DNA is paternal (most commonly diploid with a 46XX karyotype) while the mitochondrial DNA is maternal. Fluorescence in situ hybridization (FISH) can confirm the diagnosis. The rate of persistent GTD after a complete mole is 15% to 20%.
- The partial mole's origin is thought to arise from the dual fertilization of an egg by two sperm, or duplication of a paternal chromosome resulting in triploidy with 2:1 paternal to maternal DNA content. Fetal components can be seen, along with fetal vasculature and hydropic villi. FISH can aid with the diagnosis if necessary, and immunohistochemistry can add information with positive staining for p57 KIP2. Cytogenetic techniques, to include chromosomal banding and restriction fragment length polymorphism (RFLP) analysis of DNA, have allowed chromosomal patterns for partial and complete molar pregnancies differentiation. The rate of persistent GTD after partial mole is 0.5% to 5% (Table 2.32).
- Choriocarcinoma occurs in 1 of 20,000 pregnancies and is inherently a high-risk disease at diagnosis, regardless of metastasis. It should be treated aggressively. 50% of tumors follow a term gestation, 20% occur after molar gestations (both partial and complete), and 25% occur after a spontaneous or elective abortion. These tumors have diverse, nonspecific ploidies and are highly malignant. Both cytotrophoblasts and syncytiotrophoblasts are present, with syncytiotrophoblasts predominating, but there are no chorionic villi. Metastasis occurs frequently to the lung (80% with symptoms such as hemoptysis or dyspnea), vagina (30% with bleeding), brain (10% with focal neurologic deficits, headache, mass effect), and liver (10% pain, hemoperitoneum).

Table 2.32 Molar Pregnancy Classifications With Characteristics

Characteristic	Complete mole	Partial mole
Hydatidiform edematous villi	Diffuse	Focal
Trophoblastic hyperplasia	Cyto- and syncytial	Syncytial
Embryo	Absent	Present
Villous capillary	No fetal RBC	Many fetal RBC
Gestational age at diagnosis	8–16 wk	10–22 wk
Beta hCG titer mIU/mL	>50,000 mIU/mL in 75%	<50,000 mIU/mL
Malignant potential	15%–25%	0.5%–5%
Karyotype	Diploid (46XX 95%, 46XY 5%)	Triploid (69XXY) 80%
Size for dates: Small Large	33% 33%	65% 10%

- PSTT may follow a term gestation, a nonmolar abortion, a complete mole, and, in theory, a partial mole. These tumors are mostly diploid and produce very low amounts of beta hCG as well as serum human placental lactogen (HPL). This is due to the presence of intermediate cytotrophoblast cells. There is an increased proportion of free beta hCG. These tumors stain for HPL, B1-glycoprotein, and Ki-67. PSTT's grows slowly and can be seen years after any type of pregnancy. It can produce a nephrotic syndrome or hematuria. The prognosis depends on the time until diagnosis; if it presents less than 4 years since a pregnancy, the prognosis is better than if later. FIGO scoring is not used to determine treatment of PSTT. These tumor present with lung metastases in 10-29% of cases and 10% of patients develop metastases during followup. Treatment is recommended with hysterectomy and LND—ovarian conservation does not adversely affect outcomes. Adjuvant chemotherapy is recommended for: metastatic disease (also surgically remove primary tumor site) and for adverse prognostic factors such as interval from last known pregnancy greater than 2 years, deep myometrial invasion, tumor necrosis, mitotic count greater than 6/10 HPF. Recommended chemotherapy regimens are: EMA-EP or paclitaxel/cisplatin-paclitaxel/etoposide doublet.
- Quiescent GTD is the state of elevated beta hCG without documented hyperglycosylated hCG. There has never been a documented case of quiescent GTD with a beta hCG level that is higher than 230 mIU/mL. In this disease state, the residual mole lacks a cytotrophoblastic cell population. Therefore, there is no hyperglycosylated hCG production, and as a result, no invasion. Usually the residual mass of tissue dies after 6 months. In 10.4% of cases, however, quiescent GTD can activate and lead to persistent trophoblastic disease. Therefore, when a hyperglycosylated hCG is detected, the patient should be treated with chemotherapy. This is similar to a low malignant potential tumor. There are some data to suggest waiting to treat until a threshold beta hCG level of 3,000 mIU/mL is detected (1,2).
- Epithelioid trophoblastic tumor (ETT) is an extremely rare subtype derived from chorionic type intermediate trophoblast cells. Treatment is best with hysterectomy and LN dissection. Chemotherapy is recommended in addition to surgery for metastatic disease (after removal of the primary tumor site), and for adverse prognostic factors such as interval from last known pregnancy greater than 2 years, deep myometrial invasion, tumor necrosis, mitotic count greater than 6/10 HPF. EMA-EP or the paclitaxel/cisplatin-paclitaxel/etoposide doublet are chemotherapy options.

DIAGNOSIS

- Diagnosis of a mole is by ultrasound and serum beta hCG level. Invasive hydatidiform mole/GTD occurs usually after evacuation of a complete mole or partial mole.
- The diagnosis of an invasive mole/GTN is made if there is: persistent beta hCG for 6 months after evacuation of a molar pregnancy, an elevating beta hCG (a 10% rise over three values in 2 weeks), a plateauing beta hCG (a plateau of 10% over four values in 3 weeks), or evidence of metastatic disease (mainly lung). In addition, some may consider the presence of an hCG value greater than 20,000 mIU/mL 4 weeks after evacuation, diagnostic for an invasive mole. It is imperative to perform dual serum and urine hCG testing to rule out phantom hCG, which is due to heterophilic/cross-reacting antibodies in the serum hCG test.

PRE-TREATMENT WORKUP

- The pre-treatment workup of GTD is a pelvic ultrasound (which can document the primary tumor as a uterine mass and give its dimensions) and a chest x-ray. If the chest x-ray is negative, a CT of the chest can be obtained. If the lungs show metastatic disease, it is then necessary to obtain an MRI of the abdomen and the brain. Alternatively, some practitioners routinely obtain a CT of the chest, abdomen, and pelvis for initial evaluation, but only the lesions seen on the CXR should be scored. A urine beta hCG and serum beta hCG both need to be performed to confirm beta hCG presence. Serum laboratories include a quantitative beta hCG and hyperglycosylated hCG, CBC, renal function tests, liver function tests, thyroid function tests, and a physical examination. A lumbar puncture can be considered if central neurologic symptoms are present and the brain MRI is negative. The plasma to CSF ratio of hCG can be less than 60 in cases with cerebral metastasis, but this ratio is not always reliable.
- Repeat D&C is controversial. With a second D&C, the risk of needing chemotherapy is 21%; with a third D&C, the risk of needing chemotherapy more than doubles to 47%, possibly due to hematogenic metastasis induced by curettage (3).

SERUM BETA hCG

- **Serum beta hCG** is a very sensitive and specific marker for trophoblastic tissue and thus a good tumor marker for this disease. The half-life of beta hCG is 24 to 36 hours. The amount of hCG correlates to the amount of viable tissue: 5 mIU/mL is approximately equal to 10,000 to 100,000 viable cells. However, it is also produced by many other carcinomas, including lung cancer, ovarian cancer, and colon cancer. Genetic testing should be performed on refractory tumors to ensure the primary is GTD and not otherwise.

STAGING

- FIGO 2002 staging is **clinical** incorporating WHO risk factors to obtain a final modified FIGO/WHO risk score (Table 2.33 A–C).

Table 2.33A AJCC 8th Edition: T Category

T	FIGO	T Criteria
Tx		Primary tumor cannot be assessed
T0		No evidence of primary tumor
T1	I	Tumor confined to the uterus
T2	II	Tumor extends to other genital structures (ovary, tube, vagina, broad ligaments) by metastasis or direct extension

Table 2.33B AJCC 8th Edition: M Category

M	FIGO	M Criteria
M0		No distant metastasis
M1		Distant metastasis
M1a	III	Lung metastasis
M1b	IV	All other distant metastasis

Table 2.33C AJCC 8th Edition: Stage Grouping

When T is	And M is	The stage is noted with risk factor score to follow:
T1	M0	I: (risk score__)
T2	M0	II: (risk score __)
Any T	M1a	III: (risk score__)
Any T	M1b	IV: (risk score __)

Source: From Amin MB, Edge SB. (2017). *AJCC Cancer Staging Manual* 8th Edition. Chicago, IL: American Joint Committee on Cancer. With permission.

- **Prognostic factors** required for staging: patients are classified into low-risk or high-risk categories of metastatic disease based on the WHO score as calculated in Table 2.33. The scores from eight risk factors are summed and incorporated into the FIGO stage, separated by a colon (e.g., stage III:8). If the score is less than seven, they are considered low risk. If the score is seven or greater, they are considered high risk. The modified WHO prognostic scoring system is not applicable to patients with PSTT or ETT (Tables 2.34 and 2.35).

Table 2.34 WHO Prognostic Scoring System for GTD as Modified by FIGO (2002)

Score	0	1	2	4
Age	≤39	≥40		
Antecedent pregnancy	Mole	Abortion	Term	
Interval months from index pregnancy	<4	4–6	7–12	>12
Pre-treatment serum hCG level (IU/L)	$<10^3$	10^3–10^4	10^4–10^5	$>10^5$
Largest tumor size including uterus	<3 cm	3–5 cm	>5	
Site of metastasis	Lung	Spleen, kidney	GI	Brain, liver
Number of metastases	–	1–4	5–8	>8
Prior failed chemotherapy drugs	–	–	1	≥2

TREATMENT

- Molar pregnancy GTD:
  - Evacuation via suction D&C is the primary treatment. Some clinicians avoid sharp curettage due to the increased risk of uterine perforation and possible metastasis. If fertility is not desired, a hysterectomy with ovarian preservation can be the primary treatment of a molar pregnancy.
  - Medications such as Prostin have been shown to increase the need for chemotherapy due to hematogenous spread via contraction of the uterine arteries.

Table 2.35 GTD Metastatic Site Rate	
GTD metastatic sites	**Percent**
Lungs	80
Vagina	30
Pelvis	20
Brain	10
Liver	10
Bowel, kidney, spleen	5

Pitocin administered after cervical dilation can assist in uterine involution in addition to expression of uterine contents extracorporeally and not into the vascular system. RhoGAM should be given if the patient is Rh negative.

○ Some patients with molar pregnancies are considered high risk for developing persistent or metastatic disease (Table 2.36). Chemoprophylaxis with a one-time dose of single-agent chemotherapy can be considered. In these patients, data have shown the rates of persistent disease have gone from about 50% to 15%. Chemoprophylaxis in lower-risk patients can also be considered if they are seen as potentially noncompliant.

- Invasive disease/GTN:
  ○ Stage I disease can be managed surgically or with chemotherapy.
    - Surgical management:
      □ A hysterectomy with ovarian preservation can be performed if fertility is not desired. A single dose of either methotrexate or dactinomycin immediately prior to the surgical procedure can be considered for prophylaxis against embolism of tumor cells from surgical manipulation.
      □ A second uterine curettage can be performed in low risk (Score 0–6) patients understanding that there is a high risk of uterine perforation. 38% of patients treated with a second D&C instead of single-agent chemotherapy normalized their hCG within 6 months, avoiding any chemotherapy; and 6.3% were re-catagorized histologically to have PSTT.
    - Single-agent chemotherapy is administered if hysterectomy is not performed. Chemotherapy is either with methotrexate or dactinomycin. The likelihood of success of weekly methotrexate is dependent on the WHO score. Weekly IM methotrexate is successful in 70% of patients with a WHO score of 0–1, but falls to 40% in those with a score of 2–4, and 12% in those who score 5–6. Biweekly pulsed dactinomycin showed a CRR of 44% when the WHO score was 5–6 (10).
  ○ Stage II disease follows the same chemotherapy principles as those of stage I disease.
  ○ Stage III disease is categorized as either low risk or high risk based on WHO risk scoring.
    - If the patient is considered low risk, initial single-agent chemotherapy is administered.
    - If the patient is high risk, combination chemotherapy with EMA-CO should be initiated.

Table 2.36 GTD High-Risk Clinical Features for Metastatic Disease	
Clinical feature	**Percent risk of GTD**
Delayed postmolar evacuation hemorrhage	75%
Theca lutein cysts >5 cm	60%
Acute pulmonary insufficiency following molar evacuation	58%
Uterus large for dates (16-wk size)	45%
Serum hCG >100,000 mIU/mL	45%
Second molar gestation	40%
Maternal age >40	25%

- ○ Stage IV disease is high risk, by definition, and is initially managed with combination chemotherapy. Treatment is usually with EMA-CO, but the methotrexate dose is increased to 1 g/m². If there are cerebral metastases, craniotomy to prevent herniation from mass or hemorrhage may be indicated. Consideration of intrathecal methotrexate or whole brain irradiation to 30 Gy is important. Intrathecal methotrexate is dosed at 12.5 mg, followed in 24 hours with 15–30 mg of oral folinic acid. This is given once with each course of CO during EMA-CO therapy.
- Single-agent chemotherapy is continued for two to three courses beyond normalization of the beta hCG for stages I to III. For high-risk and stage IV disease or a WHO score greater than 12, three to four additional courses are recommended after normalization of the beta hCG level. This is due to data suggesting that 100,000 viable cancer cells remain when the beta hCG becomes undetectable.
- Optimal therapy for PSTT is a hysterectomy with pelvic and para-aortic LN dissection. Ovarian preservation has not been found to be detrimental. This is a relatively chemoresistant tumor, so if the disease is found to be advanced, surgery with adjuvant chemotherapy is likely the best option. Chemotherapy can consist of EMA-EP or EMA-CO. The only prognostic factor identified regarding survival, is time from the last pregnancy. If this time is less than 4 years, patients usually do well; if it is greater than 4 years, this is usually universally fatal.
- ETT is generally more aggressive than PSTT but is treated in a similar fashion.
- Choriocarcinoma by definition is high-risk disease and should be treated with combination EMA-CO therapy.

MANAGEMENT OF ACUTE DISEASE-INDUCED COMPLICATIONS

- If there is uterine hemorrhage, vaginal packing, blood transfusion, and emergent uterine artery embolization can be performed. Laparotomy may be necessary for hysterectomy.
- Respiratory failure either from tumor embolization, pulmonary embolization, tumor burden, or hemorrhage may occur. Mechanical ventilation is contraindicated due to a high risk of trauma and iatrogenic hemorrhage,

but continuous positive airway pressure (CPAP) is a good alternative. Risk factors for respiratory failure are as follows: 50% opacification of lung fields on CXR, dyspnea, anemia, cyanosis, and pulmonary hypertension. Consideration for those with a high thorax tumor burden, to decrease the risk of death from pulmonary hemorrhage or respiratory failure within the first 4 weeks of therapy, is to start with induction etoposide and cisplatin (EP) for one to two cycles, and continue thereafter with EMA-CO. Low-dose induction EP consists of etoposide 100 mg/m^2 and cisplatin 20 mg/m^2 on days 1 and 2 repeating weekly for one to two cycles before starting EMA-CO. High-risk patients receiving EP compared to patients not receiving EP had a higher, but not statistically significant, relapse rate (9% vs. 6% $p = 0.44$) and death rate (12% vs. 4%; $p = 0.88$) (4).

- If cerebral metastases are identified, vigilance for cerebral hemorrhage, edema, and herniation should be maintained. If a solitary lesion is found, site directed versus whole brain radiation therapy (WB-XRT) can be considered. If multiple lesions are identified, WB-XRT is recommended with dosing to 30 Gy in 200 cGy fractions. Premedication with 24 mg of dexamethasone twice daily during treatment with WB-XRT is important. The methotrexate dose in the EMA-CO regimen is increased to 1 g/m^2 and 30 mg of folinic acid every 12 hours for 3 days starting 32 hours after the infusion begins. Surgical excision or stereotactic XRT in selected patients can be given simultaneously with systemic chemotherapy. Cure rates with brain metastasis approach 50% to 80%.

RESISTANT DISEASE

- Diagnosis of resistance to first line therapy in low risk GTN is by: a persistent elevation over 3 consecutive samples, or an increase over 2 consecutive samples lasting > 2 weeks. For patients with a hCG < 100 IU/L, they can be considered for change to single agent dactinomycin after failing methotrexate or they can be treated with EMA-CO. For patients who fail single agent treatment with a hCG level > 100–300 IU/L, they should be treated with combination EMA-CO chemotherapy.
- In stage I resistant disease a switch to the other single-agent chemotherapy drug is indicated. A hysterectomy or local uterine resection may be considered in addition to chemotherapy if there is persistent disease.
- Stage II resistant disease is treated in a similar fashion as that for stage I resistant disease. Hysterectomy with ovarian preservation may be offered if this is the sole site of resistant disease.
- Stage III resistant disease:
  - For stage III low-risk resistant disease, treatment with MAC or EMA-CO should follow single-agent chemotherapy.
  - For high-risk stage III resistant disease, treatment with other regimens is indicated. These include MAC, CHAMOCA, VPB, VIP, or ICE.
- Stage IV resistant disease: second-line combination chemotherapy with MAC, CHAMOCA, VPB, VIP, or ICE is indicated. Hysterectomy with ovarian preservation may be indicated if this appears to be the sole site of resistant disease.

RECURRENT DISEASE

- At diagnosis, reimaging with a CT of the chest, abdomen, and pelvis and MRI of the brain should be obtained. If all are negative, it may be helpful to then perform a lumbar puncture.
- Experimental imaging techniques can be employed to include anti-hCG radio-isotope scanning and PET.
- If there are lung metastases and this appears to be the only site of resistant disease on comprehensive workup, a thoracotomy with lobectomy may be considered. If there are isolated liver metastases, a wedge resection may also be considered.

FOLLOW-UP

- For stages I to III, weekly quantitative beta hCG levels are drawn until they normalize for 3 weeks. Monthly quantitative beta hCG then continue until they are normal for 6–12 consecutive months.
- For stage IV disease it is important to follow beta hCG levels monthly for 2 years after the weekly beta hCG levels have normalized.
- Contraception with oral contraceptive pills (OCPs) (preferably) or another form of reliable contraception is important. Pregnancy may be attempted after 6 to 12 months of normal beta hCGs. IUD's are not recommended due to the risk of uterine perforation.

NOTABLE TRIALS

- GOG 55: 266 patients were randomly assigned to either OCP versus barrier method contraception after molar evacuation. The median time to spontaneous regression in the OCP group was 9 weeks, compared to the median time to regression in the barrier group of 10 weeks. Twice as many patients in the barrier group became pregnant in the immediate follow-up period; 23% of patients receiving OCPs had postmolar trophoblastic disease versus 33% of patients using barrier methods. OCPs are the preferred method of contraception after evacuation of a hydatidiform mole (5).
- GOG 79: patients with nonmetastatic GTD were initially treated with 30 mg/m^2 of weekly IM MTX. If no major toxicity was encountered, the weekly dose was escalated by 5 mg/m^2 at 3-week intervals until a maximum dose of 50 mg/m^2 each week was achieved. 81% had a complete response to weekly IM MTX. Duration of therapy ranged from 3 to 19 weeks, with a median of 7 weeks. No major dose limiting toxicity occurred, thus 50 mg/m^2 is acceptable dosing (6).
- GOG 79 follow-up study: this study evaluated 62 patients with nonmetastatic GTD who were initially treated with 40 mg/m^2 weekly of IM MTX. If no major toxicity was encountered, the weekly dose was escalated by 5 mg/m^2 at 2-week intervals until a maximum dose of 50 mg/m^2 per week was achieved; 74% had a complete response. Duration of therapy ranged from 3 weeks to 16 weeks with a median of 7 weeks. No major toxicity occurred. The 40 mg/m^2 dose of weekly IM MTX therapy is no more effective and of similar toxicity to the 30 mg/m^2 regimen (7).
- GOG 174: this trial evaluated 216 eligible patients with a WHO score of 0 to 6 and metastatic disease limited to lung lesions less than 2 cm, adnexa, or vagina, and/or histologically proven nonmetastatic choriocarcinoma. Patients were

randomized to either biweekly IV actinomycin D 1.25 mg/m^2 versus weekly IM methotrexate 30 mg/m^2. Biweekly actinomycin D was superior to weekly methotrexate (CR 70% vs. 53%; p = 0.03). If the risk score was 5 to 6, or the diagnosis was choriocarcinoma, the CR to methotrexate was 9% and the CR was 42% with actinomycin D. Primary chemotherapy should then consist of actinomycin D in these intermediate and high-risk patients (8).

- GOG 242: this was a phase II study evaluating efficacy and safety of second uterine curettage in low risk nonmetastatic gestational trophoblastic neoplasia (GTN). 64 patients were enrolled and 24 (40%) were cured after second curettage without need for any chemotherapy. One uterine perforation occurred. Surgical failure occurred in 59% of women and was found more commonly in the age extremes. Four uterine hemorrhages occurred, and one new lung metastasis was observed. At the second curettage, histopathologic discrepancy changed the diagnosis (PSTT and placental nodule) for four patients. Higher WHO score trended to lower rate of second curettage cure (9).
- GOG 275: a phase III randomized trial of pulse actinomycin-D versus multiday methotrexate for the management of low risk GTN. This is an international phase III randomized trial of pulse actinomycin D versus multiday methotrexate for treatment of low-risk GTN. Results pending.

REFERENCES

1. Cole LA, Muller CY. Hyperglycosylated hCG in the management of quiescent and chemorefractory gestational trophoblastic diseases. *Gynecol Oncol.* 2010;116(1):3–9.
2. Cole LA, Laidler LL, Muller CY. USA hCG reference service, 10-year report. *Clin Biochem.* 2010;43(12):1013–1022.
3. Pezeshki M, Hancock BW, Silcocks P, et al. The role of repeat uterine evacuation in the management of persistent gestational trophoblastic disease. *Gynecol Oncol.* 2004;95(3):423–429.
4. Alifrangis C, Agarwal R, Short D, et al. EMA/CO for high-risk gestational trophoblastic neoplasia: good outcomes with induction low-dose etoposide–cisplatin and genetic analysis. *J Clin Oncol.* January 10, 2013;31(2):280–286.
5. Curry SL, Schlaerth JB, Kohorn EI, et al. Hormonal contraception and trophoblastic sequelae after hydatidiform mole (a Gynecologic Oncology Group study). *Am J Obstet Gynecol.* 1989;160(4):805–809; discussion 809–811.
6. Homesley HD, Blessing JA, Rettenmaier M, et al. Weekly intramuscular methotrexate for nonmetastatic gestational trophoblastic disease. *Obstet Gynecol.* 1988;72(3)(pt 1): 413–418.
7. Homesley HD, Blessing JA, Schlaerth J, et al. Rapid escalation of weekly intramuscular methotrexate for nonmetastatic gestational trophoblastic disease: a Gynecologic Oncology Group study. *Gynecol Oncol.* 1990;39(3):305–308.
8. Osborne RJ, Filiaci V, Schink JC, et al. Phase III trial of weekly methotrexate or pulsed dactinomycin for low-risk gestational trophoblastic neoplasia: a Gynecologic Oncology Group study. *J Clin Oncol.* 2011;29(7):825–831.
9. Osborne RJ, Filiaci VL, Schink JC, et al. Second curettage for low-risk nonmetastatic gestational trophoblastic neoplasia. *Obstet Gynecol.* September 2016;128(3):535–542.
10. Brown J, Naumann RW, Sekl MJ et al. 15 years of progress in gestational trophoblastic disease: scoring, standardization, and salvage. *Gynecol Oncol.* 2017;144:200–207.

HEREDITARY CANCER SYNDROMES

3

Hereditary Breast and Ovarian Cancers

- Hereditary breast and ovarian cancers (HBOC) is usually attributed to the *BRCA* mutations 1 and 2. The genetic mutation is found on chromosomes 17q21 and 13q12–13 for *BRCA1* and *BRCA2*, respectively, and 80% of patients have a frame shift mutation. The mutation causes a defect in double stranded (DS) DNA repair and E3 ubiquitination. Inheritance is autosomal dominant and *BRCA* is known to be a tumor suppressor gene. Up to 30% of ovarian cancers have a genetic mutation. Many are found in the Fanconi anemia pathway. These mutated genes include: *Rad50/51/51C/51D, BRIP1, BARD1, CHEK2, MRE11A, MSH2, MLH1, MSH6, PMS2, PPM1Df, POLE, POL-D1, PALB2, 17SNPs, NBN, PALB2, TP53* (1).
- The lifetime risk of HGSTOC for *BRCA1* is 25% to 40% and for *BRCA2* is 18% to 27%. Penetrance ranges from 41% to 90% for lifetime risk. Penetrance, by definition, is the net risk in the absence of any competing risks. In the Ashkenazi Jewish population the *BRCA* mutation risk is 1/40 compared to the general population risk: *BRCA1*: 1/300; *BRCA2*: 1/800. For patients who are found to harbor *BRCA1* or *2* mutations, bilateral salpingo-oophorectomy (BSO) is recommended between the ages of 35 and 40, or when childbearing is completed. Primary fallopian tube cancer (PFTC) is seen in 2% to 17% of patients at the time of risk-reducing salpingo-oophorectomy (RRSO).
- The risk reduction for HGSTOC is with RRBSO over 80%, but there is still an inherent risk of primary peritoneal cancer, possibly due to unrecognized serous tubal intraepithelial carcinoma (STIC), which is 2% to 4.3%. Oral contraceptive pills (OCPs) administered for at least 6 years can provide a 60% risk reduction for HGSTOC for *BRCA*-positive patients (2).
- The presence of a *BRCA* mutation has been found to alter disease prognosis: the DFI after chemotherapy was 14 months for mutation carriers versus 7 months in sporadic cancer patients. The complete response (CR) was found to be 3.2 times higher if the patient was *BRCA* positive. The overall survival (OS) was found to be 101 months in *BRCA* carriers versus 51 months in sporadic cancer patients. The age of onset for patients who are *BRCA1* positive was 52 years.
- Oophorectomy may decrease the incidence of breast cancer for both *BRCA1* and *2* carriers. *BRCA*-positive women are recommended to undergo a BSO by age 40 or after childbearing is completed. *BRCA1* breast cancers are often ER negative and commonly are triple negative (ER, PR, *Her-2-neu* negative). The risk of breast cancer was decreased 56% in *BRCA1* patients who underwent a BSO, and was decreased 46% in *BRCA2* patients. There was an increase in risk reduction from breast cancer the earlier the BSO was performed (3).
- Patients who have *BRCA* mutations are categorized as "high risk." If these patients do not opt for surgical management, chemoprophylaxis with OCPs

or bilateral salpingectomy, and delayed oophorectomy can be considered. Screening with every 6- to 12-month pelvic examinations, transvaginal ultrasound, and serum CA-125 levels has not proven beneficial.

- Adnexal neoplasia is found in 5% to 6% of RRSO (high-risk women). Recurrent/metastatic disease has been seen in up to 9% of women with STIC alone. The lag time from a diagnosis of STIC to pelvic recurrence was 4 years (4).
- For those women who undergo RRSO: the Sectioning and Extensively Examining the FIMbriated End (SEE-FIM) of the Fallopian Tube pathological protocol should be applied to their tubes. The tubes should be examined at 5 micrometer sections per 2 mm thick tissue block; as occult STIC may measure 1 mm or less.
- If diagnosed with unilateral breast cancer, the cumulative risk for contralateral breast cancer by age 70 is 83% for *BRCA1* and 62% for *BRCA2*.
- Genetic screening is recommended for:
  - Histologically proven HGSTOC.
  - Individual from a family with a known *BRCA 1/2* deleterious mutation.
  - An individual with breast cancer diagnosis meeting any of the following:
    - Breast cancer at:
      - An early age of ≤45 or
      - Age ≤50 years and an additional breast cancer primary, ≥1 close blood relative with breast cancer at any age, ≥1 close relative with pancreatic cancer, ≥1 relative with prostate cancer (Gleason score ≥7), or an unknown or limited family history
      - Age ≤60 years with triple negative breast cancer
    - Diagnosed at any age and has ≥1 close blood relative with breast cancer ≤50 years, or ≥1 close blood relative with invasive HGSTOC at any age, or ≥2 close blood relatives with breast cancer and/or pancreatic cancer at any age, or and/or prostate cancer (Gleason score ≥7) from a population at increased risk
  - Personal history of pancreatic cancer at any age with ≥1 close relative with breast cancer ≤50 and/or invasive HGSTOC at any age, or two relatives with breast, pancreatic cancer, or prostate cancer (Gleason score ≥7) at any age.
  - Personal history of pancreatic cancer and Ashkenazi Jewish ancestry.
  - An individual with no personal history of cancer but with a family history of any of the following:
    - A known mutation in a cancer susceptibility gene within the family, ≥2 breast cancer primaries in a single individual, ≥2 individuals with breast cancer primaries on the same side of the family, ≥1 invasive HGSTOC primary, first or second degree relative with breast cancer ≤46 years old.
    - BRCA1/2 mutation detected by tumor profiling in the absence of germline mutation analysis.
  - Personal and/or family history of three or more of the following: pancreatic cancer, prostate cancer (Gleason score >7); sarcoma; adrenocortical carcinoma; brain tumors; endometrial cancer; thyroid cancer; kidney cancer; dermatologic manifestations and/or macrocephaly; hamartomatous polyps of the gastrointestinal (GI) tract; diffuse gastric cancer; invasive HGSTOC male breast cancer are indications for further genetic risk evaluation.

- If HBOC testing criteria are met: order genetic testing with informed consent:
  - If the deleterious familial mutations is/are known, then test for that specific mutation.
  - If a mutation is not known, then comprehensive *BRCA* gene testing of the patient or proband is recommended, or multigene testing.
- Screening and risk reduction:
  - Breast awareness counseling to start at age 18.
  - Clinical breast exam every 8 to 12 months starting at age 25; annual breast MRI or mammogram if MRI not available ages 25 to 30; annual mammogram and breast MRI screening QO6-12m ages 30 to 75; after age 75, individualize testing/management.
  - If treated for breast cancer, screening of remaining breast tissue with annual mammography and breast MRI should continue.
  - Consider risk-reducing mastectomy to include reconstruction options after completion of breast feeding. If declines: tamoxifen prophylaxis should be initiated.
  - Consider RRSO between ages 35 and 40 or after completion of childbearing. If declines: OCP prophylaxis should be initiated. Salpingectomy alone is not the standard of care. The concern is that women are still at risk for developing ovarian cancer. In premenopausal women, oophorectomy reduces the risk of developing breast cancer by 60%. Interval salpingectomy followed by oophorectomy (a staged procedure) can be considered if patients are highly concerned of early surgical menopause.
  - Management of menopausal symptoms (try to not use hormonal therapies): selective serotonin reuptake inhibitors (SSRIs), clonidine, belladonna, and other therapies.
- There was a 25% incidence of germline *BRCA1* and *2* mutations identified when a histology-based referral specific to high-grade serous ovarian subtypes was employed. This suggests the genetic assessment of all women diagnosed with high-grade serous carcinoma will improve detection rates and capture mutation carriers otherwise missed by referral based on family history alone (5).
- A 2% rate of *BRCA1* mutations was identified in uterine serous cancer patients. This is compared to the 0.06% rate of *BRCA1* mutations in the general population. Nine percent of women with a history of breast cancer, and then uterine serous cancer (USC), had a *BRCA1/2* mutation. Hysterectomy can be discussed in patients with *BRCA1* mutations although this is less than the accepted positive predictive value (6).
- Pregenetic screening, counseling, and testing can be offered to those considering children.

HEREDITARY NONPOLYPOSIS COLON CANCER

- **Characteristics: hereditary nonpolyposis colon cancer** (HNPCC) can contribute to about 10% of hereditary ovarian cancers. HNPCC is also called **Lynch II syndrome**. There is an increase in colon, endometrial, ovarian, pancreatic, central nervous system (CNS) and urothelial cancers. The mutations responsible for these cancers are *MLH1, MSH2, MSH6, PMS1, PMS2,* and *EPCAm* gene deletion. These mutations cause defects in DNA mismatch repair mechanisms.

60% of the cancers present as colon cancer, and 60% present as endometrial cancer. 20–30% of uterine cancers have *MLH1* silenced by noninherited methylation of the *MLH1* promoter.

- The 2004 **HNPCC Bethesda Guidelines** were modified to include endometrial cancer as a sentinel cancer. **Bethesda Guidelines for Lynch Syndrome (LS):** this guides tumor testing for microsatellite instability (MSI) in individuals with the following:
  - Diagnosed in a patient who is younger than 50 years of age.
  - Presence of synchronous, or metachronous, colorectal cancer (CRC) or other LS-related tumors, regardless of age.
  - CRC with IHC deficient MSI histology diagnosed in a patient who is younger than 60 years of age.
  - CRC diagnosed in a patient with one or more first-degree relatives with an LS-related cancer with one of the cancers being diagnosed before age 50 years.
  - CRC diagnosed in a patient with two or more first- or second-degree relatives with LS-related cancers regardless of age.
- **Amsterdam Criteria I:** at least three relatives with CRC; all of the following criteria should be present:
  - One should be a first-degree relative of the other two.
  - At least two successive generations must be affected.
  - At least one of the relatives with CRC must have received the diagnosis before the age of 50 years.
  - Familial adenomatous polyposis (FAP) should be excluded.
  - Tumors should be verified by pathologic examination.
- **Amsterdam Criteria II:** at least three relatives must have a cancer associated with LS (colorectal, cancer of endometrium, small bowel, ureter, or renal-pelvis); all of the following criteria should be present:
  - One must be a first-degree relative of the other two.
  - At least two successive generations must be affected.
  - At least one relative with cancer associated with LS should be diagnosed before age 50 years.
  - FAP should be excluded in the CRC case(s) (if any).
  - Tumors should be pathologically verified whenever possible.
- Patients should be screened for Lynch/HNPCC syndrome if:
  - They have an endometrial or ovarian cancer and have a synchronous or metachronous colon or other Lynch/HNPCC-associated tumors at any age to include: stomach, ovarian, pancreas, ureter, renal pelvis, biliary tract, brain glioblastoma as seen in Turcot syndrome, sebaceous gland adenomas and keratoacanthomas in Muir-Torre syndrome, carcinoma of the small bowel.
  - Patients with colorectal cancer with tumor infiltrating lymphocytes, peritumoral lymphocytes, Crohn-like lymphocytic reaction, mucinous/signet-ring differentiation, or medullary growth pattern diagnosed before the age of 60.
  - Patients with endometrial or colorectal cancer and a first-degree relative with a Lynch/HNPCC-associated tumor diagnosed before the age of 50.
  - Patients with colorectal or endometrial cancer diagnosed at any age with two or more first degree or second degree relatives with Lynch/HNPCC-associated tumors regardless of age.

- Genetic testing is for the gene **mutations** of *MLH1, MSH2, MSH6, PMS1, PMS2,* and *EPCAm* gene deletion if a familial defective gene has not been identified. Immunohistochemistry can be a first-line approach on the pathological specimen and provide baseline mutation information on the tumor itself.
- **Screening tests** and **risk reduction** usually start around age 25 years old. Screening can be divided by the type of mutation carried if identified.
  ○ *MLH1, MSH2,* and *EPCAM* **mutation carriers**:
    - Colonoscopy should start between ages 20 and 25 years old, or 2 to 5 years prior to the earliest diagnosed proband. Screening should occur every 1 to 2 years.
    - Prophylactic hysterectomy with BSO is a risk-reducing option in women. Annual endometrial biopsy (EMB) beginning at age 30 to 35 is recommended for those not having completed childbearing. Any abnormal uterine bleeding should be investigated. Progestin-based contraception should be used to decrease malignant transformation of reproductive organs.
    - Consider prophylactic total colectomy as an alternative to surveillance colonoscopy for individuals with confirmed mutations. Because of incomplete penetrance, 15% to 20% of these procedures may be unnecessary, but this risk reduction option can be discussed.
    - There are no data to support annual ovarian ultrasound and serum CA-125.
    - Esophagogastroduodenoscopy (EGD) with extended duodenoscopy should be considered every 2 to 3 years beginning at age 30 to 35 years.
    - Urinalysis should start at age 25 to 30 years and continue annually.
    - A CNS annual physical examination should also start at age 25 to 30 years, but no imaging recommendations have been made.
  ○ *MSH6* and *PMS2* carriers.
    - Colonoscopy age 25 to 30 or 2 to 5 years prior to the earliest proband colon cancer if diagnosed before age 30 and repeat every 1 to 2 years.
    - Endometrial and ovarian cancer surveillance is the same as for *MLH1, MSH2,* and *EPCAm* mutation carriers.
  ○ Pregenetic screening counseling and testing should be offered for those considering children.

LI-FRAUMENI SYNDROME

- **Characteristics:** Li-Fraumeni syndrome (LFS) occurs in individuals with a mutation in the gene *TP53*. Tumors in the LFS spectrum include soft tissue sarcoma, osteosarcoma, brain tumor, breast cancer, adrenocortical carcinoma, leukemia, and lung bronchoalveolar cancer. There are two sets of criteria for inclusion.
  ○ Classic criteria to include: the combination of an individual diagnosed at age less than 45 with cancer sarcoma, and a first or second degree relative diagnosed at age less than 45 with cancer, and an additional first or second degree relative with cancer diagnosed at age less than 45 or a sarcoma diagnosed at any age.

- ○ Chompret criteria: an individual with a tumor from the LFS tumor spectrum before age 46 and
    - ▪ At least one first or second degree relative with any of the aforementioned cancers (other than breast cancer if the proband had breast cancer) before the age of 56 years or with multiple primaries at any age, or
    - ▪ An individual with multiple tumors (except multiple breast tumors), two of which belong with the LFS tumor spectrum with the initial cancer occurring before age 46, or
    - ▪ An individual with adrenocortical carcinoma or choroid plexus carcinoma at any age of onset regardless of the family history
    - ▪ Early age (≤31 years old) onset of breast cancer
- Genetic testing should be offered if: the above criteria are met. T test is for the deleterious familial *TP53* **mutation** if known, or with comprehensive *TP53* testing of the patient or proband. *TP53* testing can be ordered alone, concurrently with *BRCA1/2* testing and other gene testing, or as a follow-up test if *BRCA1/2* testing is negative as part of multigene testing panels.
- **Screening and risk reduction**: if a *TP53* mutation is identified:
  - ○ Breast cancer screening to follow the same as HBOC patients
  - ○ Other cancer risks:
    - ▪ Alert pediatricians of the risk of childhood cancers in affected families
    - ▪ Annual comprehensive physical exam to include neurologic exam
    - ▪ Avoid therapeutic radiation therapy (XRT) when possible
    - ▪ Consider colonoscopy every 2 to 5 years starting at age 25 or 5 years before the earliest known colon cancer in the family
    - ▪ Annual dermatologic exam
    - ▪ Annual whole body noncontrast-MRI per American College of Radiology Imaging Network (ACRIN) model
    - ▪ Brain MRI annually
    - ▪ Pregenetic screening counseling and testing for patients considering children

COWDEN'S DISEASE/*PTEN* HAMARTOMA TUMOR SYNDROME

- **Characteristics:** the lifetime risk for cancer in Cowden's disease varies by site. For breast cancer, the risk is 25% to 50% at age 38 to 50 years; for thyroid cancer 30% to 68%. The cumulative lifetime estimate for any cancer is 89%. Criteria for inclusion:
  - ○ Individual from a family with a known *PTEN* mutation or
  - ○ Individual with a personal history of Bannayan-Riley-Ruvalcaba syndrome (BRRS).
  - ○ Individual meeting clinical diagnostic criteria for Cowden's Disease/*PTEN* hamartoma tumor syndrome (CS/PHTS).
  - ○ For an individual not meeting clinical diagnostic criteria for CD/PHTS with a personal history of:
    - ▪ Adult Lhermitte–Duclos disease (cerebellar tumors) or
    - ▪ Autism spectrum disorder and macrocephaly
    - ▪ Two or more biopsy proven trichilemmomas or
    - ▪ Two or more major criteria (one must be macrocephaly) or

- Three major criteria without macrocephaly or
- One major and ≥ three minor criteria or
- ≥4 minor criteria.
  - Age less than 45 at onset of breast cancer.
  - Triple negative breast cancer at age less than 60 years old.
  - Two breast cancer primaries in a single individual.
  - Breast cancer at any age and more than one relative with breast cancer less than 50 years old, more than one relative with invasive ovarian cancer, more than two relatives with breast and/or pancreatic cancer at any age, or from a population at increased risk.
  - Personal or family history of three or more of the following: pancreatic, prostate, sarcoma, adrenocortical carcinomas, brain tumors, endometrial cancer, thyroid cancer, kidney cancer, dermatologic manifestations, and/or macrocephaly, hamartomatous polyps of the GI tract, diffuse gastric cancer.
  - Individual meeting clinical diagnostic criteria for CD/PHTS or
  - Individual with a personal history of
    - Bannayan-Riley-Ruvalcaba syndrome
    - Adult Lhermitte–Duclos disease (cerebellar tumors)
    - Autism spectrum disorder and macrocephaly or
    - Two or more biopsy proven trichilemmomas
    - Two or more major criteria (one must be macrocephaly) or
    - Three major criteria without macrocephaly
    - One major and greater than three minor criteria
    - ≥4 minor criteria (Table 3.1)

Table 3.1 Major and Minor Criteria for Cowden's Disease

Major criteria	Minor criteria
Breast cancer	Autism spectrum disorder
Endometrial cancer	Colon cancer
Follicular thyroid cancer	Esophageal glycogenic acanthoses (≥3)
Multiple GI hamartomas or ganglioneuromas	Lipomas (≥3)
Macrocephaly (i.e., >97% or 58 cm in adult women)	Intellectual disability (i.e., IQ ≤75)
Mucocutaneous lesions	Thyroid structural lesions (adenoma, nodules, goiter)
Multiple trichilemmomas (≥3, with one biopsy proven)	Papillary or follicular variant of papillary thyroid cancer
Multiple (≥3) acral/palmoplantar keratosis, pits, or papules	Renal cell carcinoma
Mucocutaneous neuromas (≥3)	Single GI hamartoma or ganglioneuroma
Multifocal or extensive oral mucosal papillomatosis (≥3) or biopsy proven or dermatologist diagnosed	Vascular anomalies
Multiple cutaneous facial papules (often verrucous)	

GI, gastrointestinal.

- The genetic **mutation** for this disease is in the *PTEN* gene. There are familial mutations. If the known familial mutation is not identified, then comprehensive *PTEN* testing of the patient, or, if unaffected, testing of the family member with the highest likelihood of a mutation can be performed. Consideration of multigene testing, if appropriate, can be done.
- Screening and risk reduction:
  - Annual comprehensive physical exam starting at age 18 or 5 years before the youngest age of diagnosis of the proband.
  - Breast awareness and counseling starting at age 18. Clinical breast exam every 8 to 12 months starting at age 25. Annual breast MRI (or mammogram if MRI not available) ages 25 to 28. Mammogram and breast MRI screening every 6 to 12 months ages 30 to 75. After age 75, individualize breast testing/management. For women with a *PTEN* mutation who are treated for breast cancer, screening of remaining breast tissue with annual mammography and breast MRI should continue. Risk-reducing mastectomy with reconstruction options should be considered.
  - Risk-reducing BSO between ages 35 and 40 and after completion of childbearing should be considered. RRSO with interval bilateral oophorectomy can also be considered. Management of menopausal symptoms. Avoid using hormonal therapies.
  - Endometrial cancer screening: education for prompt response to symptoms (abnormal or postmenopausal bleeding [PMPB]). Consider annual EMB and/or pelvic ultrasound beginning at age 30 to 35 years old. Discuss options of risk-reducing hysterectomy.
  - Annual thyroid ultrasound starting at the time of PHTS diagnosis.
  - Colonoscopy starting at age 35 unless symptomatic: colonoscopy should be done every 5 years or more frequently if symptomatic or if polyps are found.
  - Renal ultrasound starting at age 40, then every 1 to 2 years.
  - Dermatologic screening.
  - Consider psychomotor assessment in children at diagnosis and brain MRI if symptomatic.
  - Pregenetic screening counseling and testing for those interested children.
- Additional cancer risks:
  - Hereditary diffuse gastric cancer syndrome (*CDH1* gene) yielding a risk of 67% to 83%.
  - Lobular cancer of the breast yielding a 39% to 52% risk.

PEUTZ-JEGHERS SYNDROME (PJS)

- Characteristics of this syndrome are breast cancer with a 44% to 50% risk, ovarian cancer 18% to 21% risk (with sex cord tumors the most common), and hamartomatous polyps and lips.
- A clinical diagnosis of PJS can be made when an individual has two or more of the following features:
  - Two or more Peutz–Jeghers-type hamartomatous polyps of the small intestine.
  - Mucocutaneous hyperpigmentation of the mouth, lips, nose, eyes, genitalia, or fingers.
  - Family history of PJS.

- The *STK11/LKB1* is the main gene mutation
- Screening and risk reduction:
  - Breast cancer: there is a 45% to 50% lifetime risk. Mammogram and annual breast MRI with clinical breast exam is recommended every 6 alternating months starting at age 25 years old.
  - Colon cancer: there is a 39% lifetime risk and colonoscopy every 2 to 3 years is recommended starting in the late teens.
  - Stomach cancer: there is a 29% lifetime risk. Upper endoscopy is recommended every 2 to 3 years starting in the late teens.
  - Small intestine cancer: there is a 13% lifetime risk. Small bowel visualization with CT or MRI enterography. A baseline test should be obtained at 8 to 10 years old with follow-up interval based on findings but at least by age 18, then every 2 to 3 years, or with symptoms.
  - Pancreatic cancer: there is an 11% to 36% lifetime risk. Magnetic resonance cholangiopancreatography or endoscopic ultrasound should be obtained every 1 to 2 years starting at age 30 to 35.
  - Gynecologic cancers: pelvic examination and Pap smear can be performed annually starting around ages 18 to 20.
    - Ovary. There is an 18% to 21% lifetime risk.
    - Cervix: there is a 10% lifetime risk.
    - Uterus: there is a 9% lifetime risk.
  - Lung: there is a 15% to 17% lifetime risk. Education about symptoms and smoking cessation should be provided. No other specific recommendations have been made.
  - Pregenetic screening, counseling, and testing can be offered to those considering children.

EFFECTIVENESS OF SCREENING AND RISK REDUCTION RECOMMENDATIONS

- MRI:
  - MRI is recommended if there is greater than 20% risk of breast cancer with any identified gene mutations or genetic syndromes.
  - The sensitivity of MRI is 77% to 94% compared to the sensitivity of mammography at 33% to 65% in the detection of breast cancer.
- Risk-reducing surgery:
  - Risk-reducing mastectomy: decreases risk by 90%.
  - RRBSO: there is an 80% reduction in ovarian cancer: there is a reduction in breast cancer risk by 50%—the younger the age at which a woman has a BSO, the lower the rates of breast cancer.
- Chemoprevention:
  - Tamoxifen: *BRCA* + women with breast cancer have a 40% chance of contralateral breast cancer at 10 years. Tamoxifen has been shown to be protective with OR = 0.38 to 0.5 for *BRCA1* mutation carriers and 0.42 to 0.63 for *BRCA2* mutation carriers.
  - OCP use: the risk reduction for *BRCA1* carriers was 45% to 50% and 60% for *BRCA2* carriers (Table 3.2).

Table 3.2 Common Cancer Gene Mutations and Risk of Ovarian Cancer

Gene	Prevalence among cases	Risk of ovarian cancer	Average age of onset
BRCA1	8%	40%	50
BRCA2	5%	20%	57
MSH2, MLH1, MSH6, PMS2	0.8%	8%	47
RAD51C	1%	9%	60
PPM1Df	1.5%	25%	69
BRIP1		Increased risk	45–50
RAD51D		Increased risk	45–50
17SNP		4% with multiple alleles	
STK11		Increased risk nonepithelial ovarian cancer	

REFERENCES

1. Walsh T, Casadei S, Lee MK, et al. Mutations in 12 genes for inherited ovarian, fallopian tube, and peritoneal carcinoma identified by massively parallel sequencing. *Proc Natl Acad Sci USA.* 2011;108(44):18032-18037. doi:10.1073/pnas.1115052108

2. Narod SA, Risch H, Moslehi R, et al. Oral contraceptives and the risk of hereditary ovarian cancer. Hereditary Ovarian Cancer Clinical Study Group. *N Engl J Med.* 1998;339(7): 424-428.

3. Eisen A, Lubinski J, Klijn J, et al. Breast cancer risk following bilateral oophorectomy in BRCA1 and BRCA2 mutation carriers: an international case-control study. *J Clin Oncol.* 2005;23(30):7491-7496.

4. Conner JR, Meserve E, Pizer E, et al. Outcome of unexpected adnexal neoplasia discovered during risk reduction salpingo-oophorectomy in women with germ-line BRCA1 or BRCA2 mutations. *Gynecol Oncol.* 2014;132(2):280-286.

5. Schrader KA, Hurlburt J, Kalloger SE, et al. Germline BRCA1 and BRCA2 mutations in ovarian cancer: utility of a histology-based referral strategy. *Obstet Gynecol.* 2012;120(2) (pt 1):235-240.

6. Pennington KP, Walsh T, Lee M, et al. BRCA1, TP53, and CHEK2 germline mutations in uterine serous carcinoma. *Cancer.* 2013;119(2):332-338.

SURGICAL CARE FOR GYNECOLOGIC CANCERS 4

Anatomy

LAYERS OF THE ABDOMEN

Layers of the abdomen (from superficial to deep): skin, Camper's fascia, Scarpa's fascia, deep fascia (composed of the aponeuroses of the external oblique, internal oblique, and transversus muscles). The transversalis fascia lies below the transversus muscle. Superior to the arcuate line, the internal oblique aponeurosis splits to envelop the rectus abdominis muscle. Inferior to the arcuate line, the internal oblique and transversus abdominis aponeuroses merge and pass superficial (i.e., anteriorly) to the rectus muscle (Figure 4.1).

LIGAMENTS

- Infundibulopelvic: contains ovarian vessels and nerves
- Round: originates from the uterine cornua, passes through the inguinal ring, the inguinal canal, and inserts into the labia majora. The male counterpart to

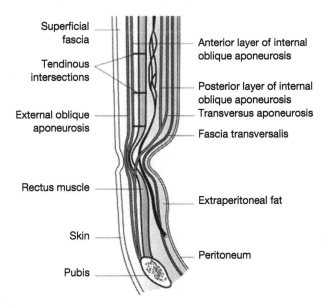

Figure 4.1 The layers of the anterior abdominal wall in transverse section.

Source: From Farthing A. Clinical anatomy of the pelvis and reproductive tract. In: *Dewhurst's Textbook of Obstetrics & Gynaecology*, Eighth Edition, Edmonds DK, ed.

© 2012 John Wiley and Sons, Ltd. Published 2012 by John Wiley and Sons, Ltd.

this ligament is the gubernaculum testis. A small evagination of peritoneum (canal of Nuck) accompanies the round ligament through the inguinal ring.

- Utero-ovarian: these contain the utero-ovarian vessels between the ovary and the uterus. They represent the proximal portion of the gubernaculum testis.
- Cardinal (Mackenrodt's ligaments): located laterally to the cervix, they originate from thickening of the endopelvic fascia. They are the main support for pelvic organs.
- Uterosacral: located posterior to the cervix, they originate from thickening of the endopelvic fascia. They insert on the anterior surface of S2 to S4.

VASCULATURE

- Ovarian vessels: travel through the infundibulopelvic ligaments. The ovarian arteries arise from the abdominal aorta, below the renal arteries. The left ovarian vein drains to the left renal vein. The right ovarian vein drains to the inferior vena cava (Figure 4.2).
- Artery of Sampson: travels through the round ligament

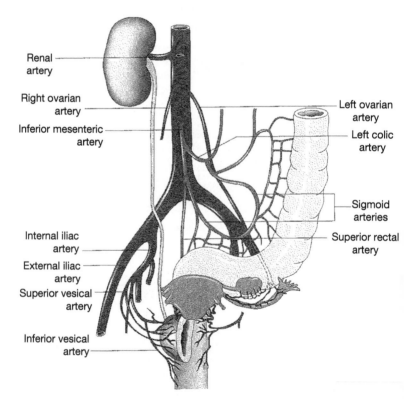

Figure 4.2 Abdomino-pelvic arterial distributions.

Source: From Holschneider CH, et al. Cytoreductive surgery: pelvis and radical oophorectomy. In: *Surgery for Ovarian Cancer, Third Edition,* Bristow RE, et al., eds. Boca Raton, FL: Taylor & Francis Group; 2016.

- External iliac artery and vein: become the femoral vessels after they pass under the inguinal ligament. There are two branches of the external iliac artery and vein: the deep circumflex iliac and the inferior epigastric.
- The internal iliac artery and vein are also known as the hypogastric. Branches of the internal iliac artery:
  o Posterior division: iliolumbar, lateral sacral (superior and inferior), superior gluteal
  o Anterior division: inferior gluteal, internal pudendal, obturator, middle rectal, uterine, vaginal, inferior vesical, superior vesical, obliterated umbilical
- Branches of the celiac trunk: left gastric, common hepatic (branches: right gastric, gastroduodenal), splenic
- Omental blood supply: right and left gastroepiploics, from the gastro-duodenal and splenic vessels, respectively
- Short gastric arteries originate from the splenic artery
- Marginal artery of Drummond: collateral blood supply for the large bowel
- Blood supply to bowel is from two main arteries, the superior and inferior mesenteric arteries.
  o Superior mesenteric artery (SMA) supplies the:
    ▪ Small bowel is supplied by the SMA
    ▪ Right colon is supplied by right colic and ileocolic arteries which are branches of the SMA
    ▪ Appendix: ileocolic branch of the SMA
    ▪ Transverse colon: middle colic branch of the SMA
  o Inferior mesenteric artery (IMA) supplies the:
    ▪ Descending colon: left colic branch of the IMA
    ▪ Sigmoid colon and rectum: sigmoid arteries, superior hemorrhoidal artery branches of the IMA

NERVES

The following nerves are composed of contributing spinal nerve roots:
- Brachial plexus: C5, C6, C7, C8, and T1
  o Injury can cause paresthesias of the radial, ulnar, or median nerves.
  o Etiology of injury is from traction on the extended arm or neck.
- Genitofemoral nerve: L1 and L2
  o It arises on the medial border of the psoas muscle. It is a sensory nerve to the medial thigh, and motor innervation to the cremaster muscle.
  o Injury can cause paresthesia or anesthesia of the labia or skin of the superior thigh.
  o Etiology of injury is transection or traction of the nerve along the psoas muscle.
- Ilioinguinal nerve: L1
  o It arises on the anterior abdominal wall between the internal oblique and transversus abdominis muscles. It supplies the skin over the pubic symphysis.
  o Injury can cause paresthesia or anesthesia of the lower abdomen. Etiology of injury is commonly from scar fibrosis.

- Lateral femoral cutaneous nerve: L2 and L3
  - Injury can cause paresthesia or anesthesia to the anterior and lateral thigh.
- Femoral nerve: L2, L3, L4
  - Injury can cause paresthesia or anesthesia to the anterior and medial thigh, groin pain, weakness of knee extension, and thigh flexion.
  - Etiology of injury is often from retractor placement, stirrup positioning, and tumor invasion.
- Obturator nerve: L2, L3, L4
  - It emerges from the medial border of the psoas muscle, traverses the obturator space.
  - Injury can cause sensory loss to the upper and medial thigh, and weakness in hip adductors.
  - Etiology of injury is commonly transection during lymph node (LN) dissection.
- Accessory obturator nerve: L3 and L4
  - It is present in 5% to 30% of patients.
- Internal pudendal nerve: S1, S2, and S3
  - Injury can cause sensory loss to the labia.
- Sciatic nerve: L5 and S1
  - Injury can cause paresthesias of the posterior leg skin and hamstring areas and difficulty with knee flexion.
  - Etiology of injury is from stretch injury from poor stirrup positioning.
- Common peroneal nerve: L4, L5, S1, S2
  - Symptoms are foot drop.
  - Etiology of injury is usually from poor stirrup positioning.
- Autonomic nerves
  - Symptoms are large bowel dysfunction and urinary retention.
  - Etiology of injury is from radical pelvic surgery or tumor invasion of the autonomic plexus.

VULVAR AND GROIN ANATOMY

- The anatomical boundaries of the groin form the femoral triangle. This is bounded superiorly by the inguinal ligament, the sartorius muscle laterally to medially, and the adductor longus muscle medially to laterally. The base of the triangle consists of the iliacus, iliopsoas, and pectineus muscles, laterally to medially.
- Through the triangle run the femoral nerve and three other smaller nerves. The femoral nerve consists of the anterior femoral cutaneous branch and the medial femoral cutaneous branches from the L1, L2, and L3 nerve roots. The lateral femoral cutaneous nerve runs on top of the iliopsoas muscle and originates from L1. The genital–femoral nerve runs medial to the psoas muscle in the abdomen and originates from the L1 and L2 nerve roots. The ilioinguinal nerve also runs through the triangle and originates in the L1 root.
- Innervation to the vulva is from branches of the genitofemoral nerve and the perineal branch of the posterior femoral cutaneous nerve (a branch of the femoral nerve). The internal pudendal nerve also provides innervation to the vulva.

- The femoral artery gives off branches to form the superficial circumflex, the external pudendal, and the superficial epigastric arteries. The femoral vein receives branches from the superficial circumflex, external pudendal, and superficial epigastric veins. These enter the femoral vein near the saphenous vein, or sometimes drain into the saphenous prior to entry into the femoral vein.
- The lymphatics drain first into the superficial inguinal LNs. Around the clitoris and prepuce, the LNs may drain directly into the deep inguinal LNs or the pelvic LN, but this has little clinical relevance. The superficial inguinal LNs lie around the branches of the femoral vein. The deep inguinal LNs lie medial to the femoral vein beneath the cribriform fascia. The most superior deep inguinal node is Cloquet's node, which is medial to the femoral vein. Jackson's node is the most distal of the external iliac nodes; thus, Jackson's node is first exiting the pelvic LNs and last entering from the groin route.
- The blood supply to the vulva is not anomalous. The internal pudendal artery (a branch of the anterior division of the internal iliac) divides to form the perineal, clitoral, and inferior rectal arteries. The superficial external pudendal (a branch of the common femoral) supplies the lower abdominal wall, pubis, and labia majora. The deep external pudendal (a branch of the common femoral) supplies the labial fat pad. The veins commonly follow arteries except that the superficial epigastric and superficial and deep external pudendal drain into or near the saphenous and may not drain directly into the femoral vein.

LYMPH NODES

- LN basins should be sampled/completely dissected in most gynecologic cancer staging surgeries.
- The node basins for uterine and cervical cancers:
  - Pelvic to include: external and internal iliac and obturator spaces to the mid-common iliac
  - Para-aortic: from the mid-common iliac to the IMA and higher to the renal vessels.
- The node basins for vulvar cancer:
  - Inguinal–femoral groin LNs in the femoral triangle.
- The node basins for tubo-ovarian cancers:
  - Pelvic to include: external and internal iliac and obturator spaces up to the mid-common iliac.
  - Para-aortic: from the mid-common iliac to the renal vessels.

POTENTIAL SPACES IN THE PELVIS

There are eight potential spaces in the pelvis: the space of Retzius, the right and left paravesical spaces, the vesicovaginal space, the right and left pararectal spaces, the rectovaginal space, and the presacral space. These potential spaces are avascular and contain loose areolar or fatty connective tissue and can be developed to aid surgical dissection (Figure 4.3).

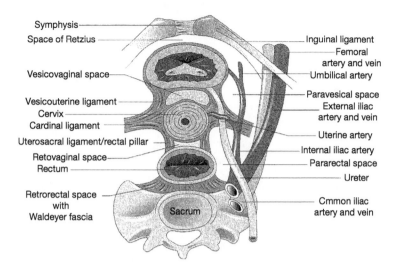

Figure 4.3 Eight potential spaces of the pelvis: retropubic spaces of Retzius, right and left paravesical spaces, vesicovaginal space, right and left pararectal spaces, rectovaginal space, and presacral space.

Source: From Holschneider CH, et al. Cytoreductive surgery: pelvis and radical oophorectomy. In: *Surgery for Ovarian Cancer, Third Edition*, Bristow RE, et al., eds. Boca Raton, FL: Taylor & Francis Group; 2016.

RECOMMENDED LABORATORIES

Recommended laboratories include: complete blood count (CBC), partial thromboplastin time (PTT), prothrombin time (PT), comprehensive metabolic panel (CMP), and liver function tests (LFTs). Other recommended studies include an EKG, a chest x-ray (CXR), and pelvic imaging as appropriate. Further workup depends on patient medical history and physical findings.

BOWEL PREPARATION

- The administration of a preoperative bowel preparation is debatable. The pros include easy palpation of the entire colon, improved exposure, a decrease in operative time due to easier handling, and the removal of solid material from the gastrointestinal (GI) tract. The cons include more anastomotic leaks from liquid stool, more sepsis due to trauma from the prep, and nonsignificant differences in operative times or facilitated exposure.
- There are a number of different preparations: polyethylene glycol (PEG) can be given in 4 L, magnesium citrate can be given in 300-mL bottles × 2 with or without a Dulcolax suppository, and antibiotic preparations. Antibiotic preparations include erythromycin base 1 g and neomycin 1 g; each given by mouth at 1, 2, and 10 p.m. the day before surgery. The erythromycin is given for both its antibiotic and its stimulant mechanisms of action. Another option is metronidazole 1 g and neomycin 1 g by mouth given at 1, 2, and 10 p.m. the day before surgery.
  - A meta-analysis of bowel preparation and outcomes was reviewed in elective colorectal surgery for effect of type of bowel preparation on anastomotic leak, surgical site infection (SSI), and ileus. Three arms were reviewed to include: preoperative mechanical bowel preparation (MBP) and antibiotics (MBP+/ABX+), MBP alone (MBP+/ABX−), and no bowel preparation (no-prep). 8,442 patients were evaluated. 27% were given no bowel preparation, 45.3% were given a mechanical bowel preparation without antibiotics (MBP+/ABX−) and 27.5% were given mechanical bowel prep with oral antibiotics (MBP+/ABX+). Patients in the MBP+/ABX+ or MBP+/ABX− had reduced ileus [MBP+/ABX+: OR = 0.57, 95% CI: 0.48–0.68; MBP+/ABX−: OR = 0.78, 95% CI: 0.68–0.91] as well as surgical site infection [MBP+/ABX+: OR = 0.39, 95% CI: 0.32–0.48; MBP+/ABX−: OR = 0.80, 95% CI: 0.69–0.93] compared to no prep. There was also a lower association with anastomotic leak for the MBP+/ABX− group compared to no prep. On multivariate analysis, the addition of antibiotics to MBP was associated with reduced anastomotic leak rates (OR = 0.57, 95% CI: 0.35–0.94), surgical site infection (OR = 0.40, 95% CI: 0.31–0.53) and postoperative ileus (OR = 0.71, 95% CI: 0.56–0.90).

Thus, MBP with oral antibiotics reduced by almost half SSI, anastomotic leak, and ileus after colorectal surgery (1).

- It is important to rehydrate with electrolytes (Gatorade) after the preparation, and care should be taken in patients with renal, heart, or liver failure.

ASA SCORE

The American Society of Anesthesiologists Score (ASA Score) provides risk information regarding surgical patients. There are five score classifications. Gynecologic oncology patients usually fall into classes 2 or 3. Class 1 is usually healthy and young persons. Class 2 patients have mild to moderate systemic disease. Class 3 patients have severe systemic disease. Class 4 patients have severe life-threatening systemic disease, and Class 5 patients are usually moribund.

CARDIAC RISK SCORE

Cardiac risk evaluation is important because 1 of 12 patients over the age of 65 will have coronary artery disease. 30% of those undergoing major elective surgery have at least one cardiac risk factor. The Goldman multifactorial index helps to stratify patients based on their history and studies ordered (Table 4.1). The index of cardiac risk factors is listed in Table 4.1.

FUNCTIONAL STATUS

It is commonly determined by metabolic equivalents (METS). The ability to climb one flight of stairs is equal to 4 METS, and considered a decent functional status.

If a patient has a diagnosis of congestive heart failure (CHF), a recent ECHO can assist in perioperative management. Normal ejection fraction (EF) is 60% to 70%. Severe CHF is less than 40%. Care with IVF should be taken in these patients as to not fluid overload them (Table 4.2).

Table 4.1 Cardiac Risk and Associated Score

Sign/Symptom	Points
S3 gallop or increased JVP	11
Myocardial infarction in last 6 months	10
More than 5 PVCs/min	7
Any rhythm other than sinus or PAC	7
Age greater than 70 years	5
Emergent noncardiac operative procedure	4
Aortic stenosis	3
Poor general health	3
Abdominal or thoracic surgery	3

JVP, jugular venous pressure; PAC, premature atrial contraction; PVC, premature ventricular contractions.

Table 4.2 Cardiac Risk Class			
Class	**Points**	**Morbidity (%)**	**Mortality (%)**
I	0–5	0.7	0.2
II	6–12	5	1.6
III	13–25	11	2.3
IV	≥26	22	55.6

SUBACUTE BACTERIAL ENDOCARDITIS

Prophylaxis for subacute bacterial endocarditis (SBE) should still be remembered. There are three categories of risk that require different levels of antibiotic protection.

- The low-risk category includes isolated secundum atrial septal defect (ASD); prior surgical repair of an ASD, ventricular septal defect (VSD), or patent ductus arteriosus (PDA) more than 6 months from surgery; a prior coronary artery bypass graft (CABG), mitral valve prolapse (MPV) without valve regurgitation; physiologic heart murmurs; prior Kawasaki disease without valve dysfunction; pacemakers and defibrillators; and prior rheumatic fever without valve dysfunction.
- The moderate-risk category includes acquired valve dysfunctions, hypertrophic cardiomyopathy, MVP with valve regurgitation or thickened leaflets, and other congenital cardiac malformations.
- The high-risk category includes patients with prosthetic cardiac valves, prior SBE, complex cyanotic congenital heart disease, tetralogy of Fallot, transposition of the great arteries, patients with a single ventricle, or surgically constructed systemic pulmonary shunts or conduits.
- Treatment is directed at the moderate- and high-risk patients. Those who are moderate risk should get ampicillin 2 g IV within 30 minutes of the procedure. If they are allergic to ampicillin, they should receive vancomycin 1 g IV over 1 hour within 2 hours of starting the procedure. High-risk patients should receive ampicillin 2 g and gentamicin 1.5 mg/kg IV 30 minutes prior to surgery and again 8 hours after the surgery. If the patient is allergic to ampicillin, the patient should then receive vancomycin 1 g and gentamicin 1.5 mg/kg IV 2 hours prior to surgery and 8 hours after surgery.

COMORBIDITY INDICES

- **Charlson comorbidity index (CCI)**: the index accounts for the patient age and 16 conditions.
- The CCI index predicts the 10-year mortality for patients presenting with one or more of the conditions in the model. This is an index used in decision making when a medical professional is presented with a treatment solution but needs to take into account the short- and long-term benefits of the treatment in a patient with other comorbid conditions to assess the long term risk. Each of the conditions listed is awarded a value-based point of 1, 2, 3, or 6 and combined with an age-based score. The more points given, the more likely the predicted adverse outcome. The total points are then summed. This CCI score is transformed by algorithm into a 10Y survival/mortality percentage taking into account that C is the score result obtained by summing the points.

○ Age—divided into five age groups of different risk:
   ▪ ≤40 years (0 points)
   ▪ Between 41 and 50 (1 point)
   ▪ Between 51 and 60 (2 points)
   ▪ Between 61 and 70 (3 points)
   ▪ ≥71 years (4 points)
• Comorbidity-based score: **1, 2, 3, or 6 points** depending on the mortality risk associated with each of the comorbidities.

➤ Myocardial infarction	➤ Congestive heart failure
➤ Peripheral vascular disease	➤ Cerebrovascular disease
➤ Dementia	➤ Chronic obstructive pulmonary disease (COPD)
➤ Connective tissue disease	➤ Peptic ulcer disease
➤ Diabetes mellitus	➤ Moderate to severe chronic kidney disease
➤ Hemiplegia	
➤ Malignant lymphoma	➤ Leukemia
➤ Solid tumor	➤ Liver disease
	➤ AIDS

○ 1 point condition—Myocardial infarction (MI), CHF, peripheral vascular disease (PVD), dementia, cerebrovascular disease, connective tissue disease, ulcer, chronic liver disease, diabetes mellitus.
○ 2 point condition—Hemiplegia, moderate to severe kidney disease, diabetes mellitus with end organ damage, solid tumor, leukemia, lymphoma.
○ 3 point condition—Moderate to severe liver disease.
○ 6 point condition—Malignant tumor, metastasis, AIDS (2).
• **The cumulative illness index rating scale (CIRS)** was developed by Linn in 1968. Fourteen systems are evaluated and scored. The scores are then summed and can range from 0 to 56. A higher score predicts a worse outcome.
• Scoring:
   ○ Less than 6 and CrCL greater than 70 mL/min (GO: suitable for treatment).
   ○ Greater than 6 and CrCL less than 70 mL/min (SLOW: suitable for reduced treatment).
   ○ Severe comorbidities and short-life expectancy (NO: suitable for supportive care).
   ○ Each system is rated as follows:
      ▪ 1 = NONE: no impairment to that organ/system.
      ▪ 2 = MILD: impairment does not interfere with normal activity; treatment may or may not be required; prognosis is excellent.
      ▪ 3 = MODERATE: impairment interferes with normal activity; treatment is needed; prognosis is good.

- 4 = SEVERE: impairment is disabling; treatment is urgently needed; prognosis is guarded.
- 5 = EXTREMELY SEVERE: impairment is life-threatening; treatment is urgent; prognosis is grave.

- **Cardiac**
  - **Level 0:** no problem.
  - **Level 1:** remote MI (>5 years ago)/occasional angina treated with PRN medicine.
  - **Level 2:** CHF compensated with medicine/daily angina medicine/left ventricular hypertrophy/atrial fibrillation/bundle branch block/daily antiarrhythmic medicine.
  - **Level 3:** previous MI within 5 years/abnormal stress test/status postpercutaneous coronary angioplasty or coronary artery bypass graft surgery.
  - **Level 4:** marked activity restriction secondary to cardiac status (i.e., unstable angina or intractable CHF).
  - CHF requiring daily medications "2"; an intermediate condition "3"; intractable CHF "4." Arrhythmias—EKG findings of atrial fibrillation, right or left bundle branch block, or the necessity of daily antiarrhythmic drugs "2"; a bifascicular block "3"; a pacemaker for cardiogenic syncope "3." Valvular disease—Detectable murmurs without MET restriction "1." Pericardial pathology—A pericardial effusion or pericarditis "3."
- Hypertension
  - **Level 0:** no problem.
  - **Level 1:** hypertension compensated with salt restriction and weight loss/ serum cholesterol greater than 200 mg/dL.
  - **Level 2:** daily antihypertensive medicine/one symptom of atersclerotic disease (angina, claudication, bruit, amaurosis fugax, absent pedal pulses)/aortic aneurysm less than 4 cm.
  - **Level 3:** two or more symptoms of atherosclerosis.
  - **Level 4:** previous surgery for vascular problem/aortic aneurysm greater than 4 cm.
  - **Hypertension**—Defined as a persistently elevated diastolic pressure greater than 90 mmHg. Managed drug free—"1"; single daily antihypertensive—"2"; two or more drugs for control or with left ventricular hypertrophy—"3."
  - **Peripheral atherosclerotic disease**—Evidence of at least one physical symptom or imaging evidence (e.g., angiogram) merits a "2," two or more symptoms "3," if a history of bypass graft or if surgery is currently indicated "4."
- Vascular
  - **Level 0:** no problem.
  - **Level 1:** hypertension compensated with salt restriction and weight loss/ serum cholesterol greater than 200 mg/dL. Serum cholesterol above normal.
  - **Level 2:** daily antihypertensive medicine/one symptom of atersclerotic disease (angina, claudication, bruit, amaurosis fugax, absent pedal pulses)/aortic aneurysm less than 4 cm.
  - **Level 3:** two or more symptoms of atherosclerosis.
  - **Level 4:** previous surgery for vascular problem/aortic aneurysm greater than 4 cm.

- ○ Hypertension—Defined previously.
- ○ Peripheral atherosclerotic disease—Defined previously.
- Respiratory (lungs, bronchi, trachea below the larynx)
  - ○ **Level 0:** no problem.
  - ○ **Level 1:** recurrent episodes of acute bronchitis, currently treated asthma with PRN inhalers, cigarette smoker greater than 10 but less than 20 pack years.
  - ○ **Level 2:** CXR evidence of COPD, requires daily theophylline or inhalers, treated for pneumonia two or more times in the past 5 years, smoked 20 to 40 pack years.
  - ○ **Level 3:** limited ambulation secondary to limited respiratory capacity, requires oral steroids for lung disease, smoked greater than 40 pack years.
  - ○ **Level 4:** requires supplemental oxygen, at least one episode of respiratory failure requiring assisted ventilation, any lung cancer.
  - ○ Chronic bronchitis, asthma, and emphysema—These conditions are rated "1" if only PRN inhalers are required, "2" if daily theophylline or inhalers are required, "3" if steroids are required, and "4" if supplemental oxygen is required. Pneumonia—Acute pneumonia treated as an outpatient would merit a "3," and if hospitalization was required a "4."
- ENT (eye, ear, nose, throat, larynx)
  - ○ **Level 0:** no problem.
  - ○ **Level 1:** corrected vision 20/40, chronic sinusitis, mild hearing loss.
  - ○ **Level 2:** corrected vision 20/60 or reads newsprint with difficulty, requires hearing aid, chronic sinonasal complaints requiring medication, requires medication for vertigo.
  - ○ **Level 3:** partially blind (requires an escort to venture out), unable to read newsprint, conversational hearing still impaired with hearing aid.
  - ○ **Level 4:** functional blindness, functional deafness, laryngectomy.
- Upper GI
  - ○ **Level 0:** no problem.
  - ○ **Level 1:** hiatal hernia, heartburn complaints treated with PRN medications.
  - ○ **Level 2:** needs daily H2 blocker or antacid, documented gastric or duodenal ulcer within 5 years.
  - ○ **Level 3:** active ulcer, guaiac positive stools, any swallowing disorder or dysphagia.
  - ○ **Level 4:** gastric cancer, history of perforated ulcer, melena or hematochezia from upper GI source.
- Lower GI (intestines, hernias)
  - ○ **Level 0:** no problem.
  - ○ **Level 1:** constipation managed with PRN meds, active hemorrhoids, status post hernia repair.
  - ○ **Level 2:** requires daily bulk laxatives or stool softeners, diverticulosis, untreated hernia.
  - ○ **Level 3:** bowel impaction in the past year, daily use of stimulant laxatives or enemas.
  - ○ **Level 4:** hematochezia from lower GI source, currently impacted, diverticulitis flare up, status postbowel obstruction, bowel carcinoma.
  - ○ Diverticular disease—A diagnosis of diverticulosis or a history of diverticulitis in the past merits a "2," an active flare-up of diverticulitis merits a "4," and an intermediate condition a "3."

- Hepatic (liver only)
  - **Level 0:** no problem.
  - **Level 1:** history of hepatitis greater than 5 years ago, cholecystectomy.
  - **Level 2:** mildly elevated LFTs (up to 150% of normal), hepatitis within 5 years, cholelithiasis, daily or heavy alcohol use within 5 years.
  - **Level 3:** elevated bilirubin (total >2), marked elevation of LFTs (>150% of normal), requires supplemental pancreatic enzymes for digestion.
  - **Level 4:** biliary obstruction, any biliary tree carcinoma, cholecystitis, pancreatitis, active hepatitis.
  - Gallbladder disease—A remote cholecystectomy merits a "1," cholelithiasis or gallstones visualized with imaging techniques merits a "2," and acute cholecystitis a "4."
  - Hepatitis—A history of hepatitis within 5 years that is inactive at present merits a "2," active hepatitis a "4."
  - Pancreatic disease—Pancreatic insufficiency requiring supplemental enzymes or chronic pancreatitis merits a "3," acute pancreatitis a "4."
  - Carcinoma—Any hepato-biliary tree carcinoma generally merits a "4."
- Renal (kidneys only)
  - **Level 0:** no problem.
  - **Level 1:** passage of kidney stone within the past 10 years or asymptomatic kidney stone, pyelonephritis within 5 years.
  - **Level 2:** serum creatinine greater than 1.5 but less than 3.0 without diuretic or antihypertensive medication.
  - **Level 3:** serum creatinine greater than 3.0 or serum creatinine greater than 1.5 in conjunction with diuretic, antihypertensive, or bicarbonate therapy, current pyelonephritis.
  - **Level 4:** requires dialysis, renal carcinoma.
- Other genitourinary (GU) (ureters, bladder, urethra, prostate, genitals)
  - **Level 0:** no problem.
  - **Level 1:** stress incontinence, hysterectomy.
  - **Level 2:** abnormal Pap smear, frequent urinary tract infections (UTIs) (three or more in the past year), urinary incontinence (nonstress) in females, current UTI, any urinary diversion procedure.
  - **Level 3:** vaginal bleeding, cervical carcinoma in situ, hematuria, urosepsis in past year.
  - **Level 4:** acute urinary retention, any GU carcinoma except as stated.
  - Urinary infections—Recurrent UTI's (three or more in the past year) merits a "1" in women. A current UTI merits a "2," a history of urosepsis in the past year a "3," and a current urosepsis a "4." Urinary diversion procedure—Patients with ileal loops, indwelling catheters, or nephrostomies would merit at least a "2."
- Musculoskeletal–integumentary (muscles, bone, skin)
  - **Level 0:** no problem.
  - **Level 1:** uses PRN medications for arthritis or has mildly limited activities of daily living (ADLs) from joint pathology, excised nonmelanotic skin cancers, skin infections requiring antibiotics within a year.
  - **Level 2:** daily anti-arthritis medications or use of assistive devices or moderate limitation in ADLs, daily medications for chronic skin conditions, melanoma without metastasis.

○ **Level 3:** severely impaired ADLs secondary to arthritis, requires steroids for arthritis condition, vertebral compression fractures from osteoporosis.

○ **Level 4:** wheelchair-bound, severe joint deformity, or severely impaired usage, osteomyelitis, any bone or muscle carcinoma, metastatic melanoma.

○ Orthopedic surgery—Since hip or knee replacements are usually performed for severe arthritis we suggest a rating of 3.

• Neurological (brain, spinal cord, nerves; does not include dementia)

○ **Level 0:** no problem.

○ **Level 1:** frequent headaches requiring PRN medications without interference with daily activities, a history of transient ischemic attacks (TIA).

○ **Level 2:** requires daily medications for chronic headaches or headaches that regularly interfere with daily activities, history of cerebrovascular accident (CVA) without residual deficit, neurodegenerative disease (Parkinson's, multiple sclerosis [MS], ALS—mild severity).

○ **Level 3:** history of CVA with mild residual deficit, any central nervous system (CNS) neurologic procedure, neurodegenerative disease—moderate severity.

○ **Level 4:** history of CVA with residual functional hemiparesis or aphasia, neurodegenerative disease—severe.

• Endocrine–metabolic (includes diabetes, diffuse infections, infections, toxicity)

○ **Level 0:** no problem.

○ **Level 1:** diabetes mellitus compensated with diet, obesity: body mass index (BMI) greater than 30, hypothyroidism requiring hormone replacement.

○ **Level 2:** diabetes mellitus requiring insulin or oral agents.

○ **Level 3:** morbid obesity BMI greater than 45.

○ **Level 4:** brittle or poorly controlled diabetes mellitus, diabetic coma in the past year, requires adrenal hormone replacement.

○ Diabetes mellitus—diet controlled, "1"; insulin or oral agents required, "2"; poorly controlled or a history of diabetic ketoacidosis or nonketotic hyperosmolar coma in the past year, "4."

○ Thyroid hormone replacement—Thyroid replacement in the elderly is common and should be rated a "1" if otherwise uncomplicated.

○ Obesity—Obesity is rated using the BMI as the current standard for measuring weight for a given height.

• Psychiatric/behavioral (includes dementia, depression, anxiety, agitation, psychosis)

○ **Level 0:** no psychiatric problem or history thereof.

○ **Level 1:** minor psychiatric condition or history thereof. Specifically: previous outpatient mental health treatment during a crisis, outpatient treatment for depression greater than 10 years ago, current usage of minor tranquilizers for episodic anxiety (occasional usage), mild early dementia (MMS > 25 < 28).

○ **Level 2:** a history of major depression (by *DSM-5* criteria within the past 10 years [treated or untreated]), mild dementia (MMS 20–25), any previous psychiatric hospitalization, any psychotic episode, substance abuse history greater than 10 years ago.

○ **Level 3:** currently meets *DSM-5* criteria for major depression or two or more episodes of major depression in the past 10 years, moderate dementia

(MMS 15–20), current usage of daily antianxiety medication, currently meets *DSM-5* criteria for substance abuse or dependence, requires daily antipsychotic medication.

- ○ **Level 4:** current mental illness requiring psychiatric hospitalization, institutionalization, or intensive outpatient management, for example, patients with severe or suicidal depression, acute psychosis or psychotic decompensation, severe agitation from dementia, severe substance abuse. Severe dementia (MMS <15).
- Hematopoietic
  - ○ **Level 0:** no problem.
  - ○ **Level 1:** hemoglobin: females >10 <12, anemia of chronic disease.
  - ○ **Level 2:** hemoglobin: females >8 <10, anemia secondary to iron, vitamin B_{12}, or folate deficiency or chronic renal failure, total white blood cell (WBC) count >2,000 but <4,000.
  - ○ **Level 3:** hemoglobin: females <8, total WBC <2,000.
  - ○ **Level 4:** any leukemia, any lymphoma.
  - ○ Malignancy—Any hematologic malignancy would merit a "4" (3).

REFERENCES

1. Kiran RP, Murray AC, Chiuzan C, et al. Combined preoperative mechanical bowel preparation with oral antibiotics significantly reduces surgical site infection, anastomotic leak, and ileus after colorectal surgery. *Ann Surg*. September 2015;262(3):416-425.
2. Charlson ME, Pompei P, Ales KL, MacKenzie CR. A new method of classifying prognostic comorbidity in longitudinal studies: development and validation. *J Chronic Dis*. 1987;40(5):373-383.
3. Miller MD, Paradis CF, Houck PR, et al. Rating chronic medical illness burden in geropsychiatric practice and research: application of the Cumulative Illness Rating Scale. *Psychiatry Res*. 1992;41(3):237-248.

LAPAROTOMY INCISIONS

- The most common vertical incision used for an exploratory laparotomy in oncology is a vertical midline incision. A less commonly used vertical incision is the paramedian incision.
- There are three common transverse skin incisions, with differences in fascial entry:
  - Pfannenstiel: dissects fascia from rectus muscles
  - Cherney: dissects the tendons of the rectus abdominis muscles from the pubic bone. A major complication with this incision is the development of osteomyelitis due to suturing of muscles back to bone.
  - Maylard: muscle cutting. Involves ligating the inferior epigastrics prior to transection of the muscle bodies. This incision does not separate the transversalis fascia from the rectus muscles.

INCISION CLOSURE

- Abdominal wall closure:
  - Mass closure: made with one continuous length of suture material; includes all body wall layers, and incorporates the peritoneum, fascia, and muscles.
  - Smead-Jones (far-near, near-far): a double loop, interrupted mattress suture technique that incorporates all the body layers in the outside suture ("far") and fascia and peritoneum in the inner suture ("near").
  - Fascial incision strength after surgery: week 1: 10%, week 2: 25%, week 3: 30%, week 4: 40%, 6 months: 80%.
- Subcutaneous tissue: if the wound is greater than 2 cm deep, subcutaneous suture or placement of a Jackson–Pratt (JP) drain is indicated.
- Skin closure:
  - Staples
  - Subcuticular suture with Monocryl or Vicryl with or without a dermabond overlay
  - Vertical mattress skin closure: useful in delayed primary closure of abdominal incisions and in perineal wound closure (place the knot lateral to the line of incision)

LYMPH NODE DISSECTION

- The boundaries for the pelvic lymph node dissection (P-LND) are the following: superiorly the distal half of the common iliac vessels, laterally the anterior and medial aspect of the external and internal iliac vessels, the ureter or the superior vesical artery medially, the circumflex iliac vein inferiorly, and the obturator nerve posteriorly.

- The boundaries for the para-aortic lymph node dissection (PA-LND) are the following: the fat pads over and lateral to the inferior vena cava and aorta, the inferior mesenteric artery (or up to renal vessels) superiorly, and the proximal half of the common iliac vessels inferiorly, and the ureters laterally (Figure 4.4).
- For a high PA-LND, the LNs up to the renal vessels are removed medial to the ureters and anterior to the great vessels.
- Sentinel LND: radiolabeled albumin with Technetium-99 is injected into the tumoral/peritumoral bed preprocedure (directly to the tumor for vulvar and cervical lesions; or into the cervix, the fundus via laparoscopic injection, or the corpus via hysteroscopic injection for uterine cancer). Lymphazurin blue or indocyanine green is then injected into the tumoral bed at initiation of surgical procedure and the first lymph node (LN) identified in the drainage basins from that tumor site is dissected and sent for frozen section. If negative, the procedure is considered complete. If positive, a complete lymphadenectomy is usually recommended. There may be more than one sentinel node and for midline structures/tumors, SLND should be evaluated bilaterally.

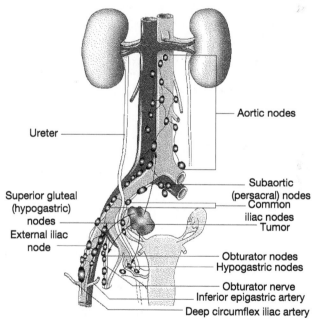

Figure 4.4 Lymphatic drainage of the ovary. The three principal routes are to (a) the para-aortic nodal basins accompanying the ovarian vessels; (b) the obturator and iliac nodal basins through the broad ligament; and (c) the external iliac and inguinal nodal basins via the round ligament.

Source: From Holschneider CH, et al. Cytoreductive surgery: pelvis and radical oophorectomy. In: *Surgery for Ovarian Cancer, Third Edition*, Bristow RE, et al., eds. Boca Raton, FL: Taylor & Francis Group; 2016.

BOWEL DIVERSION

- When an ostomy is considered preoperatively, an ostomy consult should be obtained. The consult is for patient education in addition to identification of best placement; this includes evaluation of the patient's waistline, common pant line, and any other individual body nuances.
- A mucous fistula is the distal segment of bowel remaining at the time of end ostomy. It is brought through a separate ostomy site when an end ostomy is placed. The mucous fistula is performed when the remaining distal bowel is more than 10 cm from the anus. These mucous fistulas have minimal drainage. It is important to ensure that both ends are distant enough from each other so that cross fecal contamination and infection cannot occur.
- Complications:
  - ○ Stricture: there is a 3% stricture rate for all ostomies. Dilation or surgical correction can be performed for strictures.
  - ○ Prolapse: the descending colon has the least risk of prolapse.
  - ○ Hernia
- There are two common types of ostomy:
  - ○ An end ostomy is performed when a takedown is not planned. A mucous fistula needs to be constructed in most cases. The distal end of resected bowel needs management because it still produces mucus, gas, and sloughed cells, and could become dilated and perforate. Permanent colostomies prolapse in 1% to 3%. If the resection of the colon occurs at the rectosigmoid and 5 to 10 cm remain, this remaining rectum is then called a Hartmann's pouch and functions as a mucous fistula with output through the anus.
  - ○ A loop ostomy should be performed when there are plans to take the ostomy down. The bowel is brought through the abdominal wall and opened on its antimesenteric side. Both sides of the opened bowel are sutured to the skin. A Hollister bridge or glass rod is placed under the bowel loop for temporary support until healing occurs. The proximal end functions as the colostomy and the distal opening functions as the mucous fistula. It is easier to take down because it is not mandatory to know which end is proximal and which is distal.
- Ileostomy: indications include diversion when no distal bowel is available, when small bowel is too dilated to perform an anastomosis, for protection of a distal anastomosis when an anastomotic leak is likely, or in the presence of a bowel perforation with peritonitis. These are high-output ostomies, so as distal an ostomy as possible is preferred. A Turnbull loop is recommended.
- Gastrostomy tube (G-tube): G-tubes are indicated for decompression of the stomach and intestine to avoid long-term use of a nasogastric tube. They are also used for intractable small bowel obstructions associated with carcinomatosis and fistulas. The body or antrum of the stomach is chosen. A size 18 to 20 Malecot or Foley catheter can be used. The greater curve of the stomach is incised with a scalpel 0.5 cm in length. Two pursestring sutures of 2-0 gauge silk are placed to secure the tube to the stomach. The gastrostomy site is brought to the peritoneal surface and secured with interrupted Vicryl sutures. The catheter is then exteriorized through a skin incision and secured to the skin with 2-0 gauge prolene sutures. The G-tube needs to be changed every 2 months.

BOWEL RESECTION

- Bowel anastomosis can be performed using either hand-sewn or stapled technique.
  - Types:
    - End to end: the bowel is aligned with cut ends together and hand sewn together using a two-layer technique (the inner layer using 3-0 gauge Vicryl and the outer imbricating layer using 3-0 gauge Vicryl or silk). Alternatively, using a stapler, the bowel ends are aligned on their antimesenteric borders. An enterotomy is made on the antimesenteric corner of the two bowel sections. One prong of the GIA stapler is then advanced through each enterotomy and fired. The TA stapler is then used to close the connected bowel segments to create a functional end-to-end anastomosis. The mesentery should be closed and silk stay sutures are placed along the antimesenteric borders to reduce tension.
    - Side to side: 5-mm enterotomies are made with the Bovie on each segment of the resected bowel 5 to 10 cm back from the primary transection site. One prong of the GIA stapler is then advanced through each enterotomy and the stapler is then fired. The TA stapler is then applied to close the defect transversely or longitudinally, whichever narrows the lumen least.
    - Low rectal anastomosis is often performed after a rectosigmoid resection. It is important to consider placing a diverting loop colostomy or loop ileostomy to protect the anastomosis and allow for healing. The anastomosis should preferably be performed out of the irradiated field. The largest staple cartridge available and accommodated by the patient should be used. If a very low anastomosis is performed, consider construction of a J pouch to increase reservoir capacity and to decrease tenesmus.
    - If fistula is present, consider excision of fistulous tract, pelvic rest × 6 weeks, fistulogram after healing and before takedown of diverting ileostomy or secondary reanastomosis.
  - Anastomotic leaks complicate bowel surgery in 0% to 30%. Rectal anastomosis has a higher complication rate of about 6%.
  - Requirements for a good anastomosis include the following: an adequate lumen of at least 2 to 3 cm, the anastomosis be tension free, there be adequate vascular supply from the mesentery with evidence of bleeding (viability) of the cut edges, and the presence of peristalsis.
  - Watershed areas of the bowel include the ileocecal junction/terminal ileum, the splenic flexure of colon (Griffith's point), and the rectosigmoid flexure (Sudeck's point).
- Meckel's diverticulum represents persistence of the vitelline yolk sac. It is present in 2% of people. It is twice as common in men as women. It is usually located within 2 feet of the ileocecal valve. It should be removed when found, due to the presence of ectopic gastric tissue in 2% of patients, that is, Zollinger–Ellison syndrome.

URINARY DIVERSION: STENTS, CONDUITS, AND BLADDER RECONSTRUCTIONS

- Ureteral stents should be placed in most ureteral injury cases. They can be placed via retrograde cystoscopy, retrograde cystotomy, ureterotomy, or antegrade through a percutaneous nephrostomy. A 6 French double pigtail stent or a pediatric feeding tube can be placed. These should be changed every 3 to 6 months. They can often be removed 2 to 6 weeks after surgery via cystoscopy.

- Urinary conduits/neobladders are often placed in the settings of pelvic exenteration, intractable hemorrhagic cystitis, a neurogenic bladder, or decreased bladder capacitance from surgery or radiation therapy (XRT). Decreased capacity is defined as an intravesical pressure greater than 30 cm of H_2O with minimum volume.
- Bladder reconstruction can be performed when there has been surgical resection with the urethra safely preserved.
- Principles of urinary conduits are a low-pressure system (<20-cm H_2O), high-volume, antirefluxing system to prevent ascending infection, and low water and solute reabsorption.
  - Universal techniques are needed. There has to be a wide uretero-bowel anastomosis, the intestinal segment should be isoperistaltic, the stoma should be protruding, the conduit should be stabilized within the abdominal cavity, and there should be an adequate diameter of the efferent loop with a straight path through the abdominal wall for urine outlet.
  - There are two types of conduits, incontinent and continent.
    - Incontinent types include:
      - Percutaneous nephrostomy tube.
      - Cutaneous ureterostomy. The ureters should be brought out 2 cm past the skin, and the skin incision should be an inverted "V" pointing down.
      - The right colon pouch is another incontinent conduit. It does not use nipple valves. It is made from nonirradiated, detubularized colon. It has an increased risk of ureteral obstruction, angulation of the distal ureters, fibrosis of the submucosal ureteral tunnels, devascularization, and distension of the pouch. The left ureter requires more mobilization to reach the colon.
      - The ileal conduit uses a longer intestinal segment. The Bricker type incorporates a horizontal internal orientation for the body of the reservoir. The ureters are anastomosed laterally. The Leadbetter modification orients the body of the conduit vertically. The ureters are brought to the midline for the anastomosis. The ureteroileal anastomoses are end to end. A Turnbull stoma is used to overcome the complications of nipple ischemia. A short ileal segment of 15 to 18 cm is used. The conduit is sutured at its proximal end to the sacral prominence. The Daniels modification is used for obese patients, and the Wallace modification is used for double ureters (where both ureters are split and sewn together).
      - A jejunal conduit has a higher incidence of electrolyte imbalances: hyperchloremic acidosis occurs in 25% to 65% of patients. There is reabsorption of potassium (K) and urea and a concomitant increase in aldosterone. It is more often outside the fields of XRT.
      - The sigmoid conduit has the advantages of avoiding small bowel anastomosis and fewer stomal complications. Disadvantages are that it cannot be used with inflammatory bowel syndromes or diverticulosis.

There is an increased risk of secondary cancers inside the conduit. The ureters should be tunneled submucosally if no prior XRT was given.

□ The transverse colon conduit has advantages in that it is good for the obese patient, in those with a history of whole pelvic radiation therapy (WP-XRT) as it is outside the field of XRT, and in those with short ureters.

- Continent diversions are contraindicated in persons with short life expectancies, in those with physical problems accessing/maintaining the conduit (dementia/arthritis), those with right colon diseases (prior bowel cancer, inflammatory bowel disease (IBD), cecal XRT), those with morbid obesity (making this a short system), and in those with compromised renal function.

  □ The ureterosigmoidostomy maintains continence through the anal sphincter. The ureters are directly tunneled and secured into the sigmoid colon and efflux is through the rectum. There are high rates of pyelonephritis, obstruction, hyperchloremic acidosis, nocturnal incontinence, and frequent bowel evacuation. Secondary carcinomas of the colon can occur.

  □ The ileocolic continent diversion (Indiana pouch) uses 10 to 15 cm of terminal ileum, the cecum, and 30 cm of ascending colon. The right colonic segment is detubularized. The terminal ileum is plicated over a red robin catheter to the level of the ileocolic valve—this provides the continence mechanism. The plicated ileum is brought to the abdominal wall. Intestinal integrity is reestablished after resection. Drains are placed to follow: stents for each ureter, a Malecot catheter placed into the right colon pouch and exits superior to the ileal stoma, a red robin/Foley catheter placed in the plicated ileum maintaining patency from the right colonic pouch through the abdominal wall, and a JP placed in the abdomen.

  □ The Miami pouch uses the same principles as earlier, but extends the intestinal resection to the level of the transverse colon. Postoperative maintenance includes irrigation of the Malecot every 4 to 6 hours with 40 mL normal saline, and irrigation of the ureteral stents only if plugged. Both drains are removed at 14 days after an intravenous pyelogram (IVP) and pouchogram are normal. If the patient had prior XRT, 21 days of stenting and drainage is recommended. The JP should be removed at the same time as the ureteral stents. Active catheterization every 2 hours the first week, every 3 hours the second week, every 4 hours the third week, every 5 hours the fourth week, and every 6 hours the fifth week is recommended. The pouch should be irrigated daily to weekly with 50 mL of normal saline. An IVP, pouchogram, and comprehensive metabolic panel (CMP) should be obtained at 3 months.

  □ The Kock ileal pouch is specifically contraindicated for chronic inflammatory or neoplastic disease of the colon, as well as in patients with short ureters. A portion of ileum is isolated and marked into segments measuring 17, 22, 22, and 17 cm; 15 cm of distal ileum remains at the ileocecal junction to protect the watershed area. The 22-cm (central portion) lengths are sutured together, then opened along their antimesenteric borders to make the reservoir. The pouch is then folded over. The 17-cm lengths are then each intussuscepted and secured with a GIA or TA stapler. The ureters are brought in to the proximal end. Mesh is attached to each intussusception to secure the intussuscepted nipples. A Marlex strut is attached from the distal mesh to the rectus muscle. The two ends of the ileal segment become the nipples: the afferent end prevents reflux into the kidneys and the efferent end is the continence mechanism. Complications include stone formation around staples, prolapse, extussusception, and stenosis from ischemia.

- Bladder reconstruction can be performed with:
  □ Right colon augmentation (enterocystoplasty)
  □ A hemi-Kock ileal bladder can also be constructed. With this technique no efferent nipple is constructed.
  □ The psoas hitch provides bladder reconstruction by mobilizing the bladder to reach a shortened ureter on the ipsilateral side. The bladder is distended with water, then opened along the dome. A suture is placed through the lateral side of the bladder to the psoas muscle on the affected side, at the level of the proximal external iliac artery. The ureter is anastomosed to the bladder and the cystotomy is closed in two layers.
  □ The Boari bladder flap is used in combination with the psoas hitch for a more extensively shortened ureter. The bladder is again distended, and opened in the dome with a U-shaped incision. The base of the created flap is then oriented toward the psoas muscle and the flap is rotated upward. The flap is tubularized around the ureter, and the bladder is then sutured to the psoas muscle. The bladder defect is then closed in two layers. This technique provides 3 to 5 cm of additional length for a shortened ureter.
- There are three methods for ureteral reanastomosis after transection:
  □ The ureteroureterostomy (UU), which is a primary reanastomosis.
  □ The transureteroureterostomy, which is an anastomosis to the contralateral ureter.
  □ The ureteroneocystostomy (UNC), which reimplants the ureter directly into the bladder, with or without psoas hitch or Boari flap.
  □ All ureteral injuries and diversions should be stented unless minimal crush injury is seen and immediately released.

RECONSTRUCTIVE SURGERY

Reconstructive surgery is useful in gynecologic oncology for coverage of perineal defects and for neovaginal construction. There are different methods of reconstruction.

- Split thickness skin grafts (STSG) are often used to cover epidermal/dermal defects encountered with simple vulvectomy. The Zimmer dermatome can produce an optimal graft thickness of 0.020 inches.

- Tissue expansion can be produced with inflatable balloons and the area harvested after an appropriate time.
- Skin flaps are used to reconstruct deeper resections. There are three types of flaps: rotational, advancement, and transpositional (pass over).
  - Common rotational flaps include the rhomboid and perineal thigh flaps. The rotational flap most often used is the rhomboid flap/Limberg flap. This flap can cover anterior, lateral, or posterior vulvar defects in addition to defects of the perianal region. The donor sites are the buttocks and posterior thigh. The blood supply is the inferior gluteal artery. The perineal thigh flap is used to cover a defect to the labial crural fold. The donor site is the medial thigh. This blood supply is unreliable. The length of the flap should be a ratio of 2:1 to the vulvar defect.
  - Advancement flaps are used to provide defect coverage when there is enough adjacent skin mobility. This is usually called a V–Y advancement flap.
  - Transpositional axial flaps move the flap on an axis (its vascular pedicle) to another site.
    - The Martius/bulbocavernosus flap is used for repair of vaginal fistulas, for vaginal reconstruction, and for repair of fourth-degree lacerations. The donor site is the labial fat pad and the blood supply is the superficial external pudendal artery (SEPA) and the perineal branch of the internal pudendal artery.
    - The SEPA flap is often used for vulvar reconstruction and repair of urethral defects. The donor site is the area directly above the mons pubis. This type of flap should not be performed if a groin node dissection is planned. The blood supply is related to the flap's name and originates from the common femoral artery. This is a sensate flap.
    - The superficial circumflex iliac artery (SCIA) flap is indicated for anterior perineal and vaginal defects. The donor site is the skin around the anterior superior iliac spine to 2.5 cm below the inguinal ligament. The blood supply again relates to its name.
    - The posterior labial artery flap is also known as the pudendal thigh flap and the Singapore flap. It too covers perineal defects and is good for vaginal reconstruction. The donor site is the labial crural fold and the inguinal crease. The blood supply is related to its name and originates from the deep external pudendal artery. This flap is sensate and innervation is from branches of the pudendal nerve and the posterior cutaneous nerves.
    - The inferior gluteal fasciocutaneous flap can cover vulvar, vaginal, and rectal defects. The donor site is the buttocks. The blood supply is the axial artery of the inferior gluteal artery, originating from the internal iliac artery. This flap can be up to 35 cm long. It too is a sensate flap and the nerve supply is from the posterior cutaneous nerve of the thigh.
- Myocutaneous flaps are distinguished by the number of vascular pedicles that supply the flap. There are five types. Type I flaps consist of a single vascular pedicle. Type II flaps have one dominant vascular pedicle and one or more minor vascular pedicles. Type III flaps obtain their blood supply from two dominant pedicles. Type IV flaps obtain their blood supply from three dominant pedicles. Type V flaps obtain their blood supply from four dominant

vascular pedicles. To test flap viability, IV fluorescein (10 mL of 10% solution, or a dose of 15 mg/kg administered over 5 minutes) can be given and a Wood's light can be placed over the flap site. Twice the dose should be used in patients with darker skin tones.

- ○ The rectus abdominis myocutaneous (RAM) flap is often used for vaginal/pelvic reconstruction. The blood supply is the superior and inferior epigastrics and it is a type III flap.
- ○ The gracilis myocutaneous (GMC) flap is used for vaginal, groin, or perineal reconstruction. It can be used as an island flap, or directly rotated into the defect. The blood supply is the medial femoral circumflex artery from the deep femoral artery. It is a type II flap.
- ○ The tensor fasciae latae flap is indicated for vulvar and groin defects, as well as for ischial and deep abdominal wall defects. The donor sites are the gluteus medius and sartorius muscles. The blood supply is the terminal branch of the lateral circumflex femoral artery. It is a type I flap. Side effects can be lateral instability of the knee, a long scar on the medial thigh, thigh pain, and vascular spasm from torsion. It is not a suitable flap for vaginal reconstruction after a supralevator exenteration.
- ○ The latissimus dorsi flap is a good flap for breast reconstruction. It is a type V flap.
- Neovaginal techniques are also varied. These include the following:
  - ○ McIndoe STSG: the McIndoe neovagina is constructed using an STSG formed around a mold. It is placed in the perineal defect and the patient should then be immobilized to allow the STSG to anneal. Daily dilation should follow indefinitely.
  - ○ The RAM flap is a more reliable neovaginal flap and is less likely to prolapse than other neovaginal flaps.
  - ○ Two GMC flaps are needed for neovaginal reconstruction if this procedure is performed. There can be vascular pedicle spasm with this type of flap. It does have a tendency to prolapse.
  - ○ The Martius flap is a durable and pliable flap to use for neovaginal reconstruction.
  - ○ The posterior labial artery thigh flap is a sensate flap but has a less reliable blood supply.
  - ○ The perineal thigh skin flap tends to prolapse and can stenose.
  - ○ Intestinal segments, including the cecum, small bowel, sigmoid colon, and rectum, can also be used for neovaginal reconstruction. The sigmoid colon is used the most often. It is important to detubularize it. The benefits of this type of neovagina are its large caliber, and low-volume mucous output. Risks include secondary malignancies, including human papillomavirus (HPV) related.

SPLENECTOMY

Splenectomy is often indicated with splenic trauma, or when tumor has involved this organ and optimal debulking is feasible if the spleen is removed.

- Anatomy: the splenic artery originates at the celiac trunk. The splenic vein combines with the hepatic veins to join the inferior vena cava (IVC).

- Technique: when performing a splenectomy, it is necessary to take down the splenogastric, splenocolic, and splenophrenic ligaments. The artery and vein should be clamped and ligated separately to decrease the risk of arteriovenous fistula.
- Complications: there is a risk of thrombocytosis post-splenectomy, as well as an increased risk of deep vein thrombosis (DVT).
- Necessary vaccines after splenectomy include immunization against *Meningococcus*, *Haemophilus influenzae*, and *Pneumococcus*. Ideally, these vaccines should be given 14 days prior to the anticipated splenectomy. If not done prior, they should be done as soon as possible after surgery.

DIAPHRAGMATIC STRIPPING

Diaphragmatic stripping is performed when optimal debulking can be achieved. The peritoneum is removed with varied techniques.

- The liver usually needs to be mobilized inferiorly with release of the falciform and triangular ligaments.
- Complications include pneumothorax when the diaphragm is perforated. To rectify this, a Foley or red rubber catheter is placed through the defect and connected to suction. A purse string suture is placed around the Foley catheter and the patient is placed in Trendelenburg. The anesthesiologist is asked to perform an expiratory Valsalva for the patient with the ventilator, and the catheter is removed with the suture tied. A chest tube is usually placed and a chest x-ray is checked postoperatively.

MINIMALLY INVASIVE SURGERY

Minimally invasive surgery (MIS) has emerged as a growing area in procedural medicine and specifically useful in gynecologic surgery.

- Three laparoscopic approaches are typically used: traditional laparoscopy, robotic-assisted laparoscopy, and laparoendoscopic single-site surgery.
- Advantages of MIS include a shorter hospitalization, a more rapid recovery, smaller incisions, and a trend for fewer analgesics.
- Limitations of MIS are a longer learning curve and the costs of instrumentation.

Surgical Devices

DRAINS

- **Gastric tube (G-tube):** indicated for decompression of the stomach to avoid long-term use of a nasogastric tube. It can also be used for feeding patients with swallowing difficulties. When placed to gravity, it can be used as an outlet for bowel contents to decrease nausea and vomiting in patients with bowel obstruction.
- **Chest tube:** indicated for pleural effusions, hemothorax, or pneumothorax (if >15%). When used with pleurovac, negative pressure is set at 20 cm of H_2O. A purse string stitch is placed subcutaneously to secure it to the skin. Petrolatum-impregnated gauze should be placed over the incision to make it airtight. Obtain CXR daily.
  - Pneumothorax: place to suction for 2 days, then to water seal for the third day. A CXR should be obtained daily to evaluate size of pneumothorax. Leave water sealed until the output is less than 100 mL in 24 hours, and check for the presence of an air leak daily. Pull the CT when the pneumothorax is <10%, when output is less than 100 mL in 24 hours and there is no air leak.
  - Hemothorax or pleural effusion: place to suction for 1 day and then to water seal for the second day. Pull when output is less than 100 mL in 24 hours.
  - Resolution normally occurs at 10% to 20% per day.
  - When it is ready to be pulled, the patient should take a deep breath and then Valsalva. The tube is then pulled out as the purse string stitch is secured tightly around the prior incision. A petrolatum gauze should be placed on top.
- **Jackson-Pratt:** indicated for subcutaneous or intraperitoneal wound drainage. Used to decrease the incidence of seroma and infection. It is a closed drain; placed to bulb suction.
  - Subcutaneous: removal is recommended when output is less than 30 mL per day. Subcutaneous drainage decreases the incidence of seromas and infections if not used in conjunction with a subcutaneous stitch.
  - **Peritoneal/intra-abdominal placement:** removal is recommended when the peritoneal output is less than 50 mL per day. If there was significant pre-operative ascites, discontinuation of the drain is when the fluid turns mainly serous.
- **Penrose drain and T-tubes:** indicated for drainage of pelvic or subcutaneous infections. It is a passive drain.
- **Nasogastric tube:** indicated for postoperative ileus or for bowel obstruction. It is placed to low intermittent suction or Gomco suction.

CENTRAL VENOUS CATHETERS

Used to administer systemic cytotoxic agents, blood products, antibiotics, or in patients with poor peripheral access.

- The Mediport is a subcutaneous port and catheter used for central venous access. It is accessed using a Huber needle. It needs a monthly flush with heparin. A CXR is needed after placement unless it is placed under fluoroscopic guidance.
- A peripherally inserted central catheter, or PICC line, is a central venous line placed through a peripheral vein. Indications are for systemic cytotoxic agents, antibiotic therapy TPN, or in patients with poor peripheral access. A daily flush is needed but it can be left in place for 6 months. A CXR after placement is needed.
- A Hickman catheter is a subclavian catheter used for central venous access. It has no subcutaneous pocket reservoir, so the rate of infection is higher. Indications are similar to the PICC line. It necessitates a daily flush. A CXR after placement is needed.
- A Groshong catheter has similar indications for central venous access. It is a semipermanent central venous catheter. It needs a weekly flush. A CXR after placement is needed.

PERITONEAL CATHETERS

- The Tenckhoff catheter is a type of intraperitoneal port-a-cath. It can be irrigated with 500 units of heparin in 15 mL normal saline flush QID × 3 days after placement. It needs a weekly maintenance flush.
- The Bardport or Mediport 8–9.6F nonfenestrated port can also be used for intraperitoneal placement. It does not need a flush.

CATHETER TROUBLESHOOTING

- If a blood clot obstructs the use of any vascular catheter, attempts at salvage with a thrombolytic agent are indicated. Patency can be checked by injection of Hypaque contrast or visualization under fluoroscopy. An example of a thrombolytic protocol is a urokinase flush with 5,000 units/mL solution. A 1-mL injection into the port is performed followed by a 3 mL normal saline flush. This is allowed to remain for 1 hour, then fluid withdrawal is attempted.
- Fibrin sheath: this occurs and is diagnosed when there is difficulty withdrawing blood but the flush is smooth or has only moderate resistance. Treatment is placement of a new port if difficulty continues.

INSTRUMENTS

- Robotics platforms: there are a few companies with robotic platforms. The benefits of robotics are: 3D laparoscopy, 7° of wrist movement compared to the 3° that conventional laparoscopy is capable of, minimization of tremor, and accentuated nodal dissection techniques. Although the cost of the program is high, the length of patient stay, amortization, and subjectively improved dissection techniques contribute to high-yield outcomes in oncologic surgery practices.
- 3D laparoscopy is now available to enhance depth of vision and facilitate dissection.

- Indocyanine green (ICG) dye: ICG is a medical diagnostics indicator substance. The patented technology is Firefly™. It can be injected into the bloodstream and binds to albumin, or injected into primary tumor and drains to the regional lymphatics. ICG absorbs between 600 and 900 nm and emits fluorescence between 750 and 950 nm in the near infrared spectrum. When an 803 nm wavelength laser illuminates the surgical field, the dye is excited and fluoresces, documenting lymphatic vessels and nodes. Toxicity is in one out of 42,000 cases to include anaphylactic shock, hypotension, tachycardia, dyspnea, or urticaria. ICG-supported navigation for sentinel lymph node biopsy is one of the main medical diagnostic uses in gynecologic oncology.
- Potential therapeutic oncologic uses reside in the selectivity of overheating a tumor cell: as ICG absorbs light at 805 nanometers, a laser of that wavelength that can site specifically overheat fluorescing tissue without damaging surrounding tissue could provide an in vivo therapeutic treatment index. Studies have also been performed investigating targeting specific cells by conjugating the ICG to antibodies such as daclizumab, trastuzumab, or panitumumab.

SUTURE

The smallest gauge suture needed to obtain hemostasis is used to decrease the degree of foreign body reaction (Table 4.3).

Table 4.3 Common Suture Material and Properties

	Name	Composition	Indication	Filament	Tensile strength (lb)	Absorption	Number of knots needed	Gauge	Method of degradation
Natural absorbable	Plain catgut	Collagen from animal submucosa	Tubal ligation	Monofilament	4.4–8.4	70% at 7 days; Full digestion at 70 days	3	0, 1-0	Enzyme digestion
	Chromic catgut	Collagen and chromic salts from animal submucosa	Serosal, visceral, vaginal tissues	Monofilament	4.4–8.4	50% at 10 days	3	0, 1-0	Enzyme digestion
Synthetic absorbable	Dexon	Glycolic acid	Serosal, visceral, vaginal tissues, fascia in low-risk patients	Braided	6.2–11.6	50% at 14 days; 30% at 21 days	4	0, 1-0, 2-0	Hydrolysis
	Vicryl	Polyglactin 910	Serosal, visceral, vaginal tissues, fascia in low-risk patients	Braided	6.2–11.6	50% at 14 days; 30% at 21 days	4	0, 1-0, 2-0	Hydrolysis
	Maxon	Polyglyconate	Fascia	Monofilament	6.2–11.6	90% at 7 days; 25% at 6 weeks	8–9	0, 1-0	Hydrolysis

(continued)

Table 4.3 Common Suture Material and Properties *(continued)*

	Name	Composition	Indication	Filament	Tensile strength (lb)	Absorption	Number of knots needed	Gauge	Method of degradation
Synthetic absorbable (cont.)	PDS	Polydioxanone	Fascia	Monofilament	6.2–11.6	90% at 7 days; 25% at 6 weeks	8–9	0, 1-0	Hydrolysis
	Monocryl	Poliglecaprone 25	Serosal, visceral, vaginal tissues under no tension	Monofilament	6.2–11.6	50% at 7 days; 30% at 21 days	8–9	0, 1-0	Hydrolysis
Nonabsorbable natural	Silk	Silk	Serosal, visceral tissues, inappropriate in infected tissue	Braided	3.2–6.0	50% at 1 year; full degradation at 2 years	3–4	0, 1-0, 2-0	Hydrolysis
Synthetic nonabsorbable	Neurolon	Nylon	Suture drains and catheters to skin	Braided	2.3–4.0	Degrades 15% per year	4	0, 1-0, 2-0	Hydrolysis
	Dermalon	Nylon	Suture drains and catheters to skin	Monofilament	2.3–4.0	Degrades 15% per year	8–9	0, 1-0, 2-0	Hydrolysis
	Mersilene, Dacron	Polyester	Visceral tissues	Uncoated, braided	2.3–4.0	Degrades 15% per year	4	0, 1-0, 2-0	Hydrolysis

(continued)

Table 4.3 Common Suture Material and Properties (*continued*)

	Name	Composition	Indication	Filament	Tensile strength (lb)	Absorption	Number of knots needed	Gauge	Method of degradation
Synthetic nonabsorbable (cont.)	Ethibond	Polyester	Visceral tissues, hernia repair	Polybutilate coated, braided	2.3–4.0	Degrades 15% per year	8–9	0, 1-0, 2-0	Hydrolysis
	Polydek	Polyester	Visceral tissues	Teflon coated, braided	2.3–4.0	Degrades 15% per year	8–9	0, 1-0, 2-0	Hydrolysis
	Prolene	Polypropylene	Fascia, vascular procedures, ureteral anastomosis, sacrospinous fixation	Monofilament	4.0–10.5	Degrades 15% per year	8–9	0, 1-0	Hydrolysis

VASCULAR INJURY

- Venous lacerations should be repaired using 6-0 gauge Prolene sutures, in an interrupted or running fashion. Irrigation with heparinized saline can be used to visualize the repair. If the vein is large caliber, distal and proximal control should be obtained using pressure or Judd-Allis clamps. If there is a large hole, a lesser vein can be harvested and opened using Potts scissors to create a patch and sewn in place with interrupted sutures. Omentum can be placed on top to help vascularize. If sutures start to tear through the vein, pledgets (small pieces of cellulose) can be used to avoid suture tension.
- Arterial damage should be approximated in a similar fashion. If the edges are ragged, consider complete resection and approximation. If there is a large hole, a vein graft can be used to patch the artery; 100 to 150 units/kg of IV heparin can be given before cross clamping the vessel. This dosing can continue every 50 minutes until circulation is re-established.

NERVE INJURY

The nerve should be repaired using 7-0 gauge Prolene sutures to align the fascicle bundles. Only the epineurium should be approximated. Nerve growth is estimated at 1 mm per day, or 1 inch per month.

GASTROINTESTINAL INJURY

- Small bowel injuries:
  - Serosal injuries can be observed if they are small, but should be primarily oversewn with 3-0 gauge silk or Vicryl sutures if large. If radiation therapy (XRT) has been administered, serosal injuries should always be oversewn.
  - A seromuscular injury is evident if bulging of the bowel wall is seen. Repair should be double layered with 3-0 gauge silk or Vicryl.
  - If there is luminal injury, a double-layered closure is indicated. Double-layered repair can be with 3-0 gauge Vicryl for the mucosal layer and either Vicryl or silk for the serosal layer.
- Large bowel injury should be evaluated for a transmural defect. If no transmural defect is identified, a primary single-layered repair can be performed using 3-0 gauge silk or Vicryl. If there is a transmural defect and no evidence of fecal contamination, a primary double-layer closure can be attempted. If there is an extensive defect, consideration should be given to resection with reanastomosis. If no bowel preparation was given, consideration should be given to a diverting loop or end colostomy with mucous fistula.

URINARY TRACT INJURY

- Urinary tract injury occurs in 1% to 2.5% of gynecologic surgeries. Intraoperative cystoscopy with 1 ampule of IV indigo carmine or 0.25 to 1.0 mg of fluorescein should follow most hysterectomy procedures to detect and provide early repair of these injuries (1–3).
- Bladder injury should be identified with direct visualization, IV fluorescein, or IV indigo carmine. The bladder should be closed in two layers using absorbable suture. This is usually with an inverting stitch of 2-0 gauge Vicryl or chromic for the first layer, and Vicryl for the second. If there is trigone injury, cystoscopy should be performed to ensure the ureters are intact. The bladder should be drained with a Foley catheter for 5 to 14 days.
- Ureteral injury is recognized at the time of surgery in 20% to 30% of cases. Injury can be via transection, ligation, crush injury, angulation, or ischemia. Injury is commonly at the level of the uterine artery, at the infundibulopelvic ligament, or at the level of the pelvic brim. Ureteral stenting should occur for most ureteral injuries. This is done via cystoscopy, cystotomy, or ureterotomy. A Jackson–Pratt (JP) drain should be placed in all cases. If there is concern for further ureteral leakage, the JP fluid can be checked for a creatinine level and compared to a serum creatinine. Stenting is maintained for 6 to 12 weeks followed by intravenous pyelography (IVP) after stent removal.
  - If there is a crush injury identified, the clamp should be released, and the ureter observed and mobilized. An ampule of IV indigo carmine should be given. If no extravasation is seen, consideration should be given to stenting the ureter.
  - A partial transection can be treated with stenting and primary closure using 4-0 gauge to 6-0 gauge delayed absorbable suture (PDS).
  - If there is complete transection, the ends should be dissected out, mobilized, and trimmed. The location of transection dictates repair.
    - A distal transection (below the pelvic brim) can be managed with ureteroneocystostomy/reimplantation. There is debate as to the benefit of tunneling the ureter into the bladder. Reimplantation can also be via a Boari flap, a psoas hitch, the Demel technique, or use of intestinal interposition with an ileal segment.
    - If there is middle pelvic transection, ureteroureterostomy or ureteroileoneocystostomy can be performed.
    - If the transection is above the pelvic brim, a transureteroureterostomy or ileal intestinal interposition can be performed. Care should be taken with a transureteroureterostomy as this procedure can compromise the opposite kidney.

INTRAOPERATIVE HEMORRHAGE

When there is life-threatening, severe intraoperative hemorrhage, the use of a "massive transfusion protocol" (MTP) may be indicated. This transfusion protocol decreases the use of blood components, as well as turnaround times, costs, and mortality (2).

- Initiate MTP.
  - Issue 4 units packed red blood cells (PRBC) and 4 units fresh frozen plasma (FFP) in cooler.
  - Once the first package is issued, prepare the second package as a "Stay Ahead" order and add a 6 pack (1 dose) of platelets.

Table 4.4 Massive Transfusion Protocol			
Blood component prepared			
First package	4 units PRBC	4 units FFP	
Second package	4 units PRBC	4 units FFP	1 dose platelets
	Prepare cryo after second package issued		1 dose cryoprecipitate
Third package	4 units PRBC	4 units FFP	1 dose platelets
	Prepare cryo after third package issued		1 dose cryoprecipitate
FFP, fresh frozen plasma; MTP, massive transfusion protocol; PRBC, packed red blood cells.			

- Once second package is issued (RBC, FFP, and platelets), begin preparing cryoprecipitate dose and set up next "Stay Ahead" package (RBC, FFP, platelets).
- Repeat as necessary (Table 4.4).

REFERENCES

1. Ibeanu OA, Chesson RR, Echols KT, et al. Urinary tract injury during hysterectomy based on universal cystoscopy. *Obstet Gynecol.* 2009;113:6-10.
2. O'Keeffe T, Refaai M, Tchorz K, et al. A massive transfusion protocol to decrease blood component use and costs. *Arch Surg.* 2008;143(7):686-690.
3. Doyle PJ, Lipetskaia L, Duecy E, et al. Sodium fluorescein use during intraoperative cystoscopy. *Obstet Gynecol.* March 2015;125(3):548-550.

RADICAL VULVAR SURGERY

- Drains:
  - Groin Jackson–Pratt (JP) drains should be discontinued when output is less than 30 mL per day.
  - Foley catheter: depending on site of resection and reconstruction, the Foley can be left in for 7 days with prophylactic antibiotics, or removed postoperative day (POD) 1.
- Antibiotics: oral prophylactic antibiotics can be given starting on POD 1 and until groin and vulvar wounds are well healed. Coverage for *Streptococcus* with antibiotics has been shown to decrease the incidence of lymphedema due to beta-hemolytic *Streptococcus*.
- Wound care: this is mainly pericare with soap and water squirt bottle to the perineum TID and after each bowel movement. The area can be blown dry with a hairdryer on cool setting after each cleaning.
- Deep vein thrombosis (DVT) prophylaxis: combination injectable anticoagulant and sequential compression devices (SCDs) should be employed until the patient is fully ambulatory. Ambulation should occur as soon as possible with control for pain, physical therapy consultation, and documentation of wound integrity.
- Nutrition: low-residue diet as tolerated
- Complications: lymphocysts—percutaneous drainage can be performed if symptomatic by palpation or with image guidance. If they are recurrent, they can be sclerosed with talc, tetracyclines, or alcohol.
- Follow-up: 6 weeks

RADICAL HYSTERECTOMY

- Drains:
  - JP drains: discontinue when less than 30 mL/day output.
  - Foley catheter: should be discontinued POD 3 to 4. A post-void residual should be checked immediately after the first self-void. The Foley should be replaced if the residual volume is greater than 100 mL, and the Foley then continued for 1 week. If at recheck, the post void residual is still elevated, the patient should be educated on self-catheterization. Bladder dysfunction can occur in up to 10% of patients due to denervation from cardinal and uterosacral ligament resection.
- Antibiotics: consider daily oral antibiotics for suppression when a Foley catheter is in place.

- Wound care: keep clean and dry. Staples: remove staples POD 3 for transverse or Maylard incisions. Remove staples POD 10 for midline incisions.
- Deep vein thrombosis (DVT) prophylaxis: combination injectable anticoagulant and SCDs should be used until the patient is fully ambulatory. Four weeks of postoperative anticoagulation should be considered. Ambulation should occur as soon as pain is controlled and strength permits.
- Nutrition: regular diet as tolerated
- Complications: lymphocysts: can occur in up to 25% of patients but are symptomatic in about 5% of patients. If infected or symptomatic, broad-spectrum antibiotics should be employed. Percutaneous drainage can be attempted if spontaneous resolution does not occur or if vessel or organ obstruction/compression occurs. They can also be sclerosed with talc, alcohol, or tetracyclines.
- Follow-up: 6 weeks

URINARY CONDUITS AND PELVIC EXENTERATION

- Drains:
  - If a nasogastric tube was inserted during surgery, it should be removed at the end of the operation.
  - Malecot (for continent conduits): should be placed to dependent drainage for 7 to 10 days. Irrigation every 4 to 6 hours with 40 mL of normal saline should be performed to prevent the accumulation of mucus.
  - Red rubber catheter in continent conduits: it should be left sewn in place until ready to self-catheterize at 7 to 10 days.
  - JP drains: should be left in place for 7 to 10 days or until output is less than 30 mL/day.
  - Gracilis flap JP leg drains: leave for 7 days or until output is less than 30 mL/day.
- Antibiotics: if the patient has a conduit, consider discharge home with PO prophylaxis.
- Wound and flap care: keep clean and dry. Pericare should be performed TID. The area can be blown dry with a hairdryer on cool setting after each cleaning. Staples should be left in place for 10 days, including those on the legs for gracilis flaps.
- DVT prophylaxis: combination injectable anticoagulant and SCDs should be employed until the patient is fully ambulatory. Consider 4 weeks of postoperative injectable anticoagulation. Ambulation should occur as soon as pain is controlled, strength permits, and wound integrity is documented.
- Nutrition: total parenteral nutrition (TPN) should be started postoperatively if the patient is suspected to be nothing by mouth (NPO) for greater than 7 days or if the patient was malnourished prior to surgery. Begin PO feedings with bowel sounds.
- Complications: evaluation of the urinary tract by intravenous pyelography (IVP) or ultrasound should be part of a postoperative fever workup. Stomas should be checked daily; if they are dusky, endoscopy should be performed.
- Other:
  - Ureteral stents: should be sewn in with chromic suture, which will spontaneously dissolve and separate between days 10 and 14.

- ○ Chest x-ray (CXR) on admission to the recovery room should be obtained if a central line was inserted.
- Follow-up: should occur at 2 weeks and 6 weeks. Lab tests: blood urea nitrogen (BUN) and creatinine should be obtained at each visit. Radiologic studies: an IVP should be obtained at discharge, 6 weeks, 6 months, 18 months, 3 years, and 5 years. A CT of abdomen and pelvis can be considered every 6 months to 1 year.

BOWEL RESECTION

- Drains:
  - ○ Nasogastric tube (NGT) can be removed immediately after surgery. If there was obstruction preoperatively, it can remain until bowel function returns.
  - ○ JP peritoneal drains can be placed if multiple enterotomies occurred to check for bowel leak or fistula. Leave drains in until fluid output is serosanguinous.
  - ○ Subcutaneous JP drains: these can be discontinued when the output is less than 30 mL/day.
  - ○ Foley: this can be discontinued on POD 1.
- Antibiotics: these should only be used postoperatively if gross peritoneal contamination occurs with bowel contents. They can be discontinued on POD 2 to 3 if the patient is afebrile.
- Wound care: vertical midline staples should remain for 10 days. Patients with transverse incisions can have their staples removed between days 3 and 5.
- DVT prophylaxis: combination injectable anticoagulant and SCDs should be employed until the patient is fully ambulatory. Consider 4 weeks of injectable postoperative anticoagulation. Ambulation should occur as soon as pain is controlled and strength permits.
- Nutrition: consider TPN if there is prolonged ileus for more than 7 days, postoperative obstruction occurs, or the patient was malnourished preoperatively.

OVARIAN CANCER DEBULKING

- Drains:
  - ○ If a nasogastric tube was placed due to obstruction, this can be removed when bowel function returns.
  - ○ JP peritoneal drain: these will always have output, especially if there was a large amount of ascites.
  - ○ Subcutaneous drains: discontinue when output less than 30 mL/day.
  - ○ Foley: discontinue on POD 1 if adequate urine output. Urine output is commonly low due to third spacing from surgery and ascites removal. Homeostasis tends to return by POD 3, and urine output normalizes around then.
- Antibiotics: these should only be used postoperatively if gross peritoneal contamination occurs with bowel contents. They can be discontinued on POD 2 to 3 if the patient is afebrile.
- Wound care: vertical midline staples should remain for 10 days. Patients with transverse incisions can have their staples removed between days 3 and 5.

- DVT prophylaxis: combination injectable anticoagulant and SCDs should be employed until the patient is fully ambulatory. Consider 4 weeks of postoperative injectable anticoagulation. Ambulation should occur as soon as pain is controlled and strength permits.
- Nutrition: consider TPN if there is prolonged ileus for more than 7 days, postoperative obstruction occurs, or the patient was malnourished preoperatively.

ENHANCED RECOVERY PATHWAYS

- Enhanced recovery is encouraged for most surgical patients. This includes:
  - Early ambulation.
  - Advancement of diet as tolerated.
  - Removal of the Foley catheter in uncomplicated patients by 24 hours.
  - Use of DVT prophylaxis with SCDs and q8h heparin or daily unfractioned heparin use.
  - Minimal use of NGT decompression.
  - Aggressive nausea and emesis prophylaxis.
  - Minimization of IV narcotics and early discontinuation of the patient controlled anesthesia (PCA) with transition to oral narcotics as soon as PO nutrition is tolerated.

GASTROINTESTINAL COMPLICATIONS

- Ileus
  - The etiology is often intraoperative manipulation, electrolyte abnormalities, narcotics, peritonitis, abscess, hematoma, or fistula.
  - Signs are nausea and vomiting, hypoactive or absent bowel sounds, and abdominal distension.
  - Workup is with laboratories and physical examination.
  - Treatment: the patient can be made nothing by mouth (NPO), intravenous fluid (IVF) initiated, and consideration given to a nasogastric tube (NGT). If the ileus does not resolve, imaging can be obtained with a CT scan of the abdomen and pelvis with oral Gastrografin contrast to rule out an obstruction. Abdominal imaging provides no difference in clinical treatment between obstruction and ileus as they will both be managed with NPO/NGT/electrolyte replacement upfront. If abscess is seen with CT, a percutaneous drain can be placed with antibiotics as indicated.
- **Bowel obstructions:** partial obstructions can resolve spontaneously in 50% of cases. Complete obstructions usually need surgical intervention.
  - **Small-bowel obstruction** (SBO)
    - The etiology can be adhesions or herniation from surgery, bowel kinking, tumor, radiation therapy (XRT) induced ischemia, and stricture.
    - Signs are nausea and vomiting. Bowel sounds are present and can be high pitched and hyperactive. Abdominal distension is present, and absence of flatus is common.
    - Workup is with lab tests, a physical examination, and CT scan of the abdomen and pelvis with PO Gastrografin contrast.
    - The patient should be made NPO, an NGT placed to low intermittent wall suction (LIWS), pain medication administered, and IVF should be initiated. Correction of electrolyte abnormalities is important in addition to antiemetics and pain management. Occasionally, high-dose steroids can reduce periluminal inflammation and have antiemetic properties. Partial obstructions can resolve with conservative management, but fewer than 50% of complete obstructions resolve similarly.
  - **Large-bowel obstruction** (LBO)
    - Etiology can be a mass causing obstruction intrinsically (intraluminal tumor), extrinsically (pelvic tumor compression), or stricture from transmural invasion.
    - Signs: LBO can have a delayed time to presentation with a lower amount of emesis.

- Workup is indicated with imaging:
  - □ CT scan of abdomen and pelvis with Gastrografin should be obtained. This can document the site of obstruction and may occasionally be therapeutic.
  - □ Barium enema: can occasionally be therapeutic. This study should be performed before a CT scan or small bowel follow-through.
- To manage conservatively: the patient should be made NPO, an NGT should be placed to LIWS, IV fluids and pain control should be instituted, and antiemetics should be given.
- To manage surgically:
  - □ IV second-generation cephalosporins should be given prior to surgical correction.
  - □ Resection with end-to-end anastomosis, loop, or end ostomy with mucous fistula can be performed.
  - □ Stenting may occasionally be useful if the patient is a poor surgical candidate.
- Enemas in partial LBO can either be therapeutic or can convert the obstruction to a complete obstruction by inducing colonic spasm.
  - □ If the patient chooses to forego extensive surgery, consider endoscopy with stent placement or diversion via end ostomy.
  - □ When considering whether to perform surgical reduction of an obstruction in a cancer patient, it is important to take into account the patient's social factors; the expected outcome; the patient's life expectancy; and the etiology and the extent of obstruction (e.g., recurrent cancer, XRT stenosis).
- Bowel perforation:
  - ○ Etiology: perforation can occur from an unrecognized enterotomy, intestinal devascularization, tumor infiltration of the bowel wall, bowel infarction (from thrombus, atrial fibrillation), or even certain chemotherapy agents (bevacizumab up to 1%–11%, paclitaxel 2%).
  - ○ Signs are peritonitis, pain, abdominal distension, and fever.
  - ○ Workup: imaging with abdominal x-ray or CT demonstrating free air under the diaphragm. Treatment is with emergent surgical exploration and antibiotics. Cecal perforation tends to occur if the cecum is dilated to, or greater than, 10 cm as seen on imaging.
  - ○ Treatment is with loop or end ostomy with mucous fistula, or ileostomy.
- Pneumoperitoneum after laparotomy should be considered when ruling out a bowel perforation. Table 4.5 demonstrates the time from surgery and percent of patients with residual abdominal air present.

Table 4.5 Pneumoperitoneum Duration Seen Radiologically After Surgery		
Time	Radiograph percent positive	CT scan percent positive
Postoperative day 3	53% positive	87% positive
Postoperative day 6	8% positive	50% positive

- Anastomotic bowel leak after a bowel resection can occur in up to 15% of patients. Prevention is avoidance of the bowel watershed areas. When performing an anastomosis, universal principles should be followed ensuring adequate vascularization of both ends of the bowel, absence of tumor at the anastomotic site, a tension-free anastomosis, and an adequate bowel lumen. Bowel viability can be ascertained with IV fluorescein dye and a Wood's lamp at the time of resection and reanastomosis, or with Doppler ultrasound.
  - Signs: leaks tend to present with nausea, ileus, abdominal pain, fever, and occasionally leakage of feculent material through the wound.
  - Workup: includes physical exam, lab tests, and a CT of the abdomen and pelvis with PO Gastrografin.
  - Treatment: a drain needs to be placed, the patient made NPO, broad-spectrum antibiotics given, and consideration for surgical intervention with intestinal diversion. The diversion can usually be taken down in about 2 months, after imaging with PO contrast shows no evidence of continued leakage or after completion of chemotherapy in abdominal cancer patients and no evidence of recurrent disease (6-12 months).
- Bowel fistula (enterocutaneous, enterovaginal, enterovesicle):
  - Signs: fistulae can present as feculent discharge from a surgical wound or the vagina.
  - Workup: diagnosis is with a CT of the abdomen and pelvis with PO Gastrografin contrast or a fistulagram. Oral activated charcoal or isosulfan blue can also be given to evaluate for color change that would indicate a fistula.
  - Treatment: an NGT should be placed, the patient made NPO, and total parenteral nutrition (TPN) initiated. Wound care should be performed, and consideration given to administration of somatostatin. If there is no resolution of the fistula with these conservative measures, surgical resection of the fistulous tract with bowel resection and temporary diversion or primary reanastomosis with protective loop ileostomy should be performed. Staged repair with a diverting loop colostomy, primary fistula repair, and ostomy take-down approximately 2 months later is the preferred option as massive inflammation can hamper primary anastomosis and compromise fistula repair.
- Stoma complications usually involve stomal retraction or devitalization.
  - Etiology: this occurs from tension or decreased blood flow to the distal bowel edges.
  - Signs include a dusky appearance, necrosis, or retraction.
  - Workup: evaluation of viability includes placement of a test tube or blood vial inside the stoma to assess the depth/extent of damage.
  - Treatment is based on location of devitalization. If it is limited to the distal segment above the fascia, observation and wound care are indicated. If there is necrosis beneath the fascia, surgical revision is necessary.
- Ostomy herniation or prolapse usually occurs in patients whose ostomy was placed lateral to the rectus muscles.
  - Prolapse occurs in 1% to 3% of patients with an ostomy.
    - Etiology: it is often due to a stoma that is too long or wide, increased intra-abdominal pressure, extensive weight loss, or a redundant sigmoid colon.
    - Treatment: conservative measures are placement of a rigid appliance with a tight belt. Treatment is resection of the protruding segment of colon

with nipple reconstruction. Care should be taken to rule out those with a hernia so there is no loop transection risk.

o Parastomal hernia: one half of patients with a prolapse also have a parastomal hernia.

   ▪ Etiology: parastomal hernias occur more often with loop ostomies than with end stomas. 2% to 3% of all end colostomy patients require hernia repair. Predisposing factors are often too large of an opening in the abdominal wall, placement lateral to the rectus muscle, placement in the laparotomy incision itself, or increased intra-abdominal pressure due to chronic obstructive pulmonary disease (COPD), coughing, heavy lifting, obesity.

   ▪ Repair is indicated if the hernia does not reduce easily, there is evidence of incarceration, or if the hernia interferes with appliance security. If the hernia is small, primary fascial repair without relocation can often be accomplished. If it is large, the ostomy can be placed at a different site (to a higher midrectus position, to the opposite side, or to the umbilicus) with repair of the primary ventral hernia. Mesh can otherwise be placed over part of the fascial defect to reduce the defect size (Sugarbaker) and the stoma can be brought out in between an aperture between the mesh and the skin. To initiate the repair, the skin should be elliptically excised, and a finger swept circumferentially around the bowel between it and the fascia.

• Short bowel syndrome is defined as malnutrition due to the lack of absorptive bowel length.

   o Etiology: this can occur from significant bowel resection or from XRT injury. A length of bowel, approximately 200 cm, is necessary for nutrient absorption.

   o Signs: symptoms include diarrhea, steatorrhea, fluid depletion, fatigue, and occasionally abdominal pain.

   o Diagnosis is made by malnutrition indices and weight loss.

   o Treatment is with caloric, vitamin, and mineral supplementation. Hyperalimentation with TPN or continuous gastrostomy tube (G-tube) nutrition should be considered if there is significant weight loss. Additionally, antacids, antidiarrheals, and lactase supplements should be given.

• Blind loop syndrome:

   o Etiology: occurs after bowel resection and bypass producing a nonfunctional but retained loop of bowel.

   o Signs: increased flatulence, steatorrhea, weight loss, fatigue, and malabsorption.

   o Diagnosis: a hydrogen breath test using glucose or lactulose can assist in the diagnosis. Bacterial overgrowth causes the majority of symptoms.

   o Treatment: antibiotics can reduce the bacterial load and decrease symptoms. Vitamin B_{12} supplementation is also often indicated.

HEMORRHAGE

• Blood loss from the gastrointestinal (GI) system can occur from a stomach ulcer, esophageal varices, a Mallory–Weiss tear, a Boerhaave tear, NGT/catheter erosion, or XRT enteritis.

- Inadequate hemostasis from a slipped suture, coagulopathy, or overanticoagulation.
- Tumor can spontaneously bleed from neovascularization.
- Symptoms can include tachycardia, ectopy, pain, abdominal distension, decreased perfusion with mental status changes from hypoxia, low urine output from renal compromise, or extremity cyanosis due to centralization of the blood supply. Diagnosis is geared to identification of the source.
- Workup: laboratories include complete blood count (CBC) and electrolytes. Imaging studies include CT, MRI, ultrasound, or angiography.
- Treatment is focused on the "ABCs." Resuscitation is with IVF (in a 3:1 crystalloid replacement ratio to blood loss), blood products, and oxygen. Treatment is surgical re-exploration or angiographic embolization.
- If hemorrhage is due to a large cervical tumor, vaginal packing with Monsel's solution is indicated. The packing should be changed every 24 to 48 hours. Embolization can be considered but this will decrease oxygenation needed for XRT to the primary tumor. Emergent hyperfractionated XRT can also be given.

POSTOPERATIVE FEVER

Postoperative fever is the most common postoperative complication. The definition of a fever is a temperature elevation taken two times, 6 hours apart. If the fever occurs within the first 24 hours of surgery, the temperature must be above 101.5°F (38.6°C). If the fever occurs greater than 24 hours after surgery, the temperature must be greater than or equal to 100.4°F (38.1°C).

- The source of the fever usually follows the "five W's":
  ○ Wind: this can represent atelectasis or pneumonia. Obtain a CXR.
  ○ Water: this can represent a urinary tract infection (UTI) or pyelonephritis. Obtain a urine analysis.
  ○ Wound: this can represent a superficial infection, a seroma, cellulitis, or abscess. Evaluation involves examination and occasionally opening of the incision.
  ○ Walk: this can represent a deep vein thrombosis (DVT), septic pelvic thrombophlebitis, or a pulmonary embolus (PE). Diagnosis is via examination, measurement of calf diameter, Doppler ultrasound, and occasionally CT angiogram.
  ○ Wonder drugs: this can result from drug fevers. This is a diagnosis of exclusion. After ruling out other causes, consideration of discontinuing all drugs and observing the patient may be beneficial. Evaluation of the white blood cell (WBC) differential may be helpful by assessment for the degree of eosinophilia.

WOUND INFECTION

- Surgical site infections (SSI) account for 40% of nosocomial infections. Risk factors for infection include surgery lasting longer than 2 hours, higher blood loss, preoperative anemia, hypothermia, poor nutrition, cancer, prior XRT, diabetes, obesity, peripheral vascular disease, and a history of prior surgical infections.
  ○ Whole-body cleansing with chlorhexidine can reduce bacterial skin counts, but they do not reduce the rate of wound infection. Alternatively, patients may shower normally before surgery.
  ○ Hair clipping, not shaving, reduces the rate of wound infections.

○ Antibiotics given 1 hour before the skin incision are recommended, except for vancomycin and the fluoroquines, which should be given 2 hours prior. Cefazolin has a longer half-life and a broad spectrum of coverage. Cefotetan is preferred in longer, radical gynecologic operations and in colorectal surgery. Alternatives are aztreonam and clindamycin, cefazolin plus metronidazole, or ampicillin–sulbactam. If the patient's weight is greater than 70 kg, it is important to double the dose or weight-base dose the antibiotics.

○ Repeat dosing is recommended if surgery lasts longer than 3 to 4 hours, or if there is greater than 1,000 mL blood loss. Antibiotics should be stopped within 24 hours of surgery to decrease bacterial resistance and complications.

○ Obese patients have a higher risk for postoperative complications due to their body habitus and medical comorbidities. Some providers suggest these patients have baseline pulmonary function tests (PFTs), assisted intubation, and delayed extubation until they are fully awake. Higher weight capacity hospital beds and operating room (OR) tables, specialized retractors, and extra-long instruments for surgery are important. A panniculectomy can be performed to improve surgical exposure.

• Classification of operative wound infections is standardized.

○ A clean operative wound has a 1% to 2% risk of a surgical wound infection. This means that the GI and respiratory tracts were not entered, no drains were placed, and there was no break in aseptic technique. Examples of these surgeries are elective hernia repair.

○ A clean contaminated wound has a 4% to 10% risk of a surgical wound infection in uninfected patients. The GI or respiratory tracts were entered but minimal contamination occurred. This includes hysterectomy, appendectomy, and most elective bowel surgery.

○ A contaminated operative wound has a 20% risk of surgical wound infection. This means there may have been a major break in sterile technique, the wound was made through nonpurulent inflammation, there was gross spill from the GI tract, or the wound was in or near contaminated skin. An example of this is a laparotomy in a patient with a colostomy.

○ An infected/dirty surgical wound has a 50% risk of wound infection. This occurs in a wound in which purulent infection or a perforated viscus was encountered. An example is a localized bowel perforation.

URINARY TRACT INJURY

• Unrecognized injury occurs in 70% of patients.

○ Signs of injury include flank pain, fever, ileus from urine, hematuria, an elevated creatinine, or serous wound drainage (vaginal or abdominal).

○ Diagnosis is with renal ultrasound, intravenous pyelography (IVP), CT with IV contrast, or cystoscopy with an attempt to pass ureteral stents.

○ Treatment is with antibiotics and ureteral stenting or percutaneous nephrostomy (PCN) to decompress the kidney and preserve renal function. Delay of definitive repair until 4 to 6 weeks should occur if the patient is unstable from other comorbidities. Recent data support repair at the time of diagnosis if the patient is stable.

- Postoperative fistulae can be either uretero-vaginal or vesico-vaginal. Symptoms are leakage of clear fluid vaginally. Diagnosis is with a tampon test: this is performed with retrograde filling of the bladder using indigo carmine or methylene blue and placement of a vaginal tampon. If the tampon turns blue, the fistula originates in the bladder. If the tampon does not turn blue, phenazopyridine (Pyridium) can be given PO. If the tampon then turns orange, the fistula is most likely of ureteral origin.
  - Uretero-vaginal fistulas tend to become apparent 5 to 14 days postoperatively. Attempts at retrograde stenting should be made first. PCN with antegrade stenting is the next best step. If stenting is not possible, PCN with drainage should be performed.
  - Vesico-vaginal fistulas should first be treated with prolonged bladder drainage, in an attempt to allow spontaneous healing. If this does not work, repair is vaginal or abdominal. Vaginal repairs are with a modified Latzko technique, or a bulbocavernosus flap. If prior XRT was given, a flap is needed to provide vascularized tissue.
  - Fistula that occurs from a neobladder should be managed conservatively. An abdominal drain and PCN should be placed. If surgical intervention is attempted, there is a 9% mortality rate and 53% rate of complications.

LYMPHATIC COMPLICATIONS

- Lymphedema mainly occurs from surgical lymph node dissection. It can, less commonly, be due to XRT or tumor infiltration. Woody edema is the main symptom. Treatment is with elevation of the leg, support hose, or pneumatic compression devices.
- Lymphangitis can present as acute erythema of the extremity, fever, and pain. It usually occurs after surgical lymph node dissection with superimposed infection. Treatment is with elevation of the leg, antibiotics, and nonsteroidal anti-inflammatory drugs (NSAIDs).
- Lymphocysts occur after lymph node dissection. Signs are a palpable cystic mass and pain. Diagnosis is via ultrasound, CT, or MRI. Treatment depends on symptoms. If the patient is asymptomatic, observation is enough. If there are symptoms, from pressure or mass effect, the cyst can be aspirated or sclerosed. If there are symptoms from infection, drainage with broad-spectrum antibiotics and NSAIDs are indicated.

NERVE INJURY

- Neuropathy can complicate any surgical procedure. This stems from positioning, retractors, or direct nerve injury from dissection. Symptoms are sharp or burning pain, paresthesias, and weakness in the affected muscle groups. Treatment is often supportive care with physical therapy. If there is extensive deficit, a neurology consult can be obtained and electromyograms can assist in assessment.
- Nerve transection: see Chapter 7.

Perioperative Management of Medical Comorbidities

ENHANCED RECOVERY PATHWAYS IN GYNECOLOGIC ONCOLOGY

Accelerated recovery with multimodal postoperative clinical pathways has been shown to improve outcomes. It starts in the preoperative period and continues through hospitalization.

- Bowel prep continues to be controversial: infection and anastomotic leak were reviewed in patients with a bowel preparation; results were 9.6% and 4.4%, respectively, with a preparation compared to 8.5% and 4.5%, respectively, for those without a preparation.
- Overnight fasting: longer fasting causes untoward metabolic changes and depletion of liver glycogen stores. Therefore, a 6-hour no solid food and a 2-hour no clear liquid regimen is advised.
- Intraoperative fluid management: euvolemia is the goal. 7% versus 24% of patients had cardiovascular complications when zero balance was the goal versus standard 3 kg to 7 kg increase of too much fluid. In patients with sepsis, an average 12 L of fluid overload occurred, which took 3 weeks to mobilize. Pulmonary congestion, edema, hyponatremia, and congestive heart failure (CHF) tend to occur with too much intravenous fluid (IVF).
- Postoperative pain control: epidural versus patient controlled analgesia (PCA) have shown different lengths of stay in gynecologic oncology patients favoring earlier discharge with PCA. Those with an epidural had a longer time to first ambulation, higher rate of pressor use during surgery, and pain control was equivalent to lower than those with a PCA (due to a 30% failure rate of epidural analgesia). Toradol has been shown to provide superior pain control and is equivalent to opioid relief with no increase in postoperative bleeding or anastomotic leaks.
- Prophylactic drains are not indicated except in those with very low anterior resections (an anastomosis within 6 cm of the anal verge). Nasogastric tube (NGT) drainage is contraindicated prophylactically (1).

VASCULAR THROMBOEMBOLISM

- Deep vein thrombosis and venous thromboembolism (DVT/VTE) **prophylaxis** should be given to most hospitalized patients. The gynecologic oncology patient population is a high-risk group.
  - Pneumatic sequential compression devices (SCDs) should be used. Use should start preoperatively, continue intraoperatively, and continue postoperatively.
  - A low-dose injectable anticoagulant should be considered prior to surgery. The normal dose of heparin is 5,000 units SC before surgery. Dalteparin

dosed at 5,000 units SC can be given before surgery. Enoxaparin can also be used at 40 mg SC before surgery.

- ○ **In-hospital prophylaxis** of DVT: the combination of SCDs and injectable anticoagulants is especially helpful for the prevention of VTE complications. The use of SCDs has taken the incidence of VTE from 25% to 8%. The use of combination therapy then took the VTE occurrence from 8% to 2%. Dosing is usually with unfractionated heparin (UFH) 5,000 q8 hours or enoxaparin 30 to 40 mg daily. The risk of DVT with laparoscopic surgery in high-risk cancer patients with appropriate prophylaxis is 1.2% (2). Care should be taken and SCDs not used if an active superficial or deep vein thrombosis (SVT)/DVT is present because of potential embolization. Graduated compression stockings have not been found to decrease DVTs (3). If there is a contraindication to anticoagulation prophylaxis, mechanical prophylaxis alone should be used.
  - ▪ **Contraindications to mechanical prophylaxis:**
    - ▫ Absolute: acute SVT/DVT, severe arterial insufficiency
    - ▫ Relative: large hematoma, skin ulcerations or wounds, thrombocytopenia (platelets <20,000/mcL) or petechial, mild arterial insufficiency, peripheral neuropathy
  - ▪ Contraindications to prophylactic or therapeutic **anticoagulation**:
    - ▫ Absolute: recent central nervous system bleed, intracranial or spinal lesion at high risk for bleeding, active bleeding (major) with more than two units PRBC transfused in 24 hours.
    - ▫ Relative: chronic clinically significant measurable bleeding for more than 48 hours, thrombocytopenia (platelets <50,000/mcL), severe platelet dysfunction (uremia, medications, dysplastic hematopoiesis), recent major operation at high risk for bleeding, underlying hemorrhagic coagulopathy, high risk for falls (head trauma).
- **Risk factors** for VTE include: known malignancy, surgery, surgical time greater than 2 to 3 hours, postoperative immobility, a past history of VTE, body mass index (BMI) greater than 30, hereditary coagulopathy, age 60 years or above, hypertension, renal disease, pulmonary disease, estrogen use, inflammatory bowel disease, and hereditary coagulopathies (methylenetetrahydrofolate reductase [MTHFR] deficiency, protein C/protein S deficiencies, prothrombin gene mutation, antithrombin III and factor V Leiden gene mutations, antinuclear antibodies, antiphospholipid antibodies; Table 4.6).
- Symptoms of an SVT/DVT are: leg edema, erythema, size discrepancy between the legs, pain, heaviness, persistent cramping, cyanosis of extremity, swelling in the neck of supraclavicular area.
- Positive physical signs are: the Pratt's, Homan's, and Moses's tests.
- Diagnosis is with Doppler ultrasound.
- Treatment
  - ○ **SVT** that is not close to the deep venous system or is a peripheral catheter-related clot: remove the catheter, symptomatic treatment with heating pad, anti-inflammatory medications, elevation of extremity
  - ○ SVT in close proximity to deep venous system in a surgical or oncologic patient: strongly consider therapeutic anticoagulation for 6 weeks and up to 12 weeks if close to the femoral system

Table 4.6 VTE Risk Factors in Cancer Patients: Khorana Predictive Model for Chemotherapy-Associated VTE

Patient characteristic	Risk score
Site of primary cancer	2
Very high risk: stomach, pancreas	1
High risk: lung, lymphoma, gynecologic, bladder, testicular	1
Prechemotherapy platelet count 350 × 10–9 or higher	1
Hemoglobin level less than 10 g/dL or use of red cell growth factors	1
Prechemotherapy leukocyte count higher than 11 × 10–9/L	1
BMI 35 kg/m² or higher	1

Total score	Risk category	Risk of symptomatic VTE
0	Low	0.8%–3%
1.2	Intermediate	1.8%–4%
3 or more	High	1%–41%

Source: Adapted from Refs. 4, 5.
VTE, venous thromboembolism.

○ Pelvic/iliac/inferior vena cava (IVC)/femoral/popliteal **DVT**:
  ▪ Therapeutic anticoagulation is indicated.
  ▪ If there is contraindication to anticoagulation:
    □ Placement of an IVC filter is indicated
    □ If there is a calf DVT and a contraindication to anticoagulation: follow-up for DVT progression should occur at the first week. If there is no progression, consider following clinically; if progression then treat with IVC filter.
○ **Upper extremity or superior vena cava DVT**:
  ▪ Therapeutic anticoagulation is indicated.
  ▪ If there is contraindication to anticoagulation: follow clinically until contraindication is resolved or progression of DVT.
○ **Catheter-related DVT**:
  ▪ therapeutic anticoagulation is indicated for as long as the catheter is in place. If the catheter is removed, the total duration of anticoagulation should be at least 3 months. Consider catheter-directed pharmaco-mediated thrombolysis in appropriate patients.
  ▪ If there is a contraindication to anticoagulation, remove the catheter.
• **Pulmonary embolism (PE)** can occur following a DVT. If DVT is untreated, 15% to 25% progress to PE. If treated, 1.6% to 4.5% can still progress to PE, with 0.9% being fatal.
  ○ Symptoms include tachypnea (90%), tachycardia (45%), hemoptysis (30%), cyanosis (20%), and a sense of impending doom (50%–65%).
  ○ Workup includes: CT angiogram/spiral CT of the chest, identification of the original thrombus with lower extremity Doppler (if Dopplers are negative a pelvic CT should follow), a chest x-ray (CXR), an enzyme-linked

immunosorbent assay (ELISA) D-dimer (which has a negative predictive value [NPV] 99.5%), an arterial blood gas (ABG) (the PO_2 is often <80 in 85% of patients) with calculation of the A-a gradient, cardiac enzymes to include troponin, and baseline coagulation studies.

- A normal A-a gradient is: 5 to 10 mmHg but increases with age and FiO_2. A conservative estimate is: (age in years/4) + 4.
- A-a gradient = $[(FiO_2) \times$ (Atmospheric pressure − H_2O pressure) − $(PaCO_2/0.8)]$—PaO_2
- A CXR has a sensitivity of 33%, a specificity of 59%. Signs on CXR are an elevated hemidiaphragm (50%), the Hampton's hump due to a pleural-based infiltrate pointed toward the hilum, Westmark's sign (dilated proximal vessels with a distal cutoff), a pleural effusion, and atelectasis.
- An EKG showing right bundle branch block (RBBB) or a right axis shift can be helpful. If chest spiral CT/CT angiogram is contraindicated, a V/Q scan can be obtained with probabilities of PE represented as low, intermediate, or high. If the probabilities are intermediate or high, it is important to confirm with echocardiogram (ECHO) to evaluate right heart strain.
- ECHO can contribute to primary workup in the diagnosis of PE.

- Treatment of PE is with supportive care and therapeutic anticoagulation. Oxygen is titrated to keep saturations greater than 92%. ECHO can evaluate for pulmonary hypertension and right heart failure. Cardiac support can be given with IV or PO medications. Consider thrombolytic therapy for massive PE or submassive PE with moderate to severe right heart enlargement or dysfunction. Embolectomy either via interventional radiology or surgery is another option, with IVC filter placement. Anticoagulants are dosed the same as for DVT. If there is a contraindication to anticoagulation: consider an IVC filter and embolectomy with frequent evaluation for change in clinical status, assessing for therapeutic anticoagulation. IVC filter removal is recommended if anticoagulation therapy is tolerated. Filters are only permanent for rare patients with contraindications to anticoagulation.
  - **Thrombolytic agents:**
    - Altplase (tPA) 0.5 to 1 mg/hr IV; or 100 mg IV over 2 hours
    - Reteplase 0.25 to 0.75 units/hr IV
    - Tenecteplase 0.25 to 0.5 mg/hr IV
  - **Contraindications to thrombolysis:**
    - **Absolute:** history of hemorrhagic stroke; intracranial tumor; ischemic stroke in prior 3 months; history of major trauma, surgery, or head injury in prior 3 weeks; platelet count below 100,000/mm³; active bleeding; bleeding diathesis
    - **Relative:** age greater than 75; pregnancy or first postpartum week; noncompressible puncture sites; traumatic resuscitation; refractory hypertension (HTN) greater than 180/100; advanced liver disease; infective endocarditis; gastrointestinal (GI) bleed in last 3 months; life expectancy less than 12 months.
  - An **IVC filter** can be placed to prevent re/embolization: indications are the following: absolute contradiction to therapeutic anticoagulation; a PE despite adequate anticoagulation, chronic PE with associated pulmonary HTN; the patient is status post a pulmonary embolectomy; baseline cardiopulmonary

dysfunction is severe enough to make a new or recurrent PE life-threatening; significant heparin-induced thrombocytopenia; patient noncompliance with anticoagulation. Another indication is the need for urgent surgery in a patient with a recent history of DVT, on anticoagulation, but needing temporary discontinuation for a procedure.

- **Therapeutic anticoagulation** is with: heparin, dalteparin, enoxaparin, or fondaparinux. It is important to not use SCDs when a DVT is diagnosed due to the risk of clot embolization.
  - ○ Dosing:
    - Heparin is given **IV** and dosed at 80 units/kg bolus, then 18 units/hr with a targeted activated partial thromboplastin time (aPTT) of 2 to 2.5 × hospital control.
    - Dalteparin is dosed at 200 units/kg SC every 24 hours or 100 units/kg SC every 12 hours.
    - Enoxaparin is dosed at 1 mg/kg SC every 12 hours. It is possible to convert to a daily dosing schedule of 1.5 mg/kg after 3 days of every-12-hour dosing.
    - Fondaparinux is dosed at 5 mg if less than 50 kg; 7.5 mg if 50 to 100 kg, or 10 mg if greater than 100 kg body weight SC daily.
    - Heparin **SC** 333 units/kg load then 250 units/kg every 12 hours.
    - Direct oral anticoagulants are not recommended.
- Conversion to PO anticoagulation is usually with warfarin. This is to start after 3 days of IV heparin or SC therapeutic anticoagulation with a 5-day overlap due to rebound coagulopathy. It is important to follow the INR to keep it 2 to ×3 normal. Duration of treatment is 3 to 6 months for DVT diagnosis, and 6 to 12 months for a diagnosis of PE. Consider lifetime anticoagulation if there is a diagnosis of cancer, hereditary coagulopathy, or arterial thrombosis.
- Drug interactions with Coumadin can affect the INR. These include erythromycin, sulphas, INH, fluconazole, amiodarone, corticosteroids, cimetidine, omeprazole, lovastatin, phenytoin, and propranolol. If the patient is malnourished, is vegetarian, or has liver disease, a lower dose may be needed. If the patient eats high amounts of green leafy vegetables, the patient may have increased levels of vitamin K and be more difficult to anticoagulate.
- There are data to suggest that continued injectable anticoagulation is better in patients with malignancy than warfarin (CANTHANOX and LITE studies) (6,7). There are also data to suggest better progression-free survival (PFS) and overall survival (OS) in patients receiving injectable anticoagulation (FAMOUS and CLOT studies) (8,9).
- **Postoperative** outpatient primary VTE **prophylaxis** is recommended for 4 weeks particularly for pelvic and abdominal cancer surgery patients. Dosing is: dalteparin 5,000 units SC daily, if BMI is greater than 40 consider 7,500; Enoxaparin 40 mg SC daily, if BMI is greater than 40 consider dosing q12 hours; fondaparinux 2.5 mg SC, if MBI is greater than 40 consider 5 mg SC daily; UFH 5,000 units SC every 8 hours, if BMI is greater than 40 consider 7,500 units every 8 hours.

- Duration of treatment for VTE:
  - A minimum of 3 months is recommended for patients with proximal DVT or PE.
  - In patients with advanced or metastatic cancer, or in patients with risk factors for recurrence (genetic), lifelong therapy is recommended. Low–molecular weight heparin (LMWH) is preferred for the first 6 months as monotherapy. Warfarin can then be substituted with the target INR of 2 to 3. Both therapies should be continued for at least a 5-day overlap and until the INR is greater than 2 for at least 24 hours. Direct oral anticoagulants (DOAC) are not recommended.
  - Catheter-associated thrombosis: continue anticoagulation as long as the catheter is in situ or for at least 3 months.
- Reversal of anticoagulation:
  - UFH: half-life 1 hour
    - Reversal with protamine 1 mg/100 units UFH
    - The maximum dose of protamine is 50 mg, and it can cause anaphylaxis if administered too fast.
  - LMWH: half-life 12 hours
    - Reversal with protamine:
      - If within 8 hours: 1 mg/mg of enoxaparin or 1 mg/100 units of dalteparin within 8 hours of the dose
      - If greater than 8 hours from dosing, then 0.5 mg/mg of protamine
      - If greater than 12 hours, consider the clinical scenario.
  - Warfarin: half-life 20 to 60 hours
    - INR 4.5 to 10, no bleeding: hold warfarin dose, when INR approaches therapeutic range less than 4, restart at reduced dose by 10% to 20% and recheck INR within 4 to 7 days
    - INR greater than 10, no bleeding: hold warfarin dose, consider small dose oral vitamin K 1 to 2.5 mg, follow INR every 1 to 2 days, when approaches therapeutic range less than 4, restarted at 20% dose reduction and recheck INR in 4 to 7 days.
    - **Avoid** SC administration of vitamin K because of erratic absorption, IV administration can be used for more rapid absorption than PO.
    - If urgent surgery is needed:
      - Within 24 hours; hold warfarin and administer vitamin K 1 to 2.5 mg IV over 1 hour and repeat INR pre-surgery to determine need for pro-thrombin complex concentrate (PCC). Fresh frozen plasma (FFP) is another option.
      - Within 48 hours: hold warfarin and give vitamin K 2.5 mg orally. Repeat INR at 24 and 48 hours to assess need for supplemental vitamin K, PCC, or FFP.
    - Life-threatening bleeding: hold warfarin and choose from the following options:
      - Administer vitamin K 10 mg IV, no faster than 1 mg/min
      - Administer 4-factor PCC IVP not exceeding 5 mL/min
      - Administer 3-factor PCC IVP not exceeding 10 mL/min
      - Administer rhFVIIa IVP over 2 to 5 minutes
      - For patients with a history of heparin-induced thrombocytopenia (HIT), use 3-factor PCC without heparin

- ○ Direct thrombin inhibitors (DTIs):
  - ■ Bivalirudin: half-life 25 minutes and argatroban half-life 45 minutes
    - □ Discontinue drug
    - □ Consider hemofiltration and hemodialysis
    - □ aPCC (anti-inhibitor coagulant complex vapor heated 50–100 units/kg IV) or rhFVIIa (90 mcg/kg IV, desmopressin 0.3 mcg/kg) may be considered.
  - ■ Dabigatran: half-life 14 to 17 hours:
    - □ Discontinue drug
    - □ Consider hemodialysis with or without charcoal filter
    - □ Oral charcoal if dose within 2 hours of ingestion at 50 to 100 g followed by doses every 1, 2, 4 hours equivalent to 12.5 g/hr
    - □ Consider aPCC anti-inhibitor coagulant complex, vapor heated 25 to 50 units/kg IV
    - □ Consider rhFVIIa 90 mcg/kg IV
- ○ Fondaparinux: factor Xa inhibitor half-life 17 to 21 hours
  - ■ Discontinue drug
  - ■ Consider rhFVIIa 90 mcg/kg IV
- ○ Rivaroxaban half-life 9 to 12 hours: direct factor Xa inhibitor
  - ■ Discontinue drug
  - ■ Consider oral charcoal
  - ■ rhFVIIa 10 to 120 mcg/kg IV, anti-inhibitor coagulant complex vapor heated 25 to 50 units/kg IV
  - ■ 4-factor PCC 25 to 50 units/kg, or if recent history of HIT in last 12 months, 3-factor PCC 50 units/kg
- ○ Apixaban half-life 12 hours: direct factor Xa inhibitor
  - ■ Discontinue drug
  - ■ Consider oral charcoal
  - ■ rhFVIIa 10 to 120 mcg/kg IV, anti-inhibitor coagulant complex vapor heated 25 to 50 units/kg IV
  - ■ 4-factor PCC 25 to 50 units/kg
  - ■ If recent history of HIT in last 12 months, 3-factor PCC 50 units/kg
- ○ **4-factor PCC:** dosing (based on units of factor IX per kilogram of actual body weight)
  - ■ INR 2 to 4.5: 25 units/kg maximum 2,500 units
  - ■ INR 4 to 6: 35 units/kg maximum 3,500 units
  - ■ INR greater than 6: 50 units/kg maximum 5,000 units
- ○ **FFP:** if 4-factor PCC unavailable or the patient is allergic to heparin and/or has a history of HIT in the last 12 months:
  - ■ INR less than 4: 3-factor PCC 25 units/kg + FFP 2 to 3 units
  - ■ INR greater than 4: 3-factor PCC 50 units/kg + FFP 2 to 3 units
  - ■ FFP 15 mL/kg if PCC not available
- ○ **rhFVIIa:** dosed at 25 mcg/kg (use if PCC unavailable or bleeding is not responsive to PCC)
- • Complications from anticoagulation do occur:
  - ○ Hemorrhage from over anticoagulation
  - ○ HIT

- Type I: there is a decrease in platelet count to around 20,000. This is not life-threatening but the patient should be removed from heparin treatment.
- Type II: there is a significant decrease in the platelet count, and an increased risk of both arterial and venous thrombi. There is also an increased risk of bleeding. The patient should be removed from heparin treatment.
- To diagnose HIT, heparin antibody testing should be ordered. Probability scoring should be calculated according to National Comprehensive Cancer Network (NCCN) guidelines. If the score is four or more, unfractionated and LMWHs as well as warfarin should be discontinued. The INR should be reversed with vitamin K. A DTI or fondaparinux should be administered. If the HIT antibody is positive, serotonin release assay (SRA) testing should be ordered and DTIs continued for 6 weeks if no VTE is identified, or 6 months if a VTE is found.

- Mechanisms of action:
  - Heparin binds to antithrombin III. It enhances the inhibition of thrombin, and factors Xa and IXa. It increases the PTT and the level of anticoagulation can be monitored in this fashion. Heparin does not cross the placenta. Reversal is with protamine sulfate dosed at 1 mg/100 units of heparin. FFP can also be used if there is acute bleeding.
  - Enoxaparin binds to and accelerates the action of antithrombin III. It preferentially potentiates the inhibition of factors Xa and IIa. Enoxaparin also has bleeding complications, but there is a lower incidence of induced thrombocytopenia. Monitoring is through antifactor Xa.
  - Warfarin inhibits the synthesis of vitamin K–dependent clotting factors II, VII, IX, and X. It also inhibits proteins C and S. It is usually effective in 48 hours. It does cross the placenta. It increases the PT and INR, and the level of anticoagulation can be monitored in this way. Reversal is with PO or IV vitamin K given at 1 to 10 mg depending on the INR.

- Preoperative anticoagulation:
  - Preoperative discontinuation: anticoagulants such as warfarin should be stopped 4 to 5 days prior to surgery if the desired PT is 1 to 1.5 and the patients were maintained at an INR of 2 to 3. Aspirin should be stopped 7 days prior to surgery due to the irreversible binding to platelets. Clopidogrel should be stopped 10 days prior to surgery.
  - **Perioperative management of anticoagulation** should be determined by the patient's medical comorbidities and urgency of surgery.
    - If emergent, PCC is the treatment of choice to reverse warfarin anticoagulation. It is a combination of blood clotting factors II, VII, IX, X, protein C and S. It is prepared from fresh frozen human plasma. For patients on oral factor Xa inhibitors who require immediate surgery, it is currently recommended to proceed with surgery as specific antidotes for reversal of the anticoagulant is not available and the half-life of these agents are between 5 and 13 hours, except for neurosurgical procedures. Idarucizumab (Praxbind) is a DTI for treatment of patients with dabigatran-induced anticoagulation when emergent surgical procedures, life-threatening, or uncontrolled bleeding is present. The recommended dose for idarucizumab is 5 g (2.5 g/vial) administered IV as two consecutive 2.5 g infusions or a bolus of both vials.

- For nonemergent surgery:
  - □ An IVC filter should be considered if VTE occurred within 4 weeks of the surgery.
  - □ If there is a very low risk of bleeding with surgery: continue anticoagulation.
  - □ If risk is low: no bridging is recommended.
  - □ If moderate risk (major abdominal/pelvic and thoracic surgeries fall into this category): bridging should occur and consider therapeutic dosing to restart at 24 to 48 hours after surgery.
  - □ If the risk is high: bridging is recommended and therapeutic dosing to restart at 24 to 48 hours after surgery.
  - □ Medical indications for bridging should occur in the moderate- and high-risk categories (Table 4.7):
    - – Bridging:
      - Stop chronic anticoagulation agent
        - ○ Stop warfarin 5 to 7 days before procedure: if INR is greater than 1.5, 1 to 2 days prior to procedure, give 1 mg vitamin K PO
        - ○ Stop fondaparinux 5 days before surgery
        - ○ Stop dabigatran 2 days if creatinine clearance (CrCl) is greater than 80 mL/min, 3 days if 50 to 79 mL/min, and 4 to 5 days if 31 to 49 mL/min
        - ○ Stop rivaroxaban 3 days prior if CrCl is greater than 30 mL/min
        - ○ Stop apixaban 3 days if CrCl is greater than 50 mL/min or 4 days if CrCl 30 to 49 mL/min
      - Start LMWH therapeutic dosing q12 hours, 2 days after stopping warfarin.
      - Stop LMWH 24 hours before surgery and if using the 1.5 mg/kg once daily dosing, the last dose should be half the total daily dose.
      - May give VTE prophylaxis with UFH or LMWH at 12 to 24 hours after surgery.
      - Restart:
        - ○ Warfarin with normal diet no sooner than 24 to 48 hours after surgery
        - ○ Dabigatran, rivaroxaban, apixaban, or fondaparinux no sooner than 7 days postoperation
      - If using therapeutic adjusted IV UFH: discontinue 4 to 6 hours before surgery
      - Naturopathic supplements are commonly used and it is important to discontinue the following prior to surgery as they can alter clotting time: vitamin E, garlic, gingko, and ginseng.
- **Arterial embolic** events:
  - ○ Arterial occlusion usually occurs from direct injury or trauma to a vessel or extremity. It may also represent a thrombotic insult from the left heart or a patent foramen ovale.

Table 4.7 Risk Stratification of VTE in Surgical Patients With Cardiovascular Comorbidity

VTE risk	Events/year	Mechanical heart valves	Atrial fibrillation	Recent VTE	Thrombophilia
High risk	>10%	Mitral valve prosthesis Caged ball, tilting disc, aortic valve prosthesis Stroke or TIA within 6 months	CHADS >5 Stroke or TIA within 3 months Rheumatic valvular heart disease	VTE within 3 months	Protein C deficiency Protein 2 deficiency Antithrombin deficiency Homozygous factor V Leiden gene mutation Homozygous prothrombin gene mutation Antiphospholipid syndrome
Moderate risk	5%–10%	Bileaflet aortic valv plus: Atrial fib Prior stroke or TIA HTN DM CHF Age >75	CHADS score 3 or 4	VTE within 3–12 months, recurrent DVT or PE, active cancer or cancer treatment within 6 months	Heterozygous factor V Leiden gene mutation, prothrombin gene homozygous mutation
Low risk	<5%	Bileaflet aortic valve prosthesis and no other risk factors for stroke	CHADS 0–2 and no prior stroke or TIA	Single VTE even >12 months prior and no other risk factors	Hyperhomocysteinemia elevated factors VIII, IX, XI

CHF, congestive heart failure; DM, diabetes mellitus; DVT, deep vein thrombosis; HTN, hypertension; TIA, transient ischemic attack; VTE, venous thromboembolism.

- ○ Symptoms are related to the arterial occlusion and the extremity usually has pallor, pulselessness, paresthesia, pain, and is cold. The diagnostic workup includes a Doppler and an angiogram.
- ○ Treatment is via vascular surgery with a thrombectomy, followed by anticoagulation as soon as the diagnosis is made.
- ○ Acute mesenteric ischemia is a medical emergency. Characteristics are abdominal pain out of proportion to the examination, and a history of atrial fibrillation. Diagnosis is via EKG and CT. Treatment is emergency laparotomy with bowel resection if indicated and surgical revascularization followed by anticoagulation.
- Neuraxial anesthesia/lumbar puncture and anticoagulation parameters: UFH 5,000 q12 hours and enoxaparin 40 mg daily is fine. Enoxaparin 30 to 40 mg q12 hours, fondaparinux 2.5 mg daily, and therapeutic dosing should be used with extreme caution. Placement of neuraxial catheter should be delayed for at least 12 hours after administration of prophylactic doses of enoxaparin. A post-neuraxial placement dose of enoxaparin should be no sooner than 4 hours after last dosing of enoxaparin.

NUTRITION

- Fifty percent of gynecologic oncology patients are malnourished at the time of their diagnosis and ensuing surgery. A weight loss of over 10% from the patient's normal weight usually means the patient is malnourished. There are a few ways to measure the level of malnutrition.
- ○ The prognostic nutritional index includes: measurement of the triceps skin fold, the serum albumin level, the serum transferrin level, and assessment of the delayed hypersensitivity response to mumps, TB, and *Candida* Ag.
- ○ Laboratory measurements of malnutrition can include the total lymphocyte count, or the serum albumin level (which has a half-life of 20 days). The serum albumin test is the single test with the most predictive value: levels less than 2.1 mg/dL are associated with morbidity from 10% to 65%.
- **Perioperative nutrition:** immunonutrition has been investigated to improve outcomes. Immunonutrition includes supplementation with arginine, dietary nucleotides, omega-e fatty acids.
- ○ Impact® nutritional support was initiated 5 days before the scheduled surgery, given TID. It was continued for 5 days after surgery if PO was tolerated. Patients receiving Impact had fewer wound complications (19.6% vs. 33%; $p = 0.049$). There was a 78% reduction in incidence of class 2 and 3 surgical site infections (SSI) (OR: 0.22; 95% CI: 0.05 to 0.95; $p = 0.044$). ASA classification, BMI, DM, history of XRT, length of surgery, and blood loss did affect outcomes. Insurance companies may resist coverage for this as it may be seen as a "food" (10).
- ○ A rapid postoperative feeding schedule has proven benefits and is usually encouraged in gynecologic surgeries. Clear liquids orally are started as soon as the patient is alert and without nausea, vomiting, or significant abdominal distension. Advancement to a regular diet after proven tolerance to liquids follows. Rapid postoperative feeding has been shown to decrease hospital length of stay with no additional adverse events.

- The Harris–Benedict equation calculates the daily basal caloric need: BEE = 655 + (9.6 × kg) + (1.8 × cm height) − (4.7 × age in years). Stress factors should be added to this caloric need as indicated: 1.2× for a minor insult, 1.3× for an elective surgical patient or with moderate stress (SIRS, sepsis), and 1.5× for severe stress (burn patients).
- Total parenteral nutrition (TPN) composition includes: glucose at 3.4 kcal/g to yield 70% of the calculated calories. The remaining 30% is from lipids (at 9 kcal/kg). Protein is added at 1 to 1.5 g nitrogen/kg. TPN should be considered if the patient has a nonfunctioning GI tract due to ileus or obstruction, is unable to tolerate PO for 7 days or more after surgery, has short bowel syndrome, or is severely malnourished.

ENDOCRINE MANAGEMENT

- Diabetes researchers estimate that in 50 years the incidence of diabetes in women will increase 178%, to 351%.
  - Diabetes mellitus can increase perioperative complications. It is important to get a preoperative ECHO for baseline cardiac function, renal labs, an HgA1c, and a urine analysis to check for protein.
  - Postoperative infections cause 20% of deaths in diabetics. To optimize glycemic control, the serum glucose should be maintained between 80 and 110 mg/dL using a weight-based sliding scale regimen. This yields a 46% reduction in septicemia and 34% reduction in hospital mortality. It is recommended to stop metformin and sulfonylurea medications 24 to 48 hours before surgery and restart when the patient tolerates a regular American Diabetes Association diet.
  - Hyperglycemia doubles the risk of surgical site infection and this also affects those who are prediabetic. Optimal perioperative glycemic control should reduce infectious complications 40% to 50%.
- Steroid therapy is indicated for patients who have medical comorbidities that need additional adrenal support.
  - Indications for stress dosing of steroids would be more than 3 weeks of, or an equivalent to, 20 mg of prednisone daily within 1 year of surgery.
  - Stress dosing is administered preoperatively with IV hydrocortisone or methylprednisolone 100 mg. Postoperative treatment is 100 mg IV every 8 hours for three doses. When the patient can tolerate PO, it is okay to resume scheduled dosing or to start a steroid taper. If the patient is clinically Cushingoid, the patient also then requires stress dosing (Table 4.8).
  - It is important to perform Accu-Check measures and place the patient on a sliding scale of insulin due to the risk of diabetic insult and systemic hyperglycemia.
- Thyroid disease: thyroid disease can complicate surgery. It is important to check a thyroid-stimulating hormone (TSH) and a T4 prior to surgery in patients with a known thyroid disorder, in diabetic patients, or in undiagnosed patients who are symptomatic.
  - Patients who are hypothyroid have more ileus, delirium, and infection without fever.

Table 4.8 Postoperative Steroid Taper Protocol

Steroid taper	Hydrocortisone (IV)	Prednisone (PO)
POD 0	100 mg IV q8 h	—
POD 1	100 mg IV q8 h	37.5 mg PO q12 h
POD 2	80 mg IV q8 h	30 mg PO q12 h
POD 3	60 mg IV q8 h	22.5 mg PO q12 h
POD 4	40 mg IV q 8 h	15 mg PO q12 h
POD 5	20 mg IV q8 h	7.5 mg PO q12 h
POD 6	May discontinue	
POD, postoperative day.		

- If the patient is severely hypothyroid, it is important to give IV thyroxine, and stress dose steroids. The half-life of thyroxine is 5 to 9 days.
- Patients who are hyperthyroid can have major complications as well. These can be cardiac related to both inotropic and chronotropic factors. Atrial fibrillation can occur in 10% to 20% of patients.
- Thyroid storm should be suspected if there is fever, tachycardia, confusion, cardiovascular (CV) collapse, or death. Preoperative treatment is with a beta blocker, initiation of or continuation of propylthiouracil (PTU) or methimazole, and administration of stress dose steroids.

HEPATIC DISEASE

Hepatitis is divided into acute and chronic diseases. It is important to check for coagulopathies in liver disease. It is also important to reduce narcotic dosing by 50% in these patients.

- Surgery should be delayed if there is acute hepatitis. The mortality ranges up to 58% if surgery is pursued in the acute phases.
- If the hepatitis is chronic, there is no change in mortality and surgery does not need to be delayed.
- The Child–Turcotte–Pugh classification system predicts mortality in patients with liver disease.
  - Encephalopathy—None: 1, mild to moderate: 2, severe: 3.
  - Ascites—None: 1, mild to moderate (responsive to diuretics): 2, severe (refractory to diuretics): 3.
  - Bilirubin level—Less than 2 mg/dL: 1, 2 to 3 mg/dL: 2, greater than 3 mg/dL: 3.
  - Albumin level—Less than 3.5 g/dL: 1, 2.8 to 3.5 g/dL: 2, less than 2.8 g/dL: 3.
  - INR—Less than 1.7: 1, 1.7 to 2.3: 2, greater than 2.3: 3.
  - Total points are added and the score then falls into a class. Class A: 5 to 6 points, Class B: 7 to 9 points, Class C: 10 to 15 points. Class A has a 10% postoperative mortality, Class B has 30% mortality, and Class C has 80% mortality.

NEUROLOGIC DISEASE

- There are a number of different etiologies that may explain altered mental status. Common causes include metabolic abnormalities, sepsis, meningitis, brain metastasis, or stroke. The initial treatment for a patient with acute-onset altered mental status is to maintain an airway, establish IV access, and provide oxygen, if necessary; laboratories and imaging follow.

- o Workup for metabolic causes includes complete blood count (CBC), comprehensive metabolic panel (CMP), urinalysis, urine drug screen, cardiac enzymes, pulse oximetry, and blood cultures.
- o Workup for sepsis or meningitis includes CBC, CMP, blood, and urine cultures. Lumbar puncture is appropriate for cell count, culture, and cytology, but should only be performed after a CT of the head demonstrates no brain lesions causing mass effect.
- o Workup for metastatic disease or stroke: CT of the head is usually ordered without contrast to evaluate for evidence of an acute hemorrhagic stroke. If negative, a study with contrast is better for evaluation of metastatic lesions. MRI is the most sensitive and specific study to evaluate for evidence of brain metastasis or stroke.
- Treatment for specific clinical situations:
  - o Narcotic drug overdose: naloxone: 1 ampule (0.01 mg/kg IV).
  - o Seizure: dilantin 1,000 mg load then 200 to 300 mg QD, Valium 5 mg IV.
  - o Brainstem herniation: hyperventilate PCO_2 to 25 to 30 mmHg, dexamethasone 10 mg IV then 4 mg IV q6 hours, mannitol 12 g/kg IV then 50 to 300 mg/kg IV q6 hours. Surgical intervention may be necessary.

ALCOHOL WITHDRAWAL

Alcohol withdrawal can cause significant morbidity. Patients with a history of alcohol abuse should be assessed for withdrawal. A well-lit room, social support, and reassurance are first steps. Seizures can occur 12 to 48 hours after alcohol cessation. Delirium tremens complicates 5% to 10% of alcohol withdrawal cases, and mortality can approach 15%. Beer can be ordered while a patient is hospitalized.

Clinical Institute Withdrawal Assessment (CIWA) Scoring	
Nausea and vomiting Score: 0 No nausea and no vomiting 1 Mild nausea with no vomiting 4 Intermittent nausea with dry heaves 7 Constant nausea, frequent dry heaves and vomiting	Tremor Score: 0 No tremor 1 Not visible, but can be felt fingertip to fingertip 4 Moderate, with patient's arms extended 7 Severe, even with arms not extended
Paroxysmal sweats Score: 0 No sweat visible 1 Barely perceptible sweating, palms moist 4 Beads of sweat obvious on forehead 7 Drenching sweats	Anxiety Score: 0 No anxiety, at ease 1 Mildly anxious 4 Moderately anxious, or guarded, so anxiety is inferred 7 Equivalent to acute panic states as seen in severe delirium or acute schizophrenic reactions

(continued)

Clinical Institute Withdrawal Assessment (CIWA) Scoring (*continued*)	
Agitation Score: 0 Normal activity 1 Somewhat more than normal activity 4 Moderately fidgety and restless 7 Paces during most of the interview, or constantly thrashes about	Tactile Disturbances Score: 0 None 1 Very mild itching, pins and needles, burning or numbness 2 Mild itching, pins and needles, burning or numbness 3 Moderate itching, pins and needles, burning or numbness 4 Moderately severe hallucinations 5 Severe hallucinations 6 Extremely severe hallucinations 7 Continuous hallucinations
Auditory disturbances Score: 0 Not present 1 Very mild harshness or ability to frighten 2 Mild harshness or ability to frighten 3 Moderate harshness or ability to frighten 4 Moderately severe hallucinations 5 Severe hallucinations 6 Extremely severe hallucinations 7 Continuous hallucinations	Visual Disturbances Score: 0 Not present 1 Very mild sensitivity 2 Mild sensitivity 3 Moderate sensitivity 4 Moderately severe hallucinations 5 Severe hallucinations 6 Extremely severe hallucinations 7 Continuous hallucinations
Headache, fullness in head Score: 0 Not present 1 Very mild 2 Mild 3 Moderate 4 Moderately severe 5 Severe 6 Very severe 7 Extremely severe	Orientation and Clouding of Sensorium Score: 0 Oriented and can do serial additions 1 Cannot do serial additions or is uncertain about date 2 Disoriented for date by no more than 2 calendar days 3 Disoriented for date by more than 2 calendar days 4 Disoriented for place and/or person

Cumulative Score:	
0–8	No medication is necessary
9–14	Medication is optional for patients with a score of 8–14
15–20	A score of 15 or over requires treatment with medication
>20	A score of over 20 poses a strong risk of delirium tremens
67	Maximum possible cumulative score

- Clinical Institute Withdrawal Assessment (CIWA) Scoring is a cumulative score that provides the basis of a treatment plan for patients undergoing alcohol withdrawal.
- Basic orders include seizure precautions, aspiration precautions, and restraints if the patient has safety risks. Admission lab tests include: CBC, CMP, liver

function tests (LFTs), partial thromboplastin time (PTT), INR, and a urine analysis. Blood alcohol levels should also be drawn. A urine toxicology screen is usually indicated. A CXR to evaluate for pneumonia should be considered. A daily CMP is important.

- IV fluids should be initiated with normal saline. D5 should be added if the patient is NPO but thiamine should be given first. When the patient becomes euvolemic, the IVF should be switched to one-half normal saline (or D5 one-half normal saline) at 125 mL/hr.
- Medications should include vitamins, benzodiazepines, and antipsychotics as indicated.
  - Vitamins include thiamine dosed at 100 mg IV for 3 days, then daily by mouth; folate 1 mg daily by mouth; and a multivitamin daily.
  - Benzodiazepines include chlordiazepoxide and lorazepam. Chlordiazepoxide (Librium) is dosed at 25 to 100 mg PO q4 to 6 hours. Lorazepam (Ativan) is dosed at 1 to 4 mg PO/SL/IM/IV. It may be given every 4 to 6 hours or every 15 to 30 min in cases of severe withdrawal. Lorazepam should be first choice in patients with liver compromise (AST > 200, INR > 1.5); in patients who need IV dosing and cannot take PO well; and in patients who exceed the maximum chlordiazepoxide dose of 600 mg in 24 hours.
- Treatment per CIWA score:
  - For a CIWA score of less than 8, scheduled doses of benzodiazepine should be considered. Patients should be assessed and assigned a CIWA score every 6 hours. Total benzodiazepine dose should be tapered by 25% per day after an initial 72-hour period. Initially, this can be achieved by decreasing the q6 hour dose. Once the dose is at the smallest unit interval (0.5–1 mg lorazepam, or 25 mg chlordiazepoxide), the dosing interval should be lengthened.
  - For patients in active withdrawal with a CIWA score of 8 to 25, symptom-triggered treatment should be initiated. These patients are categorized according to the severity of their current symptoms: mild = CIWA 8 to 13; moderate = CIWA 14 to 20; marked = CIWA 21 to 25. Patients should be assessed every 4 hours, in addition to 1 hour after medication administration.
  - For patients with severe withdrawal who are assigned a CIWA score greater than 25, intensive care unit (ICU) admission is required. Nursing staff assessment is every 2 hours. Treatment is with lorazepam and these patients may require a continuous infusion of lorazepam. The initial rate may be estimated by averaging the hourly dose of benzodiazepine delivered over the first 6 hours. The infusion rate should then be titrated with the goal of sedation scale of 3 to 4.
  - Treatment of disorientation or hallucinations without autonomic signs of alcohol withdrawal (such as tremor and diaphoresis): patients may benefit from the addition of haloperidol instead of additional benzodiazepine use.

BLOOD TRANSFUSION

- Transfusion is recommended in an asymptomatic patient for an hemoglobin (Hg) level below 6 g/dL. If a perioperative patient has an Hg of 7 g/dL and surgery is expected to have significant blood loss, or if the risks associated with anesthesia are high, the patient may be transfused before the procedure. For a postoperative Hg of 6 to 7 g/dL, transfusion is likely indicated. For an Hg 7 to 8 g/dL—transfusion can be considered in postoperative surgical patients, including those with stable cardiovascular disease. For an Hg of 8 to 10 g/dL, transfusion should be considered for some populations such as those with symptomatic anemia, ongoing bleeding, and acute coronary syndrome with ischemia. If the patient is expected to receive adjuvant therapies, an optimal Hg is 10 g/dL. If the patient is symptomatic with orthostatic hypotension, dizziness, or has new physical symptoms such as cardiac murmur, transfusion should be entertained. In general, the American Association of Blood Banks (AABB) guidelines have recommended that transfusion is not indicated solely for a Hg level <10 g/dL.

- The current risk of infection from transfusion:
  ○ Viral:
    HIV, 1 in 1,467,000.
    Hepatitis B, 1 in 282,000.
    Hepatitis C, 1 in 1,149,000.
    West Nile virus, uncommon.
    Cytomegalovirus, 50% to 85% of donors are carriers: leukocyte reduction is protective.
  ○ Bacterial: 1 in 2,000–3,000 (mostly platelets);
  ○ Parasitic diseases: babesiosis, Chagas, malaria: uncommon.
- Allogeneic blood transfusions are an alternative to standard transfusions, but need to be obtained 6 weeks prior to surgery and are screened in the same fashion as all other blood donations.
- Normovolemic hemodilution is an alternative to blood transfusion.
- **Potential Adverse Effects of Blood Transfusion:** immunomodulation from blood transfusion may lead to higher postoperative infections as well as increased morbidity and mortality from:
  ○ Acute hemolytic transfusion reaction (HTR): preformed antibodies to incompatible product (1:76,000).
  ○ ABO incompatibility occurs in 1:40,000 and is fatal in $1:1.8 \times 10^6$. Symptoms are chills, fever, hypotension, hemoglobinuria, renal failure, back pain, disseminated intravascular coagulation (DIC). Treatment: IVF to keep urine output greater than 1 mL/kg/hr, pressors as needed, and treatment of DIC.
  ○ Delayed HTR: the cause is an anamnestic immune response to incompatible red cell antigen. Symptoms are fever, jaundice, falling hemoglobin, newly positive antibody screen 1 to 2 weeks after transfusion. Treatment is transfusion as needed with compatible red blood cell (RBC). The offending antibody should be identified in the blood bank.
  ○ Febrile non-HTR: occurs in 0.1% to 1.0%. The cause is preformed anti- white blood cell (WBC) antibodies in the recipient. The risk is minimized with leukocyte-reduced products. Symptoms are a $\geq 1°C$ (2°F) rise in body temperature within 2 hours of transfusion initiation with no other explanation for fever. Treatment is with acetaminophen premedication if reactions are recurrent.
  ○ Allergic (urticarial) reactions: occur in 1% to 3%. The cause is an antibody to donor plasma proteins. Symptoms are urticaria, pruritus, flushing, and mild wheezing. Treatment is suspension of the transfusion and antihistamines. The transfusion may resume if the reaction resolves.

- o Anaphylactic: occur in 1:20,000 to 50,000. The cause is an antibody to donor plasma proteins (IgA, haptoglobin, C4). Symptoms are hypotension, urticaria, bronchospasm, angioedema, anxiety. Treatment is with epinephrine 1:1,000, 0.2 to 0.5 mL SC, antihistamines, and corticosteroids.

- o Transfusion-related acute lung injury (TRALI): occurs in 1:10,000; 10% to 20% are fatal. The cause is preformed human leukocyte antigen (HLA) or neutrophil antibodies in the donor product. Symptoms are hypoxemia, hypotension, bilateral pulmonary edema, transient leukopenia, and fever within 6 hours of transfusion. Treatment is supportive care.

- o Transfusion-associated graft-versus-host disease: this is rare but almost always fatal. The cause is an immunosuppressed recipient receives a transfusion from an HLA-similar donor (usually a family member). Symptoms are pancytopenia, maculopapular rash, diarrhea, hepatitis presenting 1 to 4 weeks after transfusion. Treatment: supportive care. It can be prevented by irradiating blood products (11).

- For most patients, a **restrictive transfusion strategy** (i.e., giving less blood; transfusing at a lower Hg levels; and aiming for a lower target Hg level) is preferred rather than a liberal transfusion strategy. Restrictive transfusion strategies have resulted in the following: a 39% decrease in the probability of receiving a transfusion (46% vs. 84%; RR = 0.61; 95% CI: 0.52–0.72); fewer units (1.19) transfused per patient; a trend toward a lower 30-day mortality (RR = 0.85; 95% CI: 0.70–1.03); a trend toward a lower overall infection rate (RR = 0.81; 95% CI: 0.66–1.00); although no difference was seen with pneumonia. No difference was seen in: functional recovery, hospital, or ICU length of stay. There was no increased risk of myocardial infarction (MI) when all trials were included (RR = 0.88; 95% CI: 0.38–2.04).

- A post-transfusion Hg level can be performed as early as 15 minutes following transfusion, as long as the patient is not actively bleeding.

- Acute coronary syndrome: the optimal transfusion threshold in the setting of acute coronary syndromes (ACS; i.e., acute MI, unstable angina) remains unanswered. A standard practice in patients with ACS is to transfuse when the Hg is less than 8 g/dL and to consider a transfusion when the Hg is between 8 and 10 g/dL. If the patient has ongoing ischemia or other symptoms, an Hg can be maintained ≥10 g/dL. The threshold of 8 g/dL is considered safe for asymptomatic medical patients with stable coronary artery disease.

REFERENCES

1. Nelson G, Kalogera E, Dowdy SC. Enhanced recovery pathways in gynecologic oncology. *Gynecol Oncol.* December 2014;135(3):586-594.

2. Nick AM, Schmeler KM, Frumovitz MM, et al. Risk of thromboembolic disease in patients undergoing laparoscopic gynecologic surgery. *Obstet Gynecol.* 2010;116(4):956-961.

3. Kahn SR, Shapiro S, Wells PS, et al. Compression stockings to prevent postthrombotic syndrome: a randomised placebo-controlled trial. *Lancet.* March 8, 2014;383(9920):880-888.

4. Khorana AA, Kuderer NM, Culakova E, et al. Development and validation of a predictive model for chemotherapy-associated thrombosis. *Blood.* May 15, 2008;111(10):4902-4907.

5. Tafur AJ, Kalsi H, Wysokinski WE, et al. The association of active cancer with venous thromboembolism location: a population-based study. *Mayo Clin Proc.* January 2011;86(1):25-30.

6. Meyer G, Marjanovic Z, Valcke J, et al. Comparison of low-molecular-weight heparin and warfarin for the secondary prevention of venous thromboembolism in patients with cancer: a randomized controlled study. *Arch Intern Med.* August 12–26, 2002; 162(15):1729-1735.

7. Hull RD, Pineo GF, Brant RF, et al. Long-term low-molecular-weight heparin versus usual care in proximal-vein thrombosis patients with cancer. *Am J Med.* December 2006;119(12):1062-1072.

8. Kakkar AK, Levine MN, Kadziola Z, et al. Low molecular weight heparin, therapy with dalteparin, and survival in advanced cancer: the fragmin advanced malignancy outcome study (FAMOUS). *J Clin Oncol.* May 15, 2004;22(10):1944-1948.

9. CLOTS (Clots in Legs Or sTockings after Stroke) Trial Collaboration, Dennis M, Cranswick G, Deary A, et al. Thigh-length versus below-knee stockings for deep venous thrombosis prophylaxis after stroke: a randomized trial. CLOTS (Clots in Legs Or sTockings after Stroke) Trial Collaboration. *Ann Intern Med.* November 2, 2010;153(9):553-562.

10. Chapman JS, Roddy E, Westhoff G, et al. Postoperative enteral immunonutrition for gynecologic oncology patients undergoing laparotomy decreases wound complications. *Gynecol Oncol.* June 2015;137(3):523-528.

11. Carson JL, Grossman BJ, Kleinman S, et al. Red blood cell transfusion: a clinical practice guideline from the AABB*. *Ann Intern Med.* July 3, 2012;157(1):49-58.

PULMONARY

- Complications related to pulmonary factors occur in 20% to 30% of postoperative patients. The functional residual capacity (FRC) is reduced when patients are supine, or have had a laparotomy. Vital capacity is decreased 45%, and FRC is reduced 20%.
- Risk factors are: obesity, surgery longer than 2 hours, chronic obstructive pulmonary disease (COPD), congestive heart failure (CHF), renal failure, poor mental status, immunosuppression, nasogastric tube (NGT) use, narcotics, smoking, sleep apnea, and asthma. COPD patients can benefit from a preoperative arterial blood gas (ABG) and pulmonary function testing (PFT).
- Correlation of operative time to complications has been reviewed and increased rates of: urinary tract infection (UTI), organ space surgical site infection (SSI), sepsis/septic shock, prolonged intubation, pneumonia, rate of deep vein thrombosis (DVT), deep incisional infection, and wound disruption were found. Per 1,000 cases, there were 116 occurrences per operating room hour (1).
- Atelectasis usually occurs postintubation, and is due to surgical pain with its associated decreased inspiratory effort. Dyspnea, tachypnea, and fever can be present. Examination reveals crackles at the lung bases. Diagnosis is with chest x-ray (CXR). Treatment is incentive spirometry.
- Pneumonia can present with dyspnea, tachypnea, fever, and decreased O_2 saturation. Examination reveals decreased breath sounds segmentally. Diagnosis is via CXR and documentation of infiltrate or consolidation. Treatment is with antibiotics, incentive spirometry, chest physiotherapy, and pulmonary toilet.
- Respiratory failure is defined as altered pulmonary function that yields hypercarbia, acidemia, or hypoxemia.
  - The etiology can be a decreased respiratory drive, airway obstruction, decreased pulmonary function, COPD, asthma, anaphylaxis, pulmonary edema from CHF, acute respiratory distress syndrome (ARDS), pneumonia, abscess, tuberculosis, pneumothorax, pleural effusion, hemothorax, cancer, anemia, or pulmonary embolus.
  - Diagnosis is via physical examination, imaging, and laboratories. It is important to obtain a CXR, oxygen saturation monitor, an ABG, a complete blood count (CBC), electrolytes, a CT angiogram if suspicion for a pulmonary embolism (PE) is present, and potentially an echocardiogram (ECHO) to rule out cardiogenic etiology.
- Oxygen is not as good as we think. 100% O_2 for greater than 6 hours has been shown to decrease macrophage activity, mucous velocity, cardiac output (CO), and can cause irreversible pulmonary damage if given for greater than

60 hours. Oxygen can be delivered via nasal prongs, a rebreathing face mask, a nonrebreathing face mask, continuous positive airway pressure (CPAP), bilevel positive airway pressure (BiPAP), and intubation with mechanical ventilation. Delivery via nasal prongs has been shown to be as good as a rebreathing face mask.

- Parameters
  - ○ PaO_2: arterial oxygen tension.
    - ▪ Normal: 70 to 100 mmHg
  - ○ PaO_2: alveolar oxygen tension $(FiO_2 \times 713) - (PaCO_2/0.8)$.
    - ▪ Normal: 100 mmHg
  - ○ $PaCO_2$: arterial CO_2 tension.
    - ▪ Normal: 35 to 44 mmHg
  - ○ AA gradient: alveolar – arterial O_2 tension or $[(FiO_2) \times (Atmospheric\ pressure - H_2O\ Pressure) - (PaCO_2/0.8)] - PaO_2$.
    - ▪ Normal is 3 to 16 mmHg or $(Age/4) + 4$
  - ○ Vital capacity: volume of expired air after maximal inspiration.
    - ▪ Normal: 3 to 5 L
  - ○ Tidal volume: volume of inspired air for each peak breath.
    - ▪ Normal: 6 to 7 mL/kg
  - ○ FEV1: maximum volume forcefully expired in 1 second.
    - ▪ Normal: greater than 83% of vital capacity
  - ○ PEF: peak expiratory flow rate.
    - ▪ Normal: greater than 400 L/minute
  - ○ NIF: negative inspiratory force.
    - ▪ Normal: 60 to 100 cm H_2O
- Parameters for intubation in respiratory failure: indications for mechanical ventilation include hypoxemia, hypercarbia, respiratory acidosis, the inability to maintain or protect the airway including changes in mental status, and respiratory fatigue. The largest endotracheal tube possible should be chosen: this is usually a 7.5 to 8 for women. This is to decrease airway resistance. Vitals and laboratory benchmarks are listed below (Table 4.9).

Table 4.9 Parameters for Intubation in Respiratory Failure

Mechanics	Results
PaO_2	<60 mmHg
$PaCO_2$	>55–60 mmHg
Respiratory rate	>30–35 bpm
Arterial pH	<7.25
NIF, negative inspiratory force	<20 cm H_2O
Vital capacity	<10 mL/kg
FiO_2	>60
PaO_2/FiO_2	<200
FEV1	<10 mL/kg

- The A-a gradient is calculated to determine shunt and help rule out a pulmonary embolus. The A-a gradient = $[(FiO_2) \times$ (Atmospheric pressure – H_2O pressure) – $(PaCO_2/0.8)] - PaO_2$. A normal gradient estimate = $(Age/4) + 4$.
- Ventilation by machine can be run by volume or by pressure. The volume cycled setting has a preset tidal volume. The pressure cycled setting stops the cycle at a preset pressure; this setting is useful in hypoxic patients.
  - Continuous mandatory ventilation (CMV) delivers a preset minute ventilation determined by a set respiratory rate and tidal volume. It is useful in heavily sedated patients, those given paralytic agents, and those who do not tolerate assisted ventilation.
  - Assist–control (A/C or volume controlled) ventilation presets the tidal volume, and this tidal volume is delivered when a breath is initiated by the patient. This is the most common mode of mechanical ventilation used in the intensive care unit (ICU). A control back up rate is set to prevent hypoventilation.
  - Intermittent mandatory ventilation (IMV) has a set rate and tidal volume, but allows unassisted spontaneous breaths and provides a full breath in relation to the amount of patient effort.
  - Synchronized intermittent mandatory ventilation (SIMV) delivers breaths at regular intervals that are based on a preset tidal volume and rate which are synchronized with the patient's respiratory efforts.
  - Pressure supported (PS) ventilation provides constant airway pressure, which is delivered during inspiration. It is the most frequently used mode during "weaning." In this mode, each time the patient inhales, the ventilator delivers a pressure-limited breath. The patient controls the rate, volume, and duration of the breaths.
- To initially set the ventilator, IMV or A/C cycles are usually chosen. The FiO_2 is started at 60% (maximum), and weaned down to a patient O_2 saturation of 90% to 95% and a FiO_2 of 21% (room air [RA]). The rate is usually initiated at 8 to 12 breaths per minute. The tidal volume is chosen at 8 to 12 mL/kg, but should be lower at 6 mL/kg if the patient is suspected or diagnosed with ARDS. A positive end-expiratory pressure (PEEP) of 5 cm H_2O is also chosen. It is important to check an ABG and adjust the settings further based on those results.
- Extubation should be a rapid goal. A spontaneous breathing trial or t-tube trial should be performed daily to assess patient status. Weaning settings on the ventilator are with SIMV or PS ventilation. To be extubated, the patient must be conscious and can protect the airway, the FiO_2 must be less than 50% (optimally at 21% RA), the PEEP should be less than 5 cm H_2O, the NIF should be greater than 20 cm H_2O (Table 4.10).
- Ventilator acquired pneumonia (VAP) occurs in 30% of patients after 72 hours of intubation. The mortality of VAP is 25% to 50%.
- Monitoring of pulmonary and cardiac status can be with a central line. The central venous pressure (CVP) is an assessment of volume status and crude cardiac function. It consists of multiple measurements, and is not a single number. A normal CVP is 8 to 10 cm H_2O, or 2 to 6 mmHg.
- A pulmonary artery (PA or Swan) catheter can be helpful when it is important to know critical cardiac output (CO) or fluid status. Complications of a Swan include pneumothorax, arrhythmia, line sepsis (2%), or PA rupture. CO is calculated thermodynamically. An estimation of preload is obtained by wedging

Table 4.10 Extubation Parameters

Weaning parameters	Acceptable for extubation
Respiratory rate	<30–35 (>8) bpm with FiO_2 <0.5
PaO_2	>60 mmHg with FiO_2 <0.5
$PaCO_2$	<50 with respiratory rate <25 bpm
NIF	More negative than 20–25 cm H_2O
Vital capacity	>10–15 mL/kg
Tidal volume	>3 mL/kg
The patient is awake and can protect the airway	

NIF, negative inspiratory force.

the end of the catheter into an afferent pulmonary capillary. This is called the pulmonary artery occlusion pressure (PAOP) or pulmonary capillary wedge pressure (PCWP). A normal PCWP is 6 to 12 mmHg. The PCWP is a crude reflection of the left arterial pressure. If the PCWP is elevated, then the preload is adequate or excessive; if it is low, then the patient is likely volume depleted. The mixed venous blood sample is blood obtained from the tip of the PA catheter and reflects the most desaturated blood in the body.

- ARDS occurs after a defined insult to the lungs. This can include hemorrhage, sepsis, shock, or pneumonia. An ABG should be drawn.
  - Symptoms are tachypnea, dyspnea, and respiratory failure.
  - There are several criteria for the diagnosis of ARDS:
    - Bilateral diffuse infiltrates are seen on CXR
    - CHF and iatrogenic volume overload are ruled out by ECHO (showing an EF >35%)
    - There is impaired oxygenation with documented oxygen saturation less than 92%
    - The calculated PaO_2/FiO_2 is ≤ torr for the diagnosis of ARDS
    - If the PaO_2/FiO_2 ≤ 300 torr, the diagnosis is acute lung injury (ALI)
  - The mortality of ARDS is 30% to 40%.
  - Treatment is with intubation, mechanical ventilation, antibiotics, and treatment of the underlying cause. Steroids have not been proven beneficial. Better survival has been seen with ventilatory support maintaining low tidal volumes to prevent barotrauma (6 mL/kg), and elevated PCO_2—permissive hypercapnia.

CARDIAC

- Myocardial infarction can occur at any time during hospitalization. Any chest pain, arrhythmia, SOB, persistent dyspepsia, or arm pain should be worked up with cardiac enzymes and an EKG (serially) as well as a CXR to start.
- Reinfarction can occur after a recent myocardial infarction (MI). Rates have decreased from 37% to now 5%-10% due to better medications used for reperfusion. The rate further decreases the longer the time from the initial insult. The rate is 2% to 3% after 4 to 6 months, and 1% to 2% if greater than 6 months have elapsed after a recent MI.

- Perioperative prophylactic beta blockers have been studied. Laughton, in 2005, showed there were fewer infarctions and lower mortality when used after surgery. The rates of infarction with use were 24% versus 39% without. The 2-year mortality was 16% with use versus 32% without. A more recent study, the POISE study in 2008, refutes the benefit of beta blocker use postoperatively. There were fewer MIs in the beta blocker group (4.2% vs. 5.7%; $p < 0.05$), but there were more deaths (3.1% vs. 2.3%; $p < 0.05$) and more cerebrovascular accidents (1% vs. 0.5%; $p < 0.05$) with beta blocker use (2).
- The role of a pulmonary artery catheter (Swan-Ganz) for surgery remains controversial and its use has decreased in modern clinical practice. There are no definitive studies that provide evidence of benefit in the surgical setting. The current indications are active CHF, severely depressed left ventricular (LV) function, and critical aortic stenosis.
- Parameters
  - CO: heart rate × Stroke volume.
    - Normal: 4 to 8 L/min
  - Cardiac index: CO/BSA m^2.
    - Normal: 2.5 to 4 L/min
  - MAP: mean arterial pressure = $1/3 \times$ (SBP – DBP) + DBP.
    - Normal: 70 to 105 mmHg
  - PAP Systolic: systolic pulmonary arterial pressure.
    - Normal: 15 to 30 mmHg
  - PAP Diastolic: diastolic pulmonary arterial pressure.
    - Normal: 5 to 12 mmHg
  - PAP mean: mean pulmonary arterial pressure.
    - Normal: 5 to 10 mmHg
  - PAWP: pulmonary artery wedge pressure = LA and LV filling pressure.
    - Normal: 5 to 12 mmHg
  - SVR: systemic vascular resistance (MAP – MRAP) (80)/CO.
    - Normal 900 to 1,400 dynes/sec/cm^{-5}
  - PVR: pulmonary vascular resistance (mean PAP – PAWP)/CO.
    - Normal 100 to 240 dynes/sec/cm^{-5}
  - VO_2: O_2 consumption.
    - Normal 115 to 1,165 mL/min/m^2
  - DO_2: O_2 delivery.
    - Normal 640 to 1,000 mL O_2/min
- Ischemic heart disease
  - Ischemic heart disease (IHD) (MI) can often-times be identified by its symptoms. Angina, nausea, vomiting, dyspnea, sweating, diaphoresis, shortness of breath (SOB), weakness, anxiety, elevated blood pressure (BP), tachycardia, bradycardia, jugular venous distension (JVD), or tachyarrhythmias are often present.
  - Workup includes: an electrocardiogram (EKG), cardiac enzymes × 3 q 6 to 8 hours (creatine kinase [CK], creatine kinase-MB [CKMB], troponin I), brain natriuretic peptide (BNP), CXR, and consideration of coronary angiography, especially if an ST elevation myocardial infarction (STEMI) is diagnosed.
  - Medical treatment is with transfer to the critical care unit (CCU) for telemetry. MIs are classified as: STEMI, NSTEMI, and unstable angina. Pulse oximetry should be obtained, aspirin administered, and oxygen placed to keep saturations greater than 90%. A CXR should be obtained in addition to an

EKG and laboratories. Initial stabilization should include administration of sublingual nitroglycerin (NTG) at 5 minute intervals for three doses if there is chest pain. IV morphine dosed at 4 to 8 mg repeated every 5 to 15 minutes is recommended for chest pain and to decrease the myocardial workload. Atropine can be given to increase blood pressure if hypotension is present due to bradycardia. Beta blockers should be administered in the absence of contraindications. Contraindications include: SBP less than 90, bradycardia, findings suggesting right ventricle infarction.

- Treatment of patients with **STEMI** include: IV thrombolysis within 30 minutes or cardiac catheterization with PTCA within 90 minutes of arrival or occurrence.

- Treatment of patients with **NSTEMI** include: observation and monitoring in a CCU with administration of stool softeners, stress ulcer prophylaxis, anti-pyretics, and bedrest. Beta blockers should be administered in the absence of contraindications. Angiotensin-converting enzyme (ACE) inhibitors may be additionally beneficial in limiting infarct size. If chest pain contin-ues, angiography and revascularization via PTCA, stenting, or surgery is indicated. IV NTG titrated to 10 to 200 mg/min to prevent hypotension can be given to alleviate coronary artery spasm and decrease infarct size. Thrombolytic therapy is not indicated in NSTEMI myocardial infarction.

- Treatment of patients with **unstable angina** is angiography with PTCA, stent-ing, or surgery. An EKG should be obtained with each set of enzymes. An ECHO is usually ordered as well for ejection fraction and ventricular assessment. Angiography should be considered the timing of PTCA based on refractory or recurrent angina, new or evolving signs of CHF, hemodynamic instability, new arrhythmias, a temporal change in troponins, or a history of PTCA in the last 6 months. For severe LV dysfunction and cardiogenic shock, angioplasty, thrombolysis, and revascularization with multivessel stenting may be indicated.

  ○ Interventional treatment:

  - Angioplasty is used to dilate a stenosed artery mechanically with a bal-loon catheter.

  - A stent can also be placed simultaneously. The stent can be mechanical alone or medicated (impregnated with paclitaxel). The medicated stents keep occluded arteries open and decrease local plaque. Noncardiac surgery can be performed 6 weeks after a medicated stent as antithrom-botics are needed for this duration. A nonmedicated/bare metal stent is indicated if surgery is urgent. Surgery can be performed 2 weeks after bare metal stent placement.

  - Thrombolysis is another option for removing coronary artery occlusion. This occurs after localization with angiography and if the diagnosis occurs within 6 hours of the onset of pain. The clot is lysed with antithrombotics.

- Heart failure is defined as an EF less than 35% to 40%. The etiology is most commonly a MI, but can be viral or hereditary.

  ○ Symptoms are SOB, lower extremity edema, or JVD. There can be ascites if there is significant right heart failure, progressing to anasarca if not managed.

  ○ Workup includes a CXR, which will show bilateral infiltrates, an EKG, an ECHO, cardiac enzymes × 3 every 6 to 8 hours, BNP, electrolytes, and a CBC. A spiral CT can help rule out a PE.

- Treatment is with O_2 supplementation, water restriction to 2 L/day, morphine, and diuretics (furosemide to start at 20 mg IV, doubling of the dose is indicated if minimal response is seen). If there is a need to increase the CO, inotropes such as dopamine or dobutamine can be considered. Digoxin can be administered to improve contractility (1 mg load 0.5 mg IV, then 0.25 mg q6 hours × 2, maintenance 0.125 mg/day, checking the level the first day then every 5 days). A daily weight and strict salt management (<2 g/day) are important.
- Pulmonary edema is characterized by SOB.
  - Diagnosis is with a physical examination demonstrating bilateral rales and low oxygen saturation. Confirmation is with CXR showing bilateral infiltrates. An EKG, an ECHO, cardiac enzymes × 3 every 6 to 8 hours, BNP, an ABG, and CT angiogram to rule out PE should be obtained to rule out cardiac and venous thromboembolism (VTE) etiologies.
  - Treatment is diuresis, O_2 supplementation, and correction of the underlying cause.
- Hypertension (HTN) is often not symptomatic (Table 4.11).
  - Characteristics when symptomatic are a headache or change in vision.
  - Diagnosis is via BP assessment. If symptomatic, an EKG, cardiac enzymes × 3 every 6 to 8 hours, and CT head without contrast or MRI are indicated to rule out stroke.
  - Parameters: grading of HTN is per Table 4.11.
  - Treatment for crisis-range HTN can include: nitroprusside (Nipride) 1 to 10 mcg/kg/min IV; ACE inhibitor (enalapril) 12.5 mg PO or 1.25 to 2.5 mg IV every 6 hours; a beta blocker (labetalol) 20 mg IV, repeated at 40 to 80 mg q10 minutes with a maximum dose of 300 mg and a maintenance dose of 0.5 to 2 mg/min; an alpha blocker (hydralazine) dosed at 5 to 20 mg IV.
  - Management of HTN, other than crisis range, is with single-agent or combination agents. First-line drugs are often diuretics (hydrochlorothiazide). Beta-blockers can be first- or second-line, as can be calcium channel blockers (a better response is seen with these drugs in African Americans). ACE inhibitors and angiotensin receptor blockers (ARBs) can be used if there are contraindications to other medications, or they can be used in combination.
- Arrhythmias are abnormal rhythms of the heart rate. It is important to always rule out a MI. If the patient is unstable, cardioversion should always be performed. Secondary investigation is directed at abnormal electrolytes, endocrine issues (thyroid-stimulating hormone [TSH]), and drug toxicity. Most arrhythmias are transient.

Table 4.11 Hypertension Categories and When to Treat				
Category	Systolic	Diastolic	Follow-up	Status
Mild	140–159	90–99	2 month	
Moderate	160–179	100–109	1 month	
Severe	180–209	110–119	1 week	Urgent
Crisis	210	120	Immediate	Crisis

o Atrial fibrillation is a tachyarrhythmia. Diagnosis is via EKG, which shows an irregularly irregular rhythm with no P wave. Treatment is with IV diltiazem. A beta blocker can be helpful if there is a rapid ventricular response. Amiodarone has a lower incidence of recurrent atrial fibrillation. Digoxin can also be used if low blood pressure accompanies the arrhythmia. If there is persistent atrial fibrillation, chronic anticoagulation should be considered based on the CHADS$_2$ score. The CHADS$_2$ score is based on patient risk factors. These include: HTN greater than 140/90; age greater than 75; diabetes mellitus (DM); history of CVA or TIA; or history of VTE. All risk factors are given a score of 1 except for the CVA and VTE components which are scored at 2 each. If the score is a 2, warfarin is recommended (Table 4.12).

o Atrial flutter is a tachyarrhythmia. Diagnosis is via EKG, which shows a saw tooth pattern. Aspirin (ASA) prophylaxis is indicated.

o Supraventricular tachycardia is a tachyarrhythmia. Diagnosis is via EKG, which shows tachycardia with no P waves. Treatment is initiated with vagal maneuvers. If this is unsuccessful, adenosine can be administered up to three times (given IV at 6 mg, again at 6 mg, then at 12 mg if no initial response).

o Bradycardia is defined as a pulse less than 60 bpm. Diagnosis is via EKG. If the patient is symptomatic and not stable, the patient should be paced transcutaneously until a permanent pacemaker can be placed or the etiology diagnosed. If the patient is stable, treatment is with atropine dosed at 1 mg IV.

o **Postoperative atrial fibrillation after noncardiac surgery:** the differential diagnosis includes: hypovolemia, intraoperative hypotension, trauma, pain, acute anemia, hypoxia, hypokalemia, low magnesium, hypervolemia or MI. A goal is HR 80 to 100 bpm, not rhythm control. The Atrial Fibrillation Follow-up Investigation of Rhythm Management (AFFIRM) trial was the largest trial to compare rate with rhythm control; 73% versus 80.1% (NS) of adverse events were observed in the rhythm control arm. Management pathways are determined by symptoms (3).

  ▪ Symptomatic (unstable BP, pulmonary edema, chest pain, change in level of consciousness): direct cardioversion. If the patient declines, then IV metoprolol, IV diltiazem, IV amiodarone, or IV digoxin should be administered.

  ▪ Asymptomatic: determine the ejection fraction (EF) (order ECHO). Consider direct current cardioversion (DCC). If the EF is:

Table 4.12 Annual Risk of Cerebrovascular Accidents (CVA) Based on CHADS$_2$ Score

Score	CVA risk
0	1.9
1	2.8
2	4
3	5.9
4	8.5
5	12.5
6	18.2

□ Greater than 45%: then oral metoprolol, diltiazem, amiodarone, digoxin.

□ Less than 45%: consider oral medications, or IV diltiazem, IV amiodarone, or IV digoxin. Flecainide and propafenone can be used if duration less than 7 days. Amiodarone, dofetilide, or ibutilide should be used if there are cardiac comorbidities.

- It is important to restart beta blockers or calcium channel blockers that were used as maintenance preoperatively.
- If atrial fibrillation persists greater than 48 hours, the need for chronic anticoagulation should be assessed.
- Risk scoring system: **CHA2DS2VASc** scoring system. A score ≥2 is high risk and oral anticoagulation is indicated.

Age: 65–74 >75	1 pt 2 pt
CHF 1 pt	1 pt
HTN 1 pt	1 pt
DM	1 pt
CVA	2 pts

- Postoperative patients have a high risk of hemorrhage with anticoagulation: the **HAS-BLED** surgical scoring system risk assesses for hemorrhage. A score ≥3 indicates high risk of bleeding: some versions include alcohol use and antiplatelet medications for one point each (4).

HTN	1 pt
Abnormal renal/liver function	1 pt
CVA	1 pt
Bleeding history	1 pt
Labine INR	1 pt
Age >65	1 pt

SHOCK AND SEPSIS

- Shock is defined as a decrease in tissue perfusion. There are five types of shock: septic, cardiogenic, hemorrhagic, neurogenic, and iatrogenic. Diagnosis is via physical examination, vitals, EKG, and lab tests. Treatment generally consists of intravenous fluid (IVF) and type-directed support.
  - Cardiogenic shock can be due to MI, HTN yielding a heavy afterload and severe cardiac strain, or pump failure from too much volume. Cardiogenic shock is managed by diuretics to reduce the preload, dopamine or dobutamine to increase cardiac function, norepinephrine if dopamine fails, and nitroprusside or a nitroglycerine drip for venous capacitance. Angiography with angioplasty, stent placement, left ventricular assist device (LVAD), or coronary artery bypass grafting (CABG) surgery can be employed for acute management.

- ○ Hemorrhagic shock is managed by IVF replacement (3:1 ratio of IVF to blood loss) and blood products, surgery for hemostasis, or embolization.
- ○ Neurogenic shock often occurs from embolic or hemorrhagic stroke, head trauma, or metastatic disease. It is managed by IVF, pressor support, hyperventilation with intubation if necessary, XRT with steroids to reduce local inflammation, and potential surgery if a mass effect is present.
- ○ Iatrogenic shock is usually related to anaphylaxis. Treatment is to stop the offending medication/infusion, administration of steroids, antihistamines, O_2, and pressor support as indicated.
- ○ Septic shock, see the following.
- Generally, the systemic inflammatory response syndrome (SIRS) occurs when two or more of the following are documented in the setting of a known cause of inflammation: a body temperature greater than 38°C or less than 36°C; a pulse greater than 90 bpm; a respiratory rate greater than 20 bpm or a $PaCO_2 \leq 32$; a WBC greater than 12×10^3/mcL, or less than 4×10^3/mcL, or greater than 10% band forms. In 2001, additional criteria were added for an inclusive approach to SIRS. These include: an altered mental status, oliguria, skin mottling, coagulopathy, hypoxemia, and hyperglycemia without a diagnosis of diabetes, thrombocytopenia, and altered liver function tests (LFTs).
- A high level of suspicion should be maintained for SIRS with suspicion of organ dysfunction determined by:
  - ○ Decreased perfusion: capillary refill greater than 3 seconds, skin mottling, cold extremities.
  - ○ Lactate greater than 2 mmol/L.
  - ○ Circulatory: SBP less than 90 mmHg, MAP less than 65 mmHg, decrease in SBP greater than 40 mmHg.
  - ○ Respiratory: PaO_2/FiO_2 less than 300; PaO_2 less than 70 mmHg; SaO_2 less than 90%.
  - ○ Hepatic: jaundice; total bilirubin greater than 4 mg/dL; increased LFT's; increased PT.
  - ○ Renal: creatinine greater than 0.3 mg/dL; urine output less than 0.5 mL/kg/hr for at least 2 hours.
  - ○ Central nervous system: altered consciousness, confusion, psychosis.
  - ○ Coagulopathy: international normalized ratio (INR) greater than 1.5 or a partial thromboplastin time (PTT) greater than 60 seconds, thrombocytopenia (platelets less than 100,000/mm³).
  - ○ Splanchnic circulation: absent bowel sounds.
- **Sepsis (septic shock)** is SIRS due to a known infection. Septic shock is sepsis with hypotension despite adequate fluid resuscitation. There are two stages: early hyperdynamic and late hypodynamic. The crude mortality is 28% to 50%. 3 and 6 hour time marks are used to mark and respond to interventions.
- The **SOFA** (sequential organ failure assessment) **score** is an assessment tool to determine extent of organ dysfunction. An increase in the SOFA score during the first 24 to 48 hours in the ICU predicts a mortality rate of at least 50%, up to 95%. Scores less than 9 predict mortality of 33%, and those above 11 can be predictive of mortality above 95%. The total points are tallied for the final score. The worst score in the past 24 hours is used to calculate the total score.

- **Respiratory system**

PaO$_2$/FiO$_2$ (mmHg)	SOFA score
<400	1
<300	2
<200 **and** mechanically ventilated	3
<100 **and** mechanically ventilated	4

- **Nervous system**

Glasgow coma scale	SOFA score
13–14	1
10–12	2
6–9	3
<6	4

- **Cardiovascular system**

MAP OR administration of vasopressors required	SOFA score
MAP <70 mm/Hg	1
Dopamine ≤5 or dobutamine (any dose)	2
Dopamine >5 OR epinephrine ≤0.1 OR norepinephrine ≤0.1	3
Dopamine >15 OR epinephrine >0.1 OR norepinephrine >0.1 (vasopressor drug doses are in mcg/kg/min)	4

- **Liver**

Bilirubin (mg/dL) [mcmol/L]	SOFA score
1.2–1.9 [>20–32]	1
2.0–5.9 [33–101]	2
6.0–11.9 [102–204]	3
>12.0 [>204]	4
If bilirubin is less than 1.2, the score is 0.	

- **Coagulation**

Platelets × 10^3/mcL	SOFA score
<150	1
<100	2
<50	3
<20	4
If platelet is more than 150, the score is 0.	

- **Kidneys**

Creatinine (mg/dL) [mcmol/L] (or urine output)	SOFA score
1.2–1.9 [110–170]	1
2.0–3.4 [171–299]	2
3.5–4.9 [300–440] (or <500 mL/d)	3
>5.0 [>440] (or <200 mL/d)	4

The **Quick SOFA** tool can identify patients at risk of sepsis: the presence of two or more qSOFA criteria points, of a total of three, represents organ dysfunction.
○ Altered mental status with Glasgow Coma Score less than 15.
○ Respiratory rate ≥ to 22 breaths/min.
○ Systolic BP ≤ 100 mmHg.
  - Intervention is needed with transfer or admit to the ICU.
    □ Lines: an arterial line is needed to measure the MAP; consideration of a PA catheter for measurement of the CO, a Foley catheter to measure urine output.
    □ Laboratories: an ABG to measure the $PaCO_2$ and PaO_2; CBC, serum **lactate** (≥2 mmol/L) or POC lactate, coagulation profile, d-dimer, fibrinogen, LFTs, total bilirubin, albumin, comprehensive metabolic panel (CMP), magnesium, phosphorus, calcium, 1,3 beta-D-glucan assay, mannan and antimannan antibody assays if candidiasis is in the differential diagnosis.
    □ Cultures for: bacteria, fungus, and virus. These should be obtained from blood, urine, sputum, and wound before antimicrobial therapy is initiated. A delay of ≥45 minutes is considered substandard for antibiotic initiation. At least two sets of blood cultures (aerobic and anaerobic) with at least one drawn percutaneously and one drawn through each vascular access devices, unless it was inserted less than 48 hours prior, are necessary.
    □ Imaging should be performed to rule out site of infection.
  - Goals: a CVP of 8 to 12; a MAP ≥65, CVP 8 to 12 mmHg (12–15 if intubated) a urine output ≥0.5 mL/kg/hr; a $ScvO_2$ ≥70% or a mixed venous oxygen saturation ≥65%, and a normalized lactate level if initially elevated. Goals are desired within 6 hours. If oxygen saturation goals are not met in 6 hours, it may be beneficial to transfuse packed red blood cells (PRBC) to achieve a hemoglobin greater than 10 g/dL.
  - **Management:**
    □ Antimicrobial therapy: administration of broad spectrum IV antimicrobials within the first hour of recognition of septic shock and severe sepsis without septic shock is indicated. This should include one or more drugs that have activity against all likely pathogens to include bacterial and/or fungal and/or viral. Low procalcitonin levels can assist the clinician in the discontinuation of empiric antibiotics in patients who initially appeared septic, but have no laboratory

evidence of infection. Combination empirical antimicrobial therapy should be started for neutropenic patients with severe sepsis. Empiric combination therapy should not be administered for more than 3 to 5 days. Antimicrobial regimen should be reassessed daily for potential de-escalation to the most appropriate single therapy as soon as the susceptibility profile is known. Duration of therapy is typically 10 to 14 days after negative blood cultures. Longer courses may be appropriate in patients who have a slow clinical response, undrainable foci of infection, bacteremia with *Staphylococcus aureus*, some fungal and viral infections, or immunologic deficiencies, including neutropenia. Antiviral therapy should be initiated as early as possible in patients with severe sepsis or septic shock of viral origin. For patients with difficult-to-treat, multidrug-resistant bacterial pathogens:

- *Pseudomonas aeruginosa* bacteremia infections associated with respiratory failure and septic shock, combination therapy with an extended spectrum beta-lactam and either an aminoglycoside or a fluoroquinolone.
- *Streptococcus pneumoniae* bacteremia infections: a combination of a beta-lactam and macrolide is recommended.

□ Source control: a specific anatomical diagnosis of infection requiring consideration for emergent source control should be identified or excluded as rapidly as possible, and intervention be undertaken for source control within the first 12 hours after the diagnosis is made. All catheters should be changed and cultured. Any site of infection should be explored and drained if possible (there is up to an 80% percutaneous success rate). Surgical exploration can potentially access those sites not amenable to needle drainage. Fever and leukocytosis, respectively, are absent in 35% and 5% of peritoneal infections. An eye examination should also be part of the workup.

□ Fluid therapy of severe sepsis: the fluid challenge technique can be applied where fluid administration is continued as long as there is hemodynamic improvement either based on dynamic (e.g., change in pulse pressure, stroke volume variation) or static (e.g., arterial pressure, heart rate) variables. Albumin can be used for fluid resuscitation when patients require very large amounts of crystalloids. Hydroxyethyl starches for fluid resuscitation should not be used.

□ Vasopressors: vasopressor therapy should be started to target a MAP of 65 mmHg. Norepinephrine is usually the first choice vasopressor. Epinephrine can be added or substituted for norepinephrine when an additional agent is needed to maintain adequate blood pressure. Vasopressin at 0.03 units/min can be added to norepinephrine with the intent of either raising the MAP or decreasing norepinephrine dosage. Low-dose vasopressin is not recommended as a single initial vasopressor. Vasopressin doses higher than 0.03 to 0.04 units/min should be reserved for salvage therapy. Phenylephrine is not recommended except when: norepinephrine is associated with serious arrhythmias; CO is known to be high and blood pressure persistently low; or as salvage therapy when combined inotrope/vasopressor drugs and low-dose vasopressin have failed to achieve MAP target. Low-dose dopamine should not be used for renal protection. All patients requiring vasopressors should have an arterial line placed.

☐ **Inotropic** therapy: dobutamine infusion up to 20 mcg/kg/min can be given or added to a vasopressor in the presence of:
  – Myocardial dysfunction as suggested by elevated cardiac filling pressures and low CO, or
  – Ongoing signs of hypoperfusion, despite achieving adequate intravascular volume and adequate MAP
  – The cardiac index should not be "improved" by pharmacologic or fluid infusion strategies to predetermined super-normal levels (grade 1B)

☐ Corticosteroids: if adequate fluid resuscitation and vasopressor therapy are able to restore hemodynamic stability, corticosteroids should not be used. If this is not achievable, IV hydrocortisone alone can be dosed at 200 mg/day; continuous flow. Hydrocortisone should be tapered when vasopressors are no longer required. An adrenocorticotropic hormone (ACTH) stimulation test should not be used to determine which patients to treat with steroids. Corticosteroids should not be administered for the treatment of sepsis in the absence of shock.

☐ Blood product and management: a target hemoglobin concentration is 7.0 to 9.0 g/dL in adults. A red blood cell transfusion can be considered when the Hg is less than 7.0 g/dL. A higher transfusion threshold for patients with myocardial ischemia, severe hypoxemia, acute hemorrhage, or ischemic heart disease can be considered. Platelet transfusion should only be given prophylactically when counts are less than 10,000/mm³ to reduce the risk of spontaneous bleeding in therapy-induced hypoproliferative thrombocytopenia. Prophylactic platelet transfusion can be considered when counts are less than 20,000/mm³, if the patient has a significant risk of bleeding, if there is active bleeding, or there is a planned invasive procedure. The goal is 50,000/mm³. For elective surgical patients with thrombocytopenia and platelets <50,000/mm³, it is recommended to transfuse platelets preoperatively. Erythropoietin should not be used as a specific treatment of anemia associated with severe sepsis. Fresh frozen plasma (FFP) should not be used to correct laboratory clotting abnormalities in the absence of bleeding or planned invasive procedures. Antithrombin should not be used for the treatment of severe sepsis and septic shock.

☐ Mechanical ventilation of sepsis-induced ARDS: the SpO₂ should be maintained ≥92%. Oxygen should be administered with mechanical ventilation if indicated. The tidal volume for mechanically ventilated patients with ALI/ARDS is 6 mL/kg. Plateau pressures should be measured and the initial upper limit goal for plateau pressures in a passively inflated lung should be ≤30 cm H_2O. PEEP should be applied at 5 cm H_2O to avoid alveolar collapse at end expiration (atelecto-trauma), with higher levels of PEEP for patients with moderate to severe ARDS. Prone positioning can be used in sepsis-induced ARDS patients with a

PaO_2/FiO_2 ratio ≤100 mmHg. The head of the bed should be elevated 30° to 45° to limit aspiration risk and to prevent the development of ventilator-associated pneumonia. A weaning protocol should be in place daily with daily spontaneous breathing trials. A conservative fluid strategy should be maintained for patients with established sepsis-induced ARDS who do not have evidence of tissue hypoperfusion. Beta 2-agonists are not recommended unless bronchospasm is present.

□ Sedation, analgesia, and neuromuscular blockade in sepsis: continuous or intermittent sedation should be minimized in mechanically ventilated patients. Neuromuscular blocking agents (NMBAs) should be avoided if possible in the septic patient without ARDS due to the risk of prolonged neuromuscular blockade following discontinuation. If NMBAs must be maintained, either intermittent bolus as required or continuous infusion with train-of-four monitoring of the depth of blockade should be used. A course of NMBA, not greater than 48 hours, can be used for patients with early sepsis-induced ARDS and a PaO_2/FiO_2 less than 150 mmHg.

□ Glucose control: glucose levels should be checked every 1 to 2 hours upon diagnosis. Insulin dosing should be initiated when two consecutive blood glucose levels are greater than 180 mg/dL. A target upper blood glucose is ≤180 mg/dL. Glucose values should be monitored every 1 to 2 hours until values and insulin infusion rates are stable, then every 4 hours.

□ Renal replacement therapy: continuous renal replacement therapies (CCRT) and intermittent hemodialysis have been shown to be equivalent in patients with severe sepsis and acute renal failure. The use of continuous therapies has been shown to facilitate management of fluid balance in hemodynamically unstable septic patients. CCRT is intended to be applied for 24 hr/day in an ICU and describes a variety of blood purification techniques, which differ according to the mechanism of solute transport, the type of membrane, the presence or absence of dialysate solution, and the type of vascular access. CRRT provides slower solute clearance per unit time as compared with intermittent therapies but over 24 hours may even exceed clearances with IHD. Solute removal with CRRT is achieved either by convection (hemofiltration), diffusion (hemodialysis), or a combination of both these methods (hemodiafiltration). Hemodialysis most efficiently removes small molecular weight substances such as urea, creatinine, and potassium. Middle and larger molecular weight substances are more efficiently removed using hemofiltration as compared with dialysis.

□ Bicarbonate therapy: sodium bicarbonate therapy has not been shown to improve hemodynamics or reduce vasopressor requirements in patients with hypoperfusion-induced lactic acidemia with pH ≥7.15.

□ DVT prophylaxis: a combination of pharmacologic therapy and intermittent pneumatic compression devices should be used whenever possible. Daily pharmacoprophylaxis is recommended with subcutaneous low-molecular weight heparin (LMWH) or three times daily unfractionated heparin. If the creatinine clearance is less than 30 mL/min, dalteparin is recommended. Patients who have a contraindication to heparin use (e.g., thrombocytopenia, severe coagulopathy, active bleeding, recent intracerebral hemorrhage) should receive mechanical prophylactic treatment. When the risk decreases, pharmacoprophylaxis should start.

□ Stress ulcer prophylaxis: stress ulcer prophylaxis using H_2 blocker or proton pump inhibitor should be given to patients with severe sepsis/septic shock who have risk factors for bleeding, with preference given to proton pump inhibitors.

□ Immunoglobulins and selenium are not recommended for use.

- **Algorithms:**
  - ○ Completed within **3** hours:
    - ■ Measure lactate level
    - ■ Obtain blood cultures prior to antibiotic administration
    - ■ Administer broad spectrum antibiotics
    - ■ Administer IVF 30 mL/kg for hypotension or a lactate ≥4 mmol/L
  - ○ To be completed within **6** hours:
    - ■ Remeasure lactate level if initially elevated (≥2 mmol/L).
    - ■ Administer vasopressors if still hypotensive to obtain a MAP ≥65 mmHg and assess CV status with one of the following:
      - □ Measure CVP; measure $ScvO_2$; bedside ECHO; or assess fluid responsiveness with passive leg raise or fluid challenge.
  - ○ CV management:
    - ■ MAP: <65 mmHg
      - □ NS or LR 30 mL/kg over 30 to 60 minutes fluid challenge
        - – If EF <40% reduce the volume of the fluid challenge. Consider colloid if pulmonary edema or liver failure. Repeat every 30 minutes until CVP ≥8 mmHg
      - □ If MAP still will not respond: then vasopressors should be initiated
        - – Norepinephrine 5 mcg/min titrate 2.5 mcg/min every 5 minutes or epinephrine 1 mcg/kg/min titrate by 0.5 mcg/kg/min every 5 minutes
      - □ If MAP still will not respond: consider hydrocortisone 50 mg IV every 6 hours
    - ■ CVP: <8 mmHg or <12 mmHg if intubated
      - □ NS or LR bolus over 30 minutes at 30 mL/kg
      - □ Consider albumin if pulmonary edema or liver failure
      - □ Repeat every 30 minutes until CVP ≥8 mmHg
  - ○ Pulmonary management:
    - ■ $ScvO_2$: less than 70%: check Hg: Hg ≥10 g/dL
    - ■ Yes: administer dobutamine as a continuous infusion until $ScvO_2$ ≥70%
    - ■ It is not recommended to give PRBC transfusion to maintain Hg ≥10 g/dL (5).
    - ■ Multiple organ dysfunction syndrome (MODS) is the development of the progressive physiologic dysfunction of two or more organ systems. This usually occurs after an acute threat to systemic homeostasis. Treatment is support of individual organ function and aggressive therapies aimed at correcting the underlying process.

FEBRILE NEUTROPENIA

- Definition: less than 500 neutrophils/mcL, or less than 1,000 neutrophils/mcL and a predicted decline to less than 500/mcL over the next 48 hours—and a single temperature greater than 38.3°C orally, or a temperature greater than 38.0°C orally sustained for over 1 hour (more than 2 consecutive elevations over 1 hour).
- Risk Scoring: it is important to risk stratify all patients into low or high risk categories by calculating the **Multinational Association for Supportive Care in Cancer (MASCC) risk score (Table 4.13):** a score of ≥21 is considered low risk and a score <21 as high risk (with a PPV of 91%, specificity of 68%, and sensitivity of 71%) (6).
  - **Low risk:** outpatient status at time of fever; no acute comorbid illness; anticipated short duration of severe neutropenia (<100 cells/mcL for <7 days); good performance status (ECOG 0–1); no hepatic or renal insufficiency.
  - **High risk:** any of the following risk factors: inpatient at time of fever development; clinically unstable; anticipated prolonged severe neutropenia of less than 100 cells/mcL for greater than 7 days; and significant medical comorbidity to include: hepatic insufficiency: 5× the upper limit of normal for aminotransferases; renal insufficiency: creatinine clearance of less than 30 mL/min; uncontrolled or progressive cancer; pneumonia or other complex infection at presentation; alemtuzumab use; mucositis grade 3–4.
- Management: all patients should receive **broad spectrum** antibiotics; **then the source** should be identified. If high risk: the patient needs to be hospitalized and IV therapy instituted. If the patient scores as low risk: PO or IV/sequential PO therapy can be administered. Discharge can be to home if patients are compliant and have established care. If intermediate to high risk, consider adding pneumocystispneumonia (PCP) prophylaxis.
- Site Management:
  - Abdominal pain: workup: abdominal CT, LFT's, bilirubin, amylase, lipase. Treatment is with oral vancomycin, fidaxomicin, or metronidazole if *Clostridium difficile* suspected. Ensure adequate anaerobic therapy.

Table 4.13 The Multinational Association for Supportive Care in Cancer (MASCC) Risk Index

5 points:
No to few symptoms Normal blood pressure
4 points:
No chronic obstructive pulmonary disease (COPD) Solid tumor or blood malignancy without prior fungal infection
3 points:
Moderate symptoms Normovolemic Outpatient management
2 points:
Age <60

○ Perirectal pain: workup: visual examination, consider CT abdomen/pelvis. Treatment: ensure adequate anaerobic therapy, consider enterococcal coverage, local care with sitz baths, stool softeners.

○ Diarrhea: workup: *C. difficile* PCR, consider testing for rotavirus, norovirus, consider stool bacterial and parasite cultures, consider adenovirus. Treatment: oral vancomycin, fidaxomicin, or metronidazole if highly suspected or confirmed *C. difficile*.

○ Urinary tract symptoms: workup: urine analysis and culture. Treatment based on specific pathogen identified.

○ Mouth/mucosal membrane:
  ▪ White coating: workup: thrush likely: fungal culture. Treatment: fluconazole first line, voriconazole, osaconazole, or echinocandin if refractory
  ▪ Vesicular lesions: workup: viral diagnostics. Treatment: anti-HSV therapy
  ▪ Necrotizing ulceration: workup: viral diagnostics, culture and gram stain, biopsy suspicious lesions, consider leukemic infiltrate. Treatment: ensure adequate anaerobic activity, consider anti-HSV therapy, and consider systemic antifungal activity

○ Esophagus: workup: viral diagnostics, culture suspicious oral lesions for both fungal and bacterial etiology, consider endoscopy if no response to therapy, consider CMV esophagitis. Treatment: guided by clinical findings fungal versus viral with ongoing broad spectrum antibiotics.

○ Sinus/nasal: workup: CT or MRI of the sinus or orbit, ENT/ophthalmology consultation, culture and stain, biopsy if indicated. Treatment: add vancomycin if periorbital cellulitis, add amphotericin B to cover aspergillosis and mucormycosis in high-risk patients with suspicious CT/MRI findings.

○ Cellulitis/skin and soft tissue infections: workup: aspirate or biopsy for culture. Treatment: gram-positive active agent.

○ Vascular access device: workup: if there is entry site inflammation, swab entry site drainage for culture, blood culture from each port of access device. Treatment: vancomycin initially or add if not responding within 48 hours of empiric therapy. If tunnel infection/port pocket infection, or septic phlebitis: workup: blood culture from each port. Treatment: if positive culture, remove catheter and culture surgical wound, add vancomycin.

○ Vascular lesions: workup: aspirate or scrape for VZV or HSV PCR or direct fluorescent antibody, herpes virus culture if PCR unavailable. Treatment: consider acyclovir.

○ Disseminated papules or other lesions: workup: aspirate or biopsy for bacterial, fungal, mycobacterial cultures, and histopathology, consider VZV evaluation. Treatment: consider vancomycin, consider mold, add active antifungal therapy in high-risk patients.

○ CNS symptoms: workup: CT and/or MRI, LP if possible, neurology consult. Treatment: initial empiric therapy pending ID consult. If suspected meningitis, include antipseudomonal beta-lactam agent that enters CSF plus vancomycin, plus ampicillin unless using meropenem. For encephalitis, add high-dose acyclovir.

○ For lung infiltrates: workup: blood and sputum cultures, consider nasal wash for viruses, *Legionella* urine Ag test, serum galactomannan or beta-glucan test if at risk for mold. CT of the chest should be obtained. Consider bronchial-alverolar lavage if poor response or diffuse infiltrates. Consider diagnostic lung biopsy. Treatment: azithromycin or fluoroquinolone. Consider adding mold active antifungal in moderate- to high-risk patients. Add antiviral therapy during influenza outbreaks. TMP/SMX coverage should be added if PCP is possible. Add vancomycin or linezolid if MRSA is suspected.

- **General antimicrobial recommendations:**
  - Uncomplicated patient with febrile neutropenia:
    - IV antibiotic monotherapy to include either: cefepime, imipenem/cilastatin, meropenem, piperacillin/tazobactum, ceftazidime.
    - Oral antibiotic therapy for low-risk patients to include either: ciprofloxacin and amoxicillin/clavulinate, or moxifloxacin, but none if quinolone prophylaxis was used.
  - Complicated febrile neutropenic patient: IV antibiotic monotherapy is preferred, but combination therapy should be used if resistance is identified.
- **Duration of treatment** for documented infections in cancer patients: the antibiotic regimen should be continued until the neutrophil count is greater than 500 cells/mcL and increasing.
  - Skin/soft tissue: 7 to 14 days.
  - Blood stream uncomplicated: gram negative: 10 to 14 days; gram positive: 7 to 14 days; *Staphylococcus aureus*: at least 2 weeks after first negative blood culture; yeast greater than 2 weeks after first negative blood culture. Consider catheter removal for *S. aureus, Pseudomonas aeruginosa, Corynebacterium jeikeium, Acinetobacter, Bacillus* organisms, atypical mycobacteria, yeasts, molds, *vancomycin-resistant enterococci, and Stenotrophomonas maltophilia.*
  - Bacterial sinusitis: 7 to 14 days.
  - Catheter removal for septic phlebitis, tunnel infection, or port pocket infection.
  - Pneumonia:
    - Bacterial 7 to 14 days;
    - Fungal (mold and yeast): *candida* should be treated for a minimum of 2 weeks after first negative blood culture;
    - Mold (*aspergillus ex*): minimum 12 weeks;
    - Viral HSV/VZV: uncomplicated, skin disease: 7 to 10 days; influenza: oseltamivir for 5 days if immunocompetent and healthy, 10 days if immunocompromised.

RENAL

The definition of acute renal failure is not standardized.

- A patient is usually diagnosed with a rising creatinine, or with a urine output of less than 400 mL/24 hr.
- There are three types of acute renal failure: prerenal, renal (intrinsic), and postrenal. Lab tests should be ordered to include a CMP, urine analysis for microscopy, urine electrolytes to include Na and creatinine, specific gravity (SG), and urine osmolality. The next step is to calculate the FeNa: the equation is UNa × SCr/SNa × UCr × 100%. The renal failure index is another calculation: (Urinary Na concentration × Plasma Cr concentration)/Urinary Cr concentration.
  - If the FeNa is less than 1% and the urine SG is greater than 1.025, the diagnosis is prerenal failure and often due to hypoperfusion. If the FeNa is greater

than 4% and the urine SG is less than 1.01, the diagnosis is often due to renal ischemia. It is important to remember that a FeNa cannot be calculated if diuretics, mannitol, or IV contrast material have been given.

o Prerenal failure: the etiology is often volume depletion from surgical blood loss, third spacing from removal of ascites, extensive bowel preparation and NPO status, CHF, severe liver disease, or other edematous states. Laboratory findings include: a urinary sodium concentration less than 20 mEq/L, a urine:plasma creatinine ratio greater than 30, urine osmolality greater than 500 mOsm/kg. The renal failure index is less than 1.

o Intrinsic renal failure: the etiology can be aminoglycoside antibiotics, IV contrast material, cytolytic drug exposure, statin medication, rhabdomyolysis, hyperuricemia, multiple myeloma, and streptococcal infection. Findings include: a urinary sodium concentration greater than 40 mEq/L, a urine:plasma creatinine ratio less than 20, and urine osmolality less than 400 mOsm/kg. The UA can show eosinophils (acute interstitial nephritis), red blood cell casts (glomerulonephritis or vasculitis), or renal tubular epithelial cells and muddy brown casts (acute tubular necrosis). The cause is sloughing of renal tubular cells into the lumen, demonstrating casts called Tamm–Horsfall bodies. Management is with support including volume repletion until euvolemia is reached, monitoring and restriction of potassium agents. A diuretic challenge can be offered if volume overload becomes evident. Dialysis should be considered if volume overload, acidosis, uremia, or EKG changes occur. Treatment is to stop the offending drug. A desired urinary output is ≥0.5 mL/kg/hr.

o Postrenal failure is usually obstructive. This can occur with bilateral hydronephrosis from cervical cancer, nephrolithiasis, urethral obstruction, bladder compression from tumor, or ureteral obstruction from tumor/stone/surgery. Lab tests include: serum BUN:Cr greater than 20:1, a urine osmolality less than 400 mOsm/kg, and a urinary sodium concentration greater than 40 mEq/L. The Foley catheter should be checked and flushed. A renal ultrasound can be obtained to document hydronephrosis. A CT urogram can be obtained to evaluate for ureteral obstruction from surgical injury or tumor. Nephrolithiasis and retroperitoneal fibrosis can also cause this complication. Reduction of the obstruction with surgical correction or placement of a percutaneous nephrostomy tube is indicated. It is important to follow for *postobstructive diuresis*: postobstructive diuresis is defined as diuresis of more than 200 mL/hr for at least 2 hours. Electrolytes should be checked every 8 hours and the urine output replaced with IVFs in the form of half normal saline at 80% of the hourly urine volume for the first 24 hours, then 50%. Postobstructive diuresis usually lasts 24 to 72 hours. Cardiac status should be observed for potential tachycardic failure.

• Chronic kidney disease is defined as a glomerular filtration rate (GFR) of less than 60 mL/min/1.73 m². End-stage renal disease (ESRD) is often caused by DM and HTN (68%). These patients are immunocompromised. The morbidity from surgery can be up to 54%, with a mortality of 4%. For renal patients, it is important to obtain a cardiac workup, manage fluids and electrolytes vigilantly, exercise caution for anemia and bleeding diatheses, and maintain both glycemic and blood pressure control.

- Cardiac disease causes the most deaths in patients with ESRD, and 23% to 40% have no cardiac symptoms. Patients need to be euvolemic prior to surgery. They need dialysis without heparin 24 hours prior to surgery, and they need postoperative dialysis the day of surgery if a large fluid load was given.
- It is important to check electrolytes immediately after surgery and every 6 to 8 hours until they are normalized.
- If the patient is uremic, platelets do not work well. Cryoprecipitate or dDAVP should be considered to prevent bleeding during surgery. IV estrogen can also be administered (0.6 mg/kg) 4 to 5 days prior to surgery.
- Indications for dialysis include (AEIOU): acidemia, electrolyte abnormalities (hyperkalemia resistant to prior interventions), EKG changes, intoxication with dialyzable substances (aspirin, lithium), volume overload, uremia, and mental status changes. A large central venous catheter may need to be placed if there is an acute need for dialysis.
- Daily management of renal complications include: strict I/Os, daily weight, and a low-sodium and low-nitrogen diet.
- Metabolic acidosis: the anion gap is calculated by subtracting the serum concentrations of chloride and bicarbonate (anions) from the concentrations of sodium and potassium (cations): = $([Na+] + [K+]) - ([Cl-] + [HCO_3^-])$.
  - Anion gap: the etiology is based on the mnemonic "PLUMSEEDS." These stand for: Paraldehyde, Lactate, Uremia, Methanol, Salicylates, Ethylene glycol, Ethanol, Diabetic ketoacidosis (DKA), Starvation. Another mnemonic is "MUDPILES": Methanol, Uremia (chronic renal failure), DKA, Propylene glycol, I (infection, iron, isoniazid, inborn errors in metabolism), Lactic acidosis, Ethylene glycol, Salicylates.
  - Nonanion gap: the two main causes are diarrhea or renal tubular acidosis. Other causes include acetazolamide, saline administration, hyperalimentation, and ureteral conduit.
- Metabolic alkalosis: usually occurs from renal dysfunction due to the loss of hydrochloric acid from nausea/vomiting, volume contraction, exogenous bicarbonate administration, hypokalemia, or hyponatremia.

ACID–BASE DISORDERS (Table 4.14)

Table 4.14 Acid–Base Disorders			
Disorder	Primary change	pH	Compensatory change
Metabolic acidosis	Decreased HCO_3	Decreased	Decreased pCO_2
Metabolic alkalosis	Increased HCO_3	Increased	Increased pCO_2
Respiratory acidosis	Increased PCO_2	Decreased	Increased HCO_3
Respiratory alkalosis	Decreased PCO_2	Increased	Decreased HCO_3

- Respiratory acidosis: occurs when there is a failure of ventilation usually due to mental status changes. These changes can occur because of a mass effect, medications, stroke, infection, or inappropriate mechanical ventilation settings.
- Respiratory alkalosis: occurs as a result of hyperventilation, including iatrogenic causes from excessive mechanical ventilation.

ELECTROLYTE ABNORMALITIES

- Sodium abnormalities
  - Hyponatremia (serum sodium <135 mEq/L):
    - Pseudohyponatremia: an erroneously low measurement of sodium caused by elevations of plasma lipids, sugars, or proteins.
    - Hypotonic hyponatremia: increase in free water relative to sodium in extracellular fluids.
    - Hypovolemic hyponatremia: characterized by loss of sodium and water, with a net loss of sodium relative to water. Caused by diuretics, adrenal insufficiency, diarrhea, or vomiting.
    - Isovolemic hyponatremia: characterized by increase in water with the same sodium content. Caused by inappropriate ADH secretion or psychogenic polydipsia.
    - Hypervolemic hyponatremia: characterized by excess of sodium and water, with a net gain of water relative to sodium. Caused by heart, renal, or hepatic failure.
    - Signs/symptoms: hyponatremic encephalopathy is associated with cerebral edema, increased intracranial pressure, and seizures.
    - Treatment: is based on low, normal, or high extracellular volume. Avoid rapid correction to prevent central pontine myelinolysis.
  - Hypernatremia (serum sodium >145 mEq/L):
    - Hypovolemic hypernatremia: caused by inadequate intake of water, excessive loss from urinary tract, sweating or diarrhea. Treatment: volume replacement.
    - Hypertonic syndromes: characterized by impaired renal water conservation. This can be caused by diabetes insipidus, either central or nephrogenic. Treatment: replace free water deficits.
    - Hypervolemic hypernatremia: characterized by an increase in hypertonic fluid. This is caused by excessive hypertonic saline resuscitation, sodium bicarbonate infusions, ingestion of seawater, or excessive amounts of table salt. Treat with sodium restriction or diuretic with fluid replacement.
    - It is important to avoid rapidly lowering the sodium concentration with free water to avoid cerebral edema.
- Potassium abnormalities
  - Hypokalemia (serum potassium <3.5 mEq/L):
    - Causes:
      - Transcellular shift of potassium into cells from insulin, beta agonists, furosemide, or alkalosis
      - Diminished intake
      - Increased potassium losses from GI or urinary tracts

- Signs: fatigue, myalgia, muscular weakness, hypoventilation, paralysis, and arrhythmias
- Symptoms: EKG changes include: T wave inversion, U waves, ST depression, prolonged QT interval, prolonged PR interval, widening of QRS complex
- Treatment: address the underlying cause
  - Each 0.1 mEq/L of deficiency on laboratory value needs replacement with 10 mEq of potassium chloride (KCl).
  - The maximum rate of KCl in a peripheral IV is 10 mEq/hr; for a central line the rate is 20 mEq/hr.
  - Magnesium: magnesium depletion can promote urinary loss of potassium, so it is recommended to also correct for magnesium deficit.
- Hyperkalemia (serum potassium >5.5 mEq/L):
  - Causes:
    - Pseudohyperkalemia caused by hemolysis from traumatic blood draw
    - Transcellular shift from acidosis; rhabdomyolysis; cytotoxic cell death or drugs such as digitalis or beta receptor antagonists
    - Impaired renal excretion from adrenal insufficiency or drugs such as ACE inhibitors, ARBs, NSAIDs, or potassium-sparing diuretics
    - Massive blood transfusions
  - Symptoms: cardiac toxicity, paralysis, and hypoventilation
  - Signs: EKG changes including increased T waves, peaked T waves, prolonged PR and QRS intervals, loss of P waves
  - Treatment is recommended if the serum K is greater than 6.5 mEq/L, the patient is acidotic, fluid overloaded, mental status changes are present, or EKG changes are present. Treatment:
    - Kayexalate PO 15 g daily to QID or PR 30 to 50 g q4 hours
    - Sodium bicarbonate: 44 to 132 mEq IV
    - Calcium chloride or calcium gluconate 10 to 30 mL of a 10% solution IV
    - Glucose: 50 g IV
    - Regular insulin: 10 units IV
    - Dialysis if the patient does not respond to the these measures
- Magnesium abnormalities
  - Hypomagnesemia:
    - Causes: diuretic therapy, antibiotics, alcohol-related illness, diarrhea, diabetes mellitus, acute MI, drugs such as digitalis or cisplatin.
    - Symptoms: generalized weakness and altered mentation. It is commonly associated with other electrolyte abnormalities, including hypokalemia, hypophosphatemia, hypocalcemia. It is also associated with hypokalemia that is refractory to treatment.
    - EKG changes: torsades de pointes, increased PR and QT intervals, atrial and ventricular arrhythmias.
    - Treatment: magnesium sulfate IV or magnesium oxide PO.
  - Hypermagnesemia:
    - Causes: impaired renal function or excessive administration.
    - Symptoms: hyporeflexia and EKG changes to include: first-degree AV block, complete heart block.

- Treatment: IV or PO calcium gluconate, IV fluids with Lasix, and hemodialysis if refractory.
- Calcium abnormalities
  - Hypocalcemia:
    - Causes: hypoalbuminemia, tumor lysis syndrome, renal failure, hypoparathyroidism, hypomagnesemia, hypermagnesemia, acute pancreatitis, rhabdomyolysis, or blood transfusion (due to citrate chelating calcium)
    - Symptoms/signs: tetany, Trousseau's sign, Chvostek's sign
    - Signs: EKG changes: increased QT interval, ventricular tachycardia
    - Treatment: IV calcium gluconate or calcium chloride 10 mL of a 10% solution; PO calcium carbonate; or calcium gluconate 1 to 2 g orally 3 times a day with meals
  - Hypercalcemia:
    - Causes: bone metastasis, hyperparathyroidism, clear cell cancer of ovary or cervix, small cell cancers.
    - Symptoms: GI disturbances, hypotension, polyuria, confusion, depressed consciousness, coma.
    - Signs: EKG changes: shortened QT interval.
    - Treatment: rehydration with NS or 1/2 NS IV; diuresis with Lasix 40 mg IV q2 hours after IV hydration; pamidronate (Aredia) 60 to 90 mg IV over 2 to 24 hours for 7 days; glucocorticoids such as hydrocortisone 250 to 500 mg IV q8 hours; calcitonin: lowers calcium by 1 to 3 mg/dL for 6 to 8 hours (perform skin test first to check for hypersensitivity, start at 4 IU/kg SQ or IM q12–24 hours); Mithramycin dosed at 25 mcg/kg via slow IV push daily.
- Phosphorus abnormalities
  - Hypophosphatemia:
    - Causes: impaired intestinal absorption, increased renal excretion, redistribution of phosphate into cells, DKA, glucose loading, oncogenic osteomalacia, hyperparathyroidism, and the diuretic phase of acute tubular necrosis.
    - Symptoms/signs: muscular weakness, heart and respiratory failure, anemia.
    - Treatment: sodium or potassium phosphate IV or PO.
  - Hyperphosphatemia:
    - Causes: renal failure, tumor lysis syndrome, metabolic and respiratory acidosis, hypoparathyroidism.
    - Symptoms/signs: deposition of calcium-phosphate complexes into soft tissue and tetany.
    - Treatment: promote phosphorus binding with sucralfate or aluminum-containing antacids. Dialysis for patients with renal failure.

FLUIDS AND BLOOD PRODUCTS

Total body water (TBW) = $0.5 \times$ kg body weight
Intracellular fluid = $0.4 \times$ kg body weight
Extracellular fluid = $0.2 \times$ kg body weight
Interstitial fluid = $0.15 \times$ kg body weight
Plasma volume = $0.5 \times$ kg body weight
Blood volume = 75 mL/kg

ELECTROLYTES (Tables 4.15 and 4.16)

- Daily fluid management:
  - Daily physiologic fluid intake is composed of the following: endogenous water production from oxidation (approximately 250 mL/day); healthy PO intake (approximately 2,000 to 2,500 mL/day).
  - Daily physiologic fluid losses: 2,000 to 2,500 mL. This is composed of water from the urine 800 to 1,500 mL; stool 200 mL; insensible losses to include respiratory 200 mL and skin 800 mL.
  - Daily fluid requirement: 1,500 mL/m² body surface area (BSA).
  - Daily body weight loss if maintenance is with IVF only: one-half kg/day.
  - Increased fluid is needed when the patient is febrile. There should be a 15% increase in IVF for each degree above normal body temperature.
- IV Fluids (Table 4.17):
  - D5W: 50g dextrose in 1,000 mL of fluid; provides 170 calories per liter.
  - LR: multiple electrolyte concentration, similar to that of plasma. It is used to expand the plasma volume in hypovolemic states in the first 24 hours.
  - NS (0.9% NaCl): this is an isotonic solution. It is used to expand volume and correct mild hyponatremia.
  - ½ NS (0.45% NaCl): this is a hypotonic solution. It is used for postoperative IVF replacement after the first 24 hours. It is used when volume expansion is not required.
  - NaCl 3%: this is a hypertonic solution and is used to treat severe hyponatremia.

Table 4.15 Common Electrolyte Distribution Within the Body

Electrolyte	Plasma	Interstitial	Intracellular
Na	142	145	10 mEq/L
K	4	–	156 mEq/L
Cl	104	114	2 mEq/L
HCO₃	27	31	8 mEq/L
Ca²⁺	5	0	3.3 mEq/L
Mg²⁺	2	0	26 mEq/L
Phos	2	–	95 mEq/L

Table 4.16 Body Fluid Composition

Fluid	Na	Cl	K	HCO₃	Daily production
Gastric juices	60–100	100	10	0	1,500–2,000 mL
Duodenum	130	90	5	0–10	300–2,000 mL
Bile	145	100	5	15–35	100–800 mL
Pancreatic	140	75	5	70–115	100–800 mL
Ileum	140	100	5	15–30	2,000–3,000 mL

Table 4.17 Fluid Composition

	Na	Cl	K	HCO$_3$	Ca	Glu	AA	Mg	PO$_4$	Ac	Osm
Plasma	140	102	4.0	28	5			2			290
NS	154	154									308
½ NS	77	77									154
¼ NS	34	34									78
LR	130	109	4.0	28	3						272
D5W						50 g					252
D10W						100 g					505
PPN	47	40	13			100 g	35 g	3	3.5	52	500
TMP	25	30	44			250 g	50 g	5	15	99	1,900
D50						500 g					2,520

FLUID DEFICITS

- Presurgical deficit: from being NPO there is a 2 mL/kg/hr loss.
- Intraoperative fluids: the rule of 1:3 blood loss to crystalloid fluid replacement should be followed. Blood transfusion should occur based on National Institutes of Health transfusion guidelines, medical comorbidities, and anticipated adjuvant therapies. Third spacing fluid loss: removal of significant ascites and water retained as tissue edema is difficult to quantify.
- It is usually assumed:
  o 4 mL/kg/hr for minimal surgical procedures (e.g., wide local excision).
  o 6 mL/kg/hr for moderate surgical procedures (e.g., appendectomy, hernia repair).
  o 8 mL/kg/hr for major surgical procedures (e.g., radical hysterectomy, bowel resection).
  o Insensible losses intraoperatively are 2 mL/kg/hr.
- Postoperative fluid replacement: calculation should include output from surgical drains, urine, and insensible losses. Diuresis from extensive third spacing takes 1 to 3 days. Management can be with D5LR for the first 24 hours. No potassium is added to the IVF because of the possibility of tumor cell lyses and extracellular release from operative cell destruction. Then D5½ NS is started postoperative day 2 for continued volume replacement. Serum potassium should be checked daily. 10 mEq of potassium is added for each 1,000 mL of NGT drainage obtained.

BLOOD COMPONENT THERAPY

- Whole blood: has a volume of 517 mL. It is only indicated for acute blood loss that is severe enough to cause hypovolemic shock.
- PRBC: has a volume of 300 mL. One unit can survive 21 days if refrigerated. The hematocrit increases 3% to 5% per unit. It contains: plasma (78 mL), citrate

(22 mL), plasma protein (42 g), Na (15 mEq), potassium (5 mEq), and acid (25 nanoEq). It is important to check a Ca^{2+} level after significant transfusion due to the citrate chelation of divalent ions.

- Platelets: one unit has a volume of 20 to 50 mL. One unit has $5.5 \times 1,010$ platelets. They can be stored for only 72 hours. One unit increases the platelet count 7,000/mcL in 1 hour. The guideline for transfusion is 0.1 unit/kg; so a normal transfusion is 6 to 8 units. Equivalences: one unit is equal to one pack. A six pack of platelets is equal to 1 dose.

- FFP: contains all clotting factors except platelets. FFP should be given after 10 to 12 units of blood. Components are: 250 mL of plasma; 200 units of factor VIII; and 200 units of factor IX.

- Cryoprecipitate is obtained from the thawing of FFP at 4°C. Factors VIII, XIII, and fibrinogen are the main factors in cryoprecipitate. Cryoprecipitate is mainly used for factor replacement in the treatment of hemophilia and von Willebrand's disease. It is transfused in a pack of 4 to 6 units each having a volume of 15 mL.

- Albumin: used for volume resuscitation and hypoproteinemia. It is infused as a 5% or 25% solution and 25 g are commonly infused. The volume effects last for 12 hours. It increases the intravascular volume by 500 mL.

- Artificial colloids include:
  ○ Hetastarch: this is a 6% chemically modified starch polymer in isotonic saline. The volume effects last for 24 hours. Side effects can be significant and include: pruritus secondary to extravascular starch deposits (not allergy) and anaphylaxis (rare, 0.006% infusions).
  ○ Dextran: this is composed of glucose polymers produced by a bacterium. 10% Dextran-40 has a volume effect for 6 hours. Allergic reactions occur in 0.032% of infusions (Tables 4.18 and 4.19).

Table 4.18 Blood Products: Composition and Indication			
Blood products	**Contents**	**Volume**	**Indication**
PRBC	Red cells	1 unit = 250 mL, raises Hct 3%	Acute or chronic blood loss
Platelets	Platelets	One unit = 50 mL, raises platelets by 6×10^3	Platelets <20 nonbleeding patient, <50 in bleeding patient
FFP	Fibrinogen, Factors II, VII, IX, X, XI, XII, XIII, and heat labile V and VII	1 unit = 150 – 250 mL, 11 g albumin, 500 mg fibrinogen, 0.7–1.0 units clotting factors	DIC, treatment >10 units of blood, liver disease, IgG deficiency, 1 unit raises fibrinogen by 10 mg/dL

(continued)

Table 4.18 Blood Products: Composition and Indication (*continued*)

Blood products	Contents	Volume	Indication
Cryoprecipitate	Factors VIII, XIII, von Willebrand's disease, fibrinogen	1 unit = 10 mL, 250 mg fibrinogen, 80 units Factor VIII	Hemophilia A, von Willebrand's disease, fibrinogen deficiency
PCC 3 or 4 factors	A combination of Factors II, VII, IX, and X	9–25–50 IU/kg can be given	Acute or chronic blood loss or reversal of warfarin

FFP, fresh frozen plasma; PCC, prothrombin complex concentrate; PRBC, packed red blood cells.

Table 4.19 Risk of Infection per Unit of Blood Transfused

Hepatitis C	1:2 million
Hepatitis B	1:350,000
HIV	1:2.3 million
Bacterial	1:5,000 per unit of platelets 1:1 million PRBC

PRBC, packed red blood cells.

NEUROLOGIC

- Neuromuscular blockage is often used to paralyze the patient. Pancuronium is chosen for its long-acting properties. It lasts for up to 90 minutes after an IV dose of 0.06 to 0.1 mg/kg. Continuous infusion is vagolytic and can cause a heart rate increase of 10 bpm or more. It is important to use vecuronium if the patient cannot tolerate an increased heart rate. An electronic twitch monitor is used to assess the degree of paralyzation. Acute quadriplegic myopathy is a potential adverse event causing post paralytic quadriparesis, which consists of the triad of acute paresis, myonecrosis with increased CPK, and abnormal electromyography.

- Delirium is often seen in ICU patients. Haldol can be used to counteract delirium because of its minimal anticholinergic and hypotensive effects. It is given at a loading dose of 2 to 10 mg IV q20 minutes, followed by scheduled dosing every 4 to 6 hours at 25% of the necessary loading dose.

- Sedation is used to medically control the ICU patient for rest, recovery, and safety in the ICU environment. Daily interruption of sedation is necessary. This is associated with a shortened duration of ICU stay, less post-traumatic stress disorder (PTSD), and shorter mechanical ventilation. Propofol is used often as a sedative. It has no analgesic properties. It does count as lipid calories at 1.1 kcal/mL. Care should be taken in patients with hypertriglyceridemia, and so it is necessary to monitor triglycerides (TG) after 2 days of use (Table 4.20).

Table 4.20 Glasgow Coma Scale

Response	Score
Eye opening	
Spontaneous	4
To verbal	3
To pain	2
None	1
Verbal response	
Oriented and talking	5
Disoriented and talking	4
Inappropriate talking	3
Incomprehensible	2
None	1
Motor response	
Obeys commands	6
Localizes pain	5
Normal flexion withdrawal	4
Decortical signs (flexion)	3
Decerebrate signs (extension)	2
None	1

Score
15 Normal
11 Normal if intubated
8 or less coma

ABDOMINAL COMPARTMENT SYNDROME

Abdominal compartment syndrome can occur due to ascites, bowel obstruction, ileus, peritonitis, or pancreatitis. It can also occur after massive fluid resuscitation in the setting of septic or hypovolemic shock. Diagnosis is by measurement of the intra-abdominal pressure via a Foley catheter with documentation of a pressure of greater than 12 mmHg on three or more occasions 4 to 6 hours apart, or a single pressure of 20 mmHg or greater. It can manifest as systemic hypotension, reduced urinary output, or decreased pulmonary compliance. On occasion, surgery to decompress the abdomen and temporary closure with a vacuum pack may be necessary.

RISK STRATIFICATION OF MORBIDITY AND MORTALITY

Risk stratification of morbidity and mortality in the ICU by different quantitative scales has been documented as reliable and reproducible in gynecologic oncology patients. Two scales are used the most often: the APACHE IV and the SOFA. An increase of the SOFA score during the first 48 hours of ICU admission predicts a mortality of 50% or more.

REFERENCES

1. Daley BJ, Cecil W, Clarke PC, et al. How slow is too slow? Correlation of operative time to complications: an analysis from the Tennessee Surgical Quality Collaborative. *J Am Coll Surg*. April 2015;220(4):550-558.
2. Devereaux PJ, Yang H, Yusuf S, et al. Effects of extended-release metoprolol succinate in patients undergoing non-cardiac surgery (POISE trial): a randomised controlled trial. *Lancet*. 2008;371(9627):1839-1847.
3. Saksena S, Slee A, Waldo AL, et al. Cardiovascular outcomes in the AFFIRM Trial (atrial fibrillation follow-up investigation of rhythm management). An assessment of individual antiarrhythmic drug therapies compared with rate control with propensity score-matched analyses. *J Am Coll Cardiol*. November 1, 2011;58(19):1975-1985.
4. Danelich IM, Lose JM, Wright SS, et al. Practical management of postoperative atrial fibrillation after noncardiac surgery. *J Am Coll Surg*. October 2014;219(4):831-841.
5. Dellinger RP, Levy MM, Rhodes A, et al. Surviving Sepsis Campaign: international guidelines for management of severe sepsis and septic shock, 2012. *Intensive Care Med*. February 2013;39(2):165-228.
6. Klastersky J, Paesmans M. The multinational association for supportive care in cancer (MASCC) risk index score: 10 years of use for identifying low-risk febrile neutropenic cancer patients. *Support Care Cancer*. May 2013;21(5):1487-1495.

GYNECOLOGIC CANCER TREATMENT MODALITIES

5

Chemotherapy

ONE LETTER AND COMBINATION CHEMOTHERAPY ABBREVIATIONS

A: dactinomycin/actinomycin D
ABVD: adriamycin/doxorubicin, bleomycin, vinblastine, dacarbazine
AcFucy: dactinomycin, 5-FU, cyclophosphamide
AI: aromatase inhibitor
B: bleomycin
BEP: bleomycin, etoposide, cisplatin
C: cyclophosphamide
CDDP: cisplatin; cis-diamminedichloroplatinum
CHOPP-R: cyclophosphamide, hydroxyurea, vincristine, procarbazine, prednisone, rituximab
CMFV: cyclophosphamide, methotrexate, 5-FU, vinblastine
D: doxorubicin
E: etoposide, VP-16
Epi: epirubicin
F: 5-FU
H: hydroxyurea
L: chlorambucil
Lev: levamisole
L-PAM: L-phenylalanine mustard
M: methotrexate
MAC: methotrexate, dactinomycin, cyclophosphamide or chlorambucil
MMC: mitomycin
MOPP: nitrogen mustard, vincristine, procarbazine, prednisone
MVPP: nitrogen mustard, vinblastine, procarbazine, prednisone
O: oncovin/vincristine
P: cisplatin
Pr: prednisolone
T: tamoxifen
TVPP: thiotepa, vinblastine, procarbazine, prednisone
V: vinblastine
VAC: vincristine, doxorubicin cyclophosphamide
VBM: vinblastine, bleomycin, methotrexate
VBP: vinblastine, bleomycin, cisplatin
VDC: vincristine, doxorubicin, cyclophosphamide

CHEMOTHERAPY DEFINITIONS

- Dose: amount of chemotherapy administered
- Intensity: the amount of drug administered over time
- Schedule: time interval for delivery of chemotherapy
- Chemotherapy cycle: one treatment of single or combination agents in the full course of therapy
- Chemotherapy course: sequence of cycles for treatment
- Planning of treatment: must take into consideration tumor type, extent of disease, patient's comorbidities including renal function, age, social and emotional function, or if therapy is primary or salvage

DELIVERY

Routes are intravenous (IV), intramuscular (IM), per oral (PO), intraperitoneal (IP), or regional. Most chemotherapy is administered systemically, by IV. It can be given regionally to primary tumors or their metastasis. IP chemotherapy is administration of chemotherapy directly into the abdominopelvic cavity. Regional chemotherapy can be used to treat solitary organ lesions, like liver metastasis. This occurs by obstruction of the outflow tract for a limited amount of time so that the chemotherapy can penetrate the tumor mass directly. It can also be directly administered to a cavity such as for pleural or pericardial lesions.

METABOLISM

- Pro-drugs can be bio-transformed into active metabolites. This includes cyclophosphamide. It is important to know those drugs that are activated by the liver because IP administration may have no effect.
- Excretion: hepatobiliary or renal excretion are the main routes of excretion. Drugs can be metabolized to pro-drugs, to inactive states, remain unchanged, or accumulate in body tissues.

PRINCIPLES OF CHEMOTHERAPY TUMOR KILL

The patient needs two cycles after resolution of tumor markers and/or no evidence of disease with complete clinical remission (CCR) to eliminate microscopic systemic disease.

CHEMOTHERAPY REGIMENS

- Primary: chemotherapy is the initial treatment.
- Adjuvant: chemotherapy is used following primary treatment with surgery or radiation therapy (XRT).
- Neoadjuvant: chemotherapy is used for initial treatment to be followed by surgery, XRT, or a combination of therapies.
- Secondary: any chemotherapy regimen given after primary chemotherapy.
- Salvage: chemotherapy is used in the treatment of recurrent or persistent disease after previous chemotherapy.
- Consolidation: chemotherapy that is continued/used for a defined interval after primary or adjuvant chemotherapy to decrease the chance of cancer recurrence

in patients with CCR. This is usually a short duration of treatment (4–6 more cycles).

- Maintenance: chemotherapy that is continued/used after primary or adjuvant chemotherapy for an indefinite interval to decrease the chance of cancer recurrence in patients with CCR. This is usually of a longer duration than consolidation therapy until progression or toxicity. Some protocols specify 18 cycles or 22 months after primary adjuvant therapy.

PLATINUM SENSITIVITY/RESISTANCE IN HGSTOC OR OVARIAN GERM CELL TUMORS

Tumors are classified as platinum sensitive, resistant, or refractory.

- Platinum sensitive: if the tumor recurs 6 or more months after the completion of primary platinum-based chemotherapy, it is said to be platinum sensitive.
- Platinum resistant: if the tumor recurs within 6 months of primary platinum-based chemotherapy, it is considered platinum resistant.
- Platinum refractory: if the tumor does not respond to initial platinum chemotherapy and growth continues during the primary treatment, it is considered platinum refractory.
- For germ cell tumors, the time interval is different and resistance is specified at 6 weeks. Germ cell tumors are designated as refractory if no response is seen at 4 weeks of ongoing chemotherapy.

TOXICITY

- Side effects from chemotherapy are graded according to severity. The most commonly affected organ systems are the gastrointestinal system, the hematopoietic system, and the integumentary system. Please refer to the common toxicity criteria (CTC) website for the full classification of toxicity grades. Management of toxicity due to chemotherapy is with a reduction in the total dose of drug per cycle, called a dose reduction. This is usually a 20% to 25% dose reduction, or a decrease in the area under the curve (AUC) by one level.
- Cardiac toxicity mainly occurs with doxorubicin. A history and exam can diagnose congestive heart failure (CHF). Confirmation is with an echocardiogram or with a multigated acquisition (MUGA) scan.
- Pulmonary toxicity has been seen mainly with bleomycin. A pre-treatment carbon monoxide spirometry diffusion capacity test (DLCO) is recommended. A 15% change in the forced expiratory volume (FEV) indicates toxicity. Pulmonary toxicity can also be determined clinically with an examination. Clinical symptoms such as rales, hypoinflation, or a lag in the inspiratory phase on exam, as well as dyspnea occur before a documented drop in FEV.
- Secondary malignancies can occur after the administration of chemotherapeutic agents. The rate is about 1% to 2%. Leukemias can occur from alkylating agents, which include melphalan, the podophyllotoxins, etoposide, cyclophosphamide, and the platinum compounds. The development of leukemias is dose dependent (2 g for etoposide). The median latency is 4 years after chemotherapy for epithelial ovarian cancer (EOC), with an overall incidence of 0.17% (1).

THE CELL CYCLE

- The cell cycle is broken into interphase and mitosis. Interphase consists of the G1, S, and G2 phases. G1 is a variable period, where protein, RNA, and DNA repair occur. The cell can terminally differentiate or continue in the cell cycle from this phase. S phase is when new DNA is synthesized. The G2 phase occurs after the S phase and thus the cell contains two times the amount of DNA. This is a short phase. It is the variation in the length of the G1 phase that affects the proliferative behavior of cell populations.
- Mitosis consists of five phases. Prophase, the first phase, is when chromosomes condense. Metaphase is when chromosomal division occurs. This is the most radiosensitive phase. Anaphase is when sister chromosomes move to opposite cell poles. Telophase demonstrates polarization of chromosomes and disassembly of the cytoskeleton occurs. Cytokinesis follows with division of the cell into separate daughter cells. Cell cycle times vary from 10 to 31 hours.
- Masses are usually palpated at 10^9 cells or 1 cm in size. The 1-cm size usually occurs after 30 doublings of one tumor cell.

GROWTH FRACTION

This consists of the fraction of cells in a tumor that is actively proliferating. This fraction ranges from 25% to 95%.

CELL DEATH

Cell death has been seen with some tumors. This has been documented in some breast cancers associated with febrile episodes (2) or when tumors outgrow their vascular supply.

LOG KILL

A constant fraction of cells are killed with each dose of therapy—not a constant number of cells. To achieve substantial tumor reduction, a repetitive insult has to be delivered to the tumor. Single-agent chemotherapy can be curative in this fashion, but is not as effective as multiagent chemotherapy. Multiagent chemotherapy uses different drugs that target separate cellular pathways. The effect can be additive or synergic.

CELL-CYCLE NONSPECIFIC CHEMOTHERAPEUTIC AGENTS

These agents kill cells in all phases of the cell cycle.

CELL-CYCLE SPECIFIC AGENTS

These agents depend on the proliferative fraction of the tumor and a specific cell cycle phase. These agents are usually more effective against tumors with a high proliferative rate and a high growth fraction.

CELL GROWTH

Growth is usually demonstrated via a Gompertzian log tumor growth curve.
- There are four phases to cell growth:
  - Lag growth phase
  - The log growth phase

- ○ Stable growth phase
- ○ Death phase

MECHANISMS OF CYTOTOXICITY

Chemotherapeutic agents can target cellular DNA, proteins (such as enzymes, receptors, or the metabolic respiratory chain), and RNA.

MECHANISMS OF RESISTANCE

- The Goldie–Coldman hypothesis is a mathematical model that predicts the probability of a tumor harboring drug-resistant clones. The number of drug-resistant clones depends on the mutation rate and the size of the tumor.
- Documented mechanisms of drug resistance include as follows:
  - ○ The multidrug resistance protein-1 (MDR-1) and MDR-2 P-glycoproteins, which are components of the adenosine triphosphate (ATP)-binding cassette (ABC) transporters. These proteins transport drugs out of cells.
  - ○ Cells can decrease the entry of the drug into the cell via down regulation of cellular receptors.
  - ○ Metabolic inactivation of the drug can occur via up-regulation of the gluta-thione (GSH) sulfate and dihydrofolate reductase (DHFR) enzymes.
  - ○ There can be altered binding affinity of the drug to albumin or intracellular targets.
  - ○ Genomic change can occur via:
    - ▪ Altered DNA repair mechanisms
    - ▪ Gene point mutation
    - ▪ Gene frameshift mutation
    - ▪ Gene deletion
    - ▪ Gene amplification
  - ○ Gatekeeping mutations: the initial genetic change that gives a single cell a selective growth advantage, allowing the subsequent acquisition of driver mutations, which alter the proliferation rate, invasion capability, cellular sig-naling, and DNA repair of a tumor.
  - ○ Passenger mutations: have no effect on the neoplastic process and accumu-late with age.

PRIOR TO CHEMOTHERAPY ADMINISTRATION

The patient should have adequate laboratory values; these are considered to be:

- White blood cell count (WBC) greater than 3×10^3/mcL with an absolute neu-trophil count (ANC) greater than 1.5×10^3/mcL
- Platelets greater than 100×10^3/mcL
- Normal liver function tests (LFTs)
- Creatinine less than 2 mg/dL or creatinine clearance greater than 50 mL/min
- Gynecologic Oncology Group (GOG) performance status of either 0, 1, or 2 with an estimated survival of more than 2 months

CLASSES OF CHEMOTHERAPY AGENTS AND INDEPENDENT MECHANISMS OF ACTION

ALKYLATING AGENTS

These work by intercalating or cross-linking DNA—making DNA adducts. They are cell-cycle nonspecific.

- **Carboplatin (Paraplatin):** a platinum compound. It is dosed with the following equation: carboplatin total dose (mg) = AUC × (GFR + 25). It can be given at an AUC of 7 as single agent or at an AUC of 5 to 6 in combination therapy. Its mechanism of action is intercalation with DNA and is administered via the IV or IP route. It is eliminated via the renal system. Its toxicities are primarily thrombocytopenia, hypersensitivity reactions, leukopenia, nausea, and vomiting. The platelet nadir is usually around 21 days. Secondary toxicities can include nephrotoxicity 7%, peripheral neuropathy 6%, and ototoxicity 1%. Vitamin B_6 can prevent some neurotoxicity. Hypersensitivity can occur in 25% of patients if more than six cycles are received. There is an increased risk of leukemia with a relative risk of 6.5. Amifostine can reduce the amount of thrombocytopenia at a dose of 910 mg/m^2.

- **Cisplatin (Platinol):** a platinum compound that works by intercalating with DNA and creating G–G adducts. It is administered either IV or IP. It can be given as a single agent to radiosensitize certain tumors at 40 to 50 mg/m^2 weekly. It can be given as single-agent therapy at 50 to 100 mg/m^2, or at 75 mg/m^2 in combination with other drugs every 3 weeks. 90% is eliminated by the renal system and 10% by the hepatic/biliary system. Primary toxicities are leukopenia and anemia. Nephrotoxicity occurs in 21%, ototoxicity in 10%, and some patients have peripheral or autonomic neuropathy. Secondary toxicities are allergic reactions, low sodium (Na), potassium (K), calcium (Ca), and magnesium (Mg). The pancytopenia nadir occurs between 18 and 23 days. To reduce some nephrotoxicity, prehydrate with normal saline intravenous fluid (IVF) and consider mannitol diuresis with an additional 3 g of $MgSO_4$.

- **Cyclophosphamide (Cytoxan):** it is a pro-drug that is activated by liver metabolism and then the active drug intercalates with DNA. It is administered either IV or PO. It can be given as a single agent or in combination with other agents. The dosing is usually 10 to 50 mg/kg IV every 1 to 4 weeks or 600 to 1,000 mg/m^2 every 4 weeks. 85% is eliminated by the liver and 15% by the renal system. Primary toxicities include pancytopenia (this is the most marrow-suppressive drug), nausea, vomiting, and alopecia. Secondary toxicities are hemorrhagic cystitis from the acrolein metabolite, syndrome of inappropriate secretion of antidiuretic hormone (SIADH) if the dose is greater than 50 mg/kg, interstitial pneumonia, cardiomyopathy, and leukemia with a relative risk of 5.4 after 10 years. The nadir occurs at days 8 to 14. To diagnose hemorrhagic cystitis, obtain a urine analysis: confirmation is with gross hematuria or 20 red blood cells per high power field (RBC/HPF). Mesna should be coadministered to decrease the incidence of hemorrhagic cystitis. Methylene blue bladder irrigation can also decrease the complications of hemorrhagic cystitis.

- **Dacarbazine (DTIC):** administered IV usually at a dose of 2 to 4.5 mg/kg/day for 5 to 10 days every 4 weeks. Elimination is via the renal system. Primary toxicities include pancytopenia, nausea, vomiting, and alopecia. Secondary toxicities include mucositis, stomatitis, myalgias, and hepatotoxicity. The nadir occurs 2 to 4 weeks after administration.

- **Ifosfamide (Ifex):** also a pro-drug; it is activated by hepatic metabolism and is administered IV at a dose of 1.2 to 1.6 g/m^2/day for 5 days every 3 to 4 weeks, 700 to 900 mg/m^2/day for 5 days every 3 weeks, or 1,000 mg/m^2 on days 1 and 2 every 28 days as part of the ifosfamide–carboplatin–etoposide (ICE) protocol. Elimination is via the renal system for 73% of the drug. Primary toxicities are hemorrhagic cystitis, pancytopenia, nausea, vomiting, and alopecia. Secondary toxicities are nephrotoxicity, SIADH, and central nervous system (CNS) toxicity. CNS toxicity is increased with baseline dementia or a low serum albumin. The neurotoxin chloroacetaldehyde is a byproduct of this drug. The nadir is days 5 to 10 after administration and this drug also needs coadministration of mesna to decrease the incidence of hemorrhagic cystitis.

- **Melphalan (Alkeran):** cross links DNA and can be administered IV, PO, or IP. Dosing occurs at 16 mg/m^2 IV every 2 weeks for four doses then at 4-week intervals, or 1 mg/kg IV every 4 weeks. The PO dose is 6 mg/day for 2 to 3 weeks followed by a 4-week holiday. There is 63 times greater exposure via the IP route. Elimination is 99% renal. Primary toxicity is pancytopenia with secondary toxicities to include nausea, vomiting, and leukemia (11.2% cumulative 10-year risk). The nadir occurs at days 28 to 35 and there is increased drug bioavailability if taken after fasting for 8 hours. Drug resistance is via increased intracellular glutathione S-transferase (GST), and buthionine sulfoximine (BSO) can reverse this resistance.

- **Temozolomide (Temodar):** a triazene analog of dacarbazine with antineoplastic activity. As a cytotoxic alkylating agent, temozolomide is converted at physiologic pH to the short-lived active compound, monomethyl triazeno imidazole carboxamide (MTIC). The cytotoxicity of MTIC is due primarily to methylation of DNA at the O6 and N7 positions of guanine, resulting in inhibition of DNA replication. Unlike dacarbazine, which is metabolized to MTIC only in the liver, temozolomide is metabolized to MITC at all sites. Temozolomide is administered orally and penetrates well into the CNS. Dosing: varies by tumor protocol but commonly is calculated: BSA × 75 then rounded to the nearest 5 mg PO BID days 1 to 14. Another regimen is 150 mg/m^2 IV daily for 5 days of a 28 day cycle.

- **Altretamine (Hexalen, Hexamethylmelamine):** this is a pro-drug that is metabolically activated by the liver. It is important to not take supplements with B_{12} because this inactivates the drug. It is administered PO at a dose of 260 mg/m^2/day in four daily divided doses for 14 to 21 days every 4 weeks. 85% is eliminated via the renal system. Primary toxicities are pancytopenia, neuropathy, nausea, vomiting, and nephrotoxicity. Secondary toxicities include rash, neurotoxicity, and seizures. The nadir occurs at days 21 to 28.

ANTITUMOR ANTIBIOTICS

These agents intercalate with DNA, inhibit RNA synthesis, and interfere with DNA repair. They are cell-cycle nonspecific except for bleomycin.

- **Bleomycin (Blenoxane):** complexes with iron to form an oxidase and produces free radicals. These free radicals produce DNA strand breaks in the G2 and

M phases. It can be administered either IV, IM, or intracavitary for effusions. Dosing is calculated at 1 unit = 1 mg. The IV dose is bolused at 30 mg/week for 12 weeks, or 10 mg/m^2/day for 4 days every 4 weeks. Do not exceed 400 mg total lifetime dose. For pleural effusions, 60 to 120 mg can be instilled into the cavity. 70% is eliminated by the kidneys. Primary toxicities are interstitial pneumonitis (10%), pulmonary fibrosis (1%), alopecia, mucositis, and nonneutropenic fever. Secondary toxicities are nausea, vomiting, pancytopenia, hyperpigmentation, and allergic reactions. The nadir occurs at day 12. Pulmonary toxicity occurs due to the iron free radicals targeting first the type I alveoli, followed by the type II alveoli. DLCO (carbon monoxide diffusion capacity spirometry) is the test to determine pulmonary toxicity. A 15% change from pre-treatment value signifies toxicity and thus the need to discontinue treatment. A CXR should be obtained prior to each course along with a DLCO, but it is important to rely on physical examination and patient symptoms. Risk factors for pulmonary toxicity are prior mediastinal irradiation, age greater than 70, and hyperoxia during surgical anesthesia. Steroid therapy may help with acute pneumonitis.

- **Doxorubicin (Adriamycin):** inhibits the strand passing activity of topoisomerase-II and also intercalates with DNA. It is administered via IV and chelates with iron and copper. These heavy metal chelations contribute to the cardio toxicity of the drug. It is dosed at 60 to 75 mg/m^2 as a single agent or 40 to 60 mg/m^2 in combination every 3 to 4 weeks. Elimination is hepatobiliary for 40% of the drug. It is a vesicant. Primary toxicity is pancytopenia and secondary toxicities are XRT recall, cardiomyopathy, and palmar plantar erythema (PPE). To avoid PPE, consider treatment with vitamin B$_6$, avoid hot tubs and high friction activities. The nadir is at days 10 to 14. With a total dose greater than 500 mg/m^2, the patient has an 11% risk of cardiomyopathy. If the total dose is greater than 600 mg/m^2, there is a 30% risk. Dexrazoxane (Zinecard) is a cardioprotective agent. It is administered at a 10:1 ratio, but if there is renal compromise, it should be dose reduced (to a 5:1 ratio). Risk factors for development of cardiomyopathy are age greater than 70 years, prior cardiac disease, and prior mediastinal XRT. Pre-treatment tests include a baseline MUGA scan or echocardiogram, EKG, and a CXR. If symptoms present during treatment, obtain a MUGA scan or an echocardiogram.

- **Liposomal Doxorubicin (Doxil):** the mechanism of action is similar to the nonliposomal form. It is given IV every 4 weeks at 40 to 50 mg/m^2. It is not a vesicant. The drug is found highly concentrated in tumor tissue (four times the serum amount). Toxicity is primarily pancytopenia. Secondary toxicity is palmar planter erythroddysesthesia (PPE).

- **Dactinomycin (Actinomycin D):** the mechanism of action is DNA intercalation and it is administered IV. Dosing can be 9 to 13 mcg/kg IV per day for 5 days every 2 weeks or 1.25 mg/m^2 every 2 weeks for nonmetastatic gestational trophoblastic disease (GTD); 90% is eliminated via the hepatobiliary system. Primary toxicities are pancytopenia, nausea, vomiting, and mucositis. Secondary toxicity is alopecia. The nadir is days 7 to 10. The mode of resistance is via MDR P-glycoprotein.

- **Mitomycin C (Mutamycin):** a pro-drug that crosslinks DNA. It is selectively activated by hypoxic cells. It is administered IV and dosed as a single agent at 10 to 20 mg/m^2 or in combination at 10 mg/m^2 every 6 to 8 weeks. Elimination is by the hepatobiliary system for 90% of the drug. Primary toxicity is pancytopenia and secondary toxicities are nausea, vomiting, nephrotoxicity, microangiopathic hemolytic anemia, hemolytic uremic syndrome (HUS), and multiorgan failure. The nadir is 4 to 6 weeks. There is cumulative myelosuppression so the total lifetime dose should be less than 60 mg/m^2.

- **Mitoxantrone (Novantrone):** inhibits topoisomerase-II and is administered IV or IP at a dose of 12 to 14 mg/m^2 IV, or 10 mg/m^2 in 2 L of NS IP every 3 weeks. Elimination is hepatobiliary and primary toxicities are nausea, vomiting, diarrhea, and myelosuppression. The nadir is day 10. This drug may cause the "Smurf" syndrome and can turn the bowel and sclera blue.

- **Levamisole (Ergamisol):** a synthetic imidazothiazole derivative initially used for helminthic infections. It is administered PO at a dose of 50 mg PO TID × 3 days per week, weekly for 1 year in combination with chemotherapy (5-fluorouracil [5-FU]). It is eliminated via the renal system. Primary toxicities are stomatitis, diarrhea, nausea, vomiting, and a metallic taste. Secondary toxicities are fever, chills, fatigue, myalgias, agranulocytosis, telangiectasia, seizures, edema, and chorea. The nadir is days 7 to 10. The tablets contain lactose: lactaid may be necessary in those with lactose intolerance.

ANTIMETABOLITES

These drugs antagonize folate, purines, pyrimidines, or ribonucleotide reductase. They therefore interfere with DNA synthesis. These agents are cell cycle specific for the S phase.

- **5-FU (Efudex):** a pro-drug that is metabolized to FUDR. FUDR is a pyrimidine antimetabolite that inhibits thymidylate synthase and is incorporated into DNA and RNA. Administration is IV or topical. Dosing as a single agent is with a loading dose of 12 mg/kg (maximum of 800 mg) IV daily for 4 to 5 days, then after 28 days, a weekly maintenance dose of 200 to 250 mg/m^2 every other day for 4 days, every 4 weeks. It can also be dosed at 800 to 1,000 mg/m^2 IV daily for 4 days, repeated every 3 to 4 weeks. Oral dosing as capecitabine, of 15 to 20 mg/kg/day for 5 to 8 days can be used. Topical/vaginal application is given as a 5% cream; apply ½ vaginal applicator of 5% 5-FU (2.5 g) deep in the vagina at bedtime every 2 to 3 weeks. Elimination is 80% by the liver and 15% by the kidneys. Primary toxicities are granulocytopenia, thrombocytopenia, mucositis, nausea, vomiting, alopecia, and hyperpigmentation. Secondary toxicities are photosensitivity, cerebellar syndrome from the metabolite fluorocitrate, palmar plantar erythrodysesthesia (occurs in 42%–82% and can be reversed with vitamin B$_6$ dosed at 50 to 150 mg), and cardiotoxicity. The nadir is days 9 to 14. Patients with a genetic deficiency of DHFR should not receive this drug.

- **Capecitabine (Xeloda):** a pro-drug that is metabolized to 5-FU. It is administered PO with a starting dose of 1,250 mg/m^2 administered as a divided BID dose. A reduced starting dose (950 mg/m^2 BID) is required for patients with a creatinine clearance equal to 30 to 50 mL/min. It is given for 14 days of a 21-day cycle. Elimination is renal and primary toxicities are diarrhea, nausea, and vomiting. Secondary toxicities are hand-and-foot syndrome, rash, dry skin, and fatigue. If the patient is taking warfarin concomitantly, frequent monitoring of the international normalized ratio (INR) is recommended.

- **Methotrexate (Trexall):** blocks DHFR and can be administered IV, PO, IM, or intrathecally. The dose can be weekly at 30 to 50 mg/m² IM or IV; 0.4 mg/kg IV or IM daily × 5 days every 14 days; 1 mg/kg IM or IV, days 1, 3, 5, and 7 with leucovorin given 15 mg orally on days 2, 4, 6, and 8 every 14 days; or 100 mg/m² IV bolus followed by 200 mg/m² 12-hour continuous IV infusion with leucovorin given 15 mg orally every 12 hours × 4 doses (beginning 24 hours after start of methotrexate infusion) every 14 days; or 12 to 15 mg/m²/week intrathecally. Elimination is mainly renal. Primary toxicities are nausea, vomiting, pancytopenia, mucositis, and hepatotoxicity. Secondary toxicities are nephrotoxicity, alopecia, and interstitial pneumonitis. The nadir is days 4 to 7. Resistance is via elevated DHFR or mutated transport mechanisms into the tumor cells. Methotrexate accumulates in pleural effusions, so it is necessary to drain effusions before administration. It is also helpful to alkalinize the urine with 3 g or 40–50 mEq per L of IVF, of sodium bicarbonate 12 hours before therapy.
- **Hydroxyurea (Hydrea):** S-phase specific and inhibits ribonucleotide reductase. It is administered IV or PO. Dosing is 1 to 3 mg/m²/day every 2 to 6 weeks; 80 mg/kg twice weekly; or 2 to 3 g/m² twice weekly. Elimination is mainly renal and toxicity is myelosuppression. The nadir occurs at 10 days.
- **Gemcitabine (Gemzar):** a synthetic nucleoside analog. It is a pro-drug and is metabolized to its active diphosphate and triphosphate states by the liver. These metabolites are then incorporated into DNA and cause masked chain termination. In addition, it is a radio-sensitizing agent and can cause radiation recall. Dosing is IV. It can be given as a single agent at 800 to 1,000 mg/m² IV weekly for 7 weeks of an 8-week cycle; 1,000 mg/m² weekly for 3 weeks of a 4-week cycle; or at 1,000 to 1,250 mg/m² days 1 and 8 with cisplatin at 75 to 100 mg/m² on day 1 of a 3-week cycle. Elimination is 90% renal. Primary toxicities are neutropenia, elevated LFTs, alopecia, and mucositis. Secondary toxicities are subcutaneous edema, HUS, and acute respiratory distress syndrome (ARDS).

PLANT ALKALOIDS

These agents inhibit microtubule function and arrest cells in M phase. They are cell-cycle specific.

- **Etoposide (VP-16, VePesid):** the mechanism of action is inhibition and stabilization of topoisomerase-II. It arrests cells in the G2 phase. There are multiple regimens but it can be given at a dose of 100 mg/m² days 1 to 5 the first week of a 3 week cycle or 50 mg/m²/day × 21 days PO. Elimination is primarily renal with 98% being cleared by the kidneys. Primary toxicities are pancytopenia, nausea, and vomiting. Secondary toxicities are alopecia, neurotoxicity, and hypotension; therefore, give over 30 minutes. It can also cause secondary leukemia above a total dose of 2 gm². The nadir is day 16.
- **Paclitaxel (Taxol):** stabilizes microtubules and promotes their formation. It can be given IV or IP and should be administered before platinum agents. Single-agent dosing is usually 175 to 250 mg/m² but in combination it is usually

dosed at 175 mg/m^2 every 3 weeks or 80 mg/m^2 weekly every 3 weeks. Dose reduction is usually to 135 mg/m^2. Elimination is 90% hepatic/biliary and 10% renal. Primary toxicities are neurotoxicity (distal extremities), pancytopenia, hypersensitivity reactions to the vehicle cremophor, arrhythmias, and alopecia. Secondary toxicities are nausea, vomiting, mucositis, arthralgias, and an abnormal EKG. The nadir is days 8 to 11. Always premedicate before chemotherapy with dexamethasone 20 mg PO 12 and 6 hours prior to administration, Benadryl 50 mg IV/PO, and cimetidine 300 mg IV both 30 minutes before initiation.

- **Albumin-Bound Paclitaxel (Abraxane, ABI-007):** stabilizes microtubules and promotes their formation. The albumin-bound drug has a superior toxicity profile because it lacks the castor oil-base that paclitaxel is mixed with. Dosing is 260 mg/m^2 IV every 3 weeks without needed premedications. Cardiotoxicity occurs in 3% of patients, neutropenia occurs in 9% of patients, and neuropathy is dose dependent.

- **Topotecan (Hycamtin):** inhibits topoisomerase-I and is usually given IV. Dosing as a single agent is 1.25 to 1.5 mg/m^2/day for 3 to 5 days/week every 3 weeks. Elimination is both renal and hepatic. Primary toxicities are myelosuppression and alopecia with secondary toxicity being asthenia. The nadir is days 9 to 15.

- **Irinotecan (Camptosar):** a pro-drug and inhibits topoisomerase-I. It is given IV at doses of: 125 mg/m^2 every week, 240 mg/m^2 every 3 weeks, or 350 mg/m^2 every 3 weeks. Elimination is hepatobiliary. Primary toxicities are anemia, nausea, vomiting, elevated liver enzymes, and alopecia. Secondary toxicity is diarrhea. Use antimotility agents (e.g., loperamide at 16 mg/day) as soon as diarrhea appears. The nadir is days 15 to 27.

- **Docetaxel (Taxotere):** inhibits the depolymerization of tubulin and stabilizes microtubules. It is given IV as a single agent at 60 to 100 mg/m^2 every 3 weeks; or in combination at 85 to 100 mg/m^2 every 3 weeks. Its elimination is primarily hepatobiliary at 99.4%. Primary toxicities are neutropenia, edema, and hypersensitivity reactions. Secondary toxicity is a maculopapular rash. The nadir occurs at 5 to 9 days. To decrease the rate of hypersensitivity reactions and third spacing edema, premedicate with corticosteroids 8 mg BID starting 1 day prior to, and continuing up to 4 days after, administration.

- **Vinblastine (Velban):** inhibits microtubule assembly by binding to tubulin and is given IV at a dose of 0.1 to 0.5 mg/kg/week (4 to 20 mg/m^2); 6 mg/m^2 days 1 and 15 every 3 weeks; or 0.15 mg/kg days 1 and 2 every 3 weeks. It is eliminated via both the renal (30%) and the hepatobiliary (20%) systems. Primary toxicities are pancytopenia, constipation, abdominal pain, and adynamic ileus. Secondary toxicities are nausea, vomiting, mucositis, alopecia, neurotoxicity, Raynaud's syndrome, and transient hepatitis. The nadir is days 4 to 10.

- **Vincristine (Oncovin):** inhibits microtubule assembly. It is administered IV at a dose of: 1 mg/m^2 or 0.01 to 0.03 mg/m^2 given every 1 to 2 weeks. Elimination is primarily renal (90%), with hepatobiliary elimination at 10%. Primary toxicities are neurotoxicity, and alopecia. Secondary toxicities are pancytopenia, constipation, and SIADH. The nadir is day 7.

- **Vinorelbine (Navelbine):** inhibits microtubule assembly and is given IV as a single agent at a dose of 30 mg/m^2 every week, or in combination at 25 mg/m^2 weekly.

Elimination is hepatobiliary. Primary toxicities are granulocytopenia, neurotoxicity, nausea, vomiting, alopecia, and chest pain. Secondary toxicities are arthralgias, shortness of breath (SOB), and constipation. The nadir is days 7 to 14. It is incompatible with 5-FU, mitomycin C, thiotepa, antibiotics, antivirals, and can exacerbate pulmonary toxicity.

HORMONAL AGENTS

These agents bind hormone receptors and either stimulate or inhibit DNA transcription depending on the agonist/antagonist properties of the drug. They are cell-cycle nonspecific.

- **Leuprolide Acetate (Lupron):** a gonadotropin-releasing hormone (GnRH) superagonist administered as a depot IM injection. Dosing can be 3.5 to 7.5 mg monthly or 11.25 to 22.5 mg every 3 months. Elimination is renal. Primary toxicity is hot flashes with secondary toxicities of headache, edema, and bone pain.
- **Megestrol (Megace):** a progestin given PO at doses of 160 to 380 mg daily. Elimination is renal. Primary toxicity is edema and weight gain. Secondary toxicities are deep venous thrombosis (DVT)/venous thromboembolism (VTE) and a Cushing-like syndrome.
- **Tamoxifen (Nolvadex):** an estrogen receptor agonist/antagonist administered PO at a dose of 20 mg/day. Elimination is hepatobiliary and primary toxicity is hot flashes. Secondary toxicities are vaginal bleeding, DVT/VTE, rash, and endometrial cancer.
- **Anastrozole (Arimidex):** a nonsteroidal aromatase inhibitor given PO. The dose is 1 mg/day. Elimination is renal. Primary toxicities are anorexia, vaginal dryness, and hot flashes. Secondary toxicities are DVT/VTE, osteopenia, and osteoporosis.
- **Letrozole (Femara):** a nonsteroidal aromatase inhibitor. It is given PO at a dose of 2.5 mg/day. Primary toxicities are bone pain and hot flashes, arthralgias, and dyspnea in 20% of patients. It does not increase serum follicle-stimulating hormone (FSH) and does not impact adrenal steroid synthesis.
- **Exemestane (Aromasin):** a steroidal aromatase inhibitor. It is an irreversible inhibitor. It is dosed at 25 mg/day. Primary toxicity is hot flashes, fatigue, and arthralgias.

NOVEL DRUGS

- **Eribulin (Halaven):** this is a halaven microtubule dynamics inhibitor. It is the mesylate salt of a synthetic analogue of halichondrin B, a substance derived from a marine sponge (*Lissodendoryx sp.*) It binds to the vinca domain of tubulin and inhibits the polymerization of tubulin and the assembly of microtubules, resulting in inhibition of mitotic spindle assembly, of vascular remodeling, reversal of epithelial–mesenchymal transition, suppression of migration and invasion, induction of cell cycle arrest at the G2/M phase, and, potentially, tumor regression. Dosing: 1.4 mg/m^2 IV day 1 and 8 of a 21 day cycle.
- **Trabectedin (Yondelis):** this is a tetrahydroisoquinoline alkaloid isolated from the marine tunicate *Ecteinascidia turbinata* that binds to the minor groove of DNA and interferes with the transcription-coupled nucleotide excision repair machinery to induce lethal DNA strand breaks and block the cell cycle in the

G2 phase. It also inhibits the differentiation of monocytes into macrophages. Dosing: 1.5 mg/m^2 IV over 24 hours once every 21 days.

- **Ixabepilone (Ixempra):** this is a microtubule-stabilizing agent that evades paclitaxel resistance via retention of tumor binding affinity despite upregulation of class III beta-tubulin and maintenance of intracellular concentrations as a nonsubstrate for the p-glycoprotein drug efflux pump. It is an orally bioavailable semisynthetic analogue of epothilone B with antineoplastic activity. Ixabepilone binds to tubulin and promotes tubulin polymerization and microtubule stabilization, thereby arresting cells in the G2-M phase of the cell cycle and inducing tumor cell apoptosis. This agent demonstrates antineoplastic activity against taxane-resistant cell lines. Dosing: 40 mg/m^2 IV every 3 weeks usually in combination therapy.

PROTECTIVE AGENTS

These agents protect against the cytotoxic effects of chemotherapeutic drugs.

- **Leucovorin:** has two mechanisms of action. It is protective against MTX and it modulates and prolongs the effects of 5-FU. Dosing is: 370 mg/m^2/day for 5 days during 5-FU infusion plus an additional infusion of 500 mg/m^2/day beginning 24 hours before the first dose of 5-FU and continuing 12 hours after completion of 5-FU therapy; or 5 to 15 mg PO or 10 to 20 mg/m^2 given IV 10 minutes before 5-FU infusion. It is eliminated by the renal system. Primary toxicities are pancytopenia, nausea, and vomiting. The nadir is days 7 to 14.
- **Dexrazoxane (Zinecard):** chemoprotective against doxorubicin-induced cardiomyopathy. It chelates divalent heavy metals and is administered IV, 30 minutes prior to chemotherapy at a dose of 10:1 (500 mg/m^2 dexrazoxane to 50 mg/m^2 of doxorubicin). Consider administration when the cumulative dose of doxorubicin rises to 300 mg/m^2. Elimination is primarily renal with toxicities of granulocytopenia, nausea, vomiting, and alopecia.
- **Amifostine:** a radioprotective and cytoprotective compound. It has a highly selective transport mechanism into normal cells and there it scavenges free radicals. It can reduce the renal toxicity of cisplatin as well as the neurotoxicity of other agents. It is administered IV 30 minutes prior to chemotherapy at a dose of 740 to 910 mg/m^2. Toxicity is mucositis, nausea, vomiting, arterial hypotension, and hypocalcemia. The dosing interval is with chemotherapy and elimination is renal.
- **Sodium thiosulfate:** protects against cisplatin-induced nephrotoxicity. It is administered IV at a dose of 16 to 20 mg/m^2 given 2 hours after cisplatin. The dose interval is with chemotherapy and elimination is renal.
- **Mesna:** chemoprotective against hemorrhagic cystitis and it inactivates the metabolite acrolein. It can be administered IV or SC at a dose that is 20% of the total cytotoxic alkylator dose. Dosing is prior to chemotherapy with two additional doses 4 and 8 hours after chemotherapy treatment. Elimination is renal.
- **Buthionine sulfoximine (BSO):** enhances the cytotoxicity of alkylator agents by modifying GSH and GST, thus depleting intracellular levels of GSH. It is administered IV. Dosing is with a loading dose of 3 g/m^2 over 30 minutes, followed by three consecutive 24-hour infusions at 18 mg/m^2. Chemotherapy should be given after 48 hours of BSO. Elimination is via the renal system.

ANTIANGIOGENESIS, TARGETED THERAPIES, AND IMMUNOTHERAPY

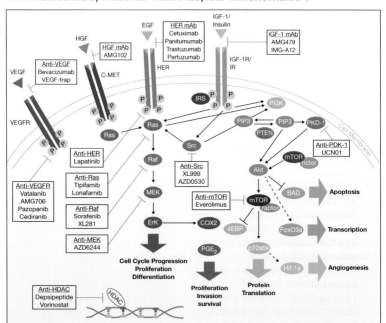

Figure 5.1 Overview of interlinked cellular signaling pathways involved in the proliferation and progression of colorectal cancer.

Source: From Siena S et al. Biomarkers Predicting Clinical Outcome of Epidermal Growth Factor Receptor–Targeted Therapy in Metastatic Colorectal Cancer. *J Nat Can Inst.* 2009;101(19):1308–1324.

Antiangiogenesis

Antiangiogenesis therapy: all members of the vascular endothelial growth factor (VEGF) family of ligands stimulate cellular responses by binding to tyrosine kinase receptors on the cell surface and causing dimerization and activation through transphosphorylation. Vascular endothelial growth factor receptors (VEGFR)-1,2,3 are membrane bound receptors and have an extracellular portion consisting of seven immunoglobulin (Ig)-like domains, a single transmembrane spanning region, and an intracellular portion containing the split tyrosine kinase domain. Inhibition can be direct or indirect (Figure 5.1).

- Direct VEGF inhibitor:
  - Bevacizumab (Avastin): a recombinant humanized monoclonal antibody directed against the VEGFR-1,2,3. Bevacizumab binds to VEGF and inhibits VEGF receptor binding, preventing the activation of the VEGFR-1,2,3 by sequestering it. Dosing: 5 to 7.5 mg/kg IV q 2 weeks or 7.5 to 15 mg/kg every 3 weeks. Elimination is renal. Primary toxicities are HTN (28%), nephrotic syndrome, gastrointestinal perforation (1% to 11%), wound dehiscence, and CHF.

- ○ Cediranib (Recentin): is an anti-angiogenic multi-tyrosine kinase inhibitor targeting VEGFR-1,2,3. It competes with adenosine triphosphate, and binds to and inhibits VEGFR-1,2,3 thus blocking the VEGF signaling, angiogenesis, and tumor cell growth. Dosing: 30 mg PO daily for a 28 day cycle.
- Indirect:
  - ○ Aflibercept (Zaltrap): a VEGF trap. It is a fusion protein that prevents VEGF receptor binding. This protein is comprised of segments of the extracellular domains of human VEGFR-1 and -2 fused to the constant region (Fc) of human IgG1 with potential antiangiogenic activity. Aflibercept functions as a soluble decoy receptor, binding to pro-angiogenic VEGFs, preventing VEGFs from binding to their cell receptors. Disruption of the binding of VEGFs to their cell receptors results in the inhibition of tumor angiogenesis, metastasis, and ultimately tumor regression. Dosing: 4 mg/kg IV every 2 weeks.
  - ○ Trebananib (AMG 386): a peptide-Fc fusion protein neutralizing peptibody that inhibits binding of angiopoietin 1 and 2 to the Tie2 receptor. Trebananib targets and binds to Ang1 and Ang2, preventing the interaction of the angiopoietins with their target Tie2 receptors. This inhibits angiogenesis and may lead to inhibition of tumor cell proliferation. Dosing: 15 mg/kg IV weekly (3).
- Vascular disrupting agents
  - ○ CA4P (Fosbretabulin): a pro-drug either in a disodium salt or a tromethamine salt form derived from the African willow bush (*Combretum caffrum*). After administration, the pro-drug fosbretabulin is dephosphorylated to its active metabolite, the microtubule-depolymerizing agent combretastatin A4, which binds to the colchicine binding site of beta-tubulin dimers and prevents microtubule polymerization, resulting in mitotic arrest and apoptosis in endothelial cells. This agent also disrupts the engagement of the endothelial cell-specific junctional molecule vascular endothelial-cadherin (VE-cadherin) and the ensuing activity of the VE-cadherin/β-catenin/AKT signaling pathway, which may result in the inhibition of endothelial cell migration and capillary tube formation. As a result of fosbretabulin's dual mechanism of action, the tumor vasculature collapses, resulting in ischemic necrosis of tumor tissue. Dosing: 45 to 60 mg/m^2 IV weekly for 3 weeks of a 4 week cycle for a total of six maximum cycles.

Targeted Therapies

- Multiple target therapies:
  - ○ Nintedanib (Vargatef/OVEF): an orally bioavailable multitargeted receptor tyrosine kinase (RTK) inhibitor with potential antiangiogenic and antineoplastic activities. It selectively binds to and inhibits VEGFR, fibroblast growth factor receptor (FGFR), and platelet-derived growth factor receptor (PDGFR) tyrosine kinases, which results in the induction of endothelial cell apoptosis; a reduction in tumor vasculature; and the inhibition of tumor cell proliferation and migration. In addition, this agent also inhibits members of the Src family of tyrosine kinases, including Src, Lck, Lyn, and FLT-3 (fms-like tyrosine kinase 3). Dosing: 200 mg PO BID.

○ Pazopanib (Voltrient): it is the hydrochloride salt of a small molecule inhibitor of multiple protein tyrosine kinases and selectively inhibits VEGFR-1,2,3, c-kit, and PDGF-R, which results in inhibition of angiogenesis in tumors in which these receptors are upregulated. Dosing: 800 mg PO BID.

○ Sorafenib (Nexavar): it blocks the enzyme RAF kinase, a critical component of the RAF/MEK/ERK signaling pathway that controls cell division and proliferation; it also inhibits the VEGFR-2/PDGFR-beta signaling cascade, thereby blocking tumor angiogenesis. Dosing: 400 mg PO q12 hours (4).

○ Rebastinib: this peptibody is an orally bioavailable small-molecule inhibitor of multiple tyrosine kinases. It inhibits angiopoietin-1 ang 1 binding to the Tie2 receptor. It binds to and inhibits the Bcr–Abl fusion oncoprotein by changing the conformation of the folded protein to disallow ligand-dependent and ligand-independent activation. It also binds to and inhibits Src family kinases LYN, HCK, and FGR and the RTKs TIE-2 and VEGFR-2. Rebastinib may exhibit more potent activity against T315I Bcr-Abl gatekeeper mutant kinases than other Bcr-Abl kinase inhibitors. The TIE-2 and VEGFR-2 RTKs regulate angiogenesis, respectively, while the Src family kinases Abl, LYN, and HCK Src regulate a variety of cellular responses including differentiation, division, adhesion, and the stress response. Dosing: 150 mg PO BID.

○ Vandetanib (Caprelsa): this is an orally bioavailable 4-anilinoquinazoline that selectively inhibits the tyrosine kinase activity of VEGFR-2. It blocks VEGF-stimulated endothelial cell proliferation and migration and reduces tumor vessel permeability. This agent also blocks the tyrosine kinase activity of epidermal growth factor receptor (EGFR). Dosing: 300 mg PO daily (5).

○ Volasertib: a dihydropteridinone derivative and cell-cycle kinase inhibitor with selectivity for Polo-like kinase 1 (Plk1) and half maximal inhibitory activity for Plk2/3. It can induce G2-M arrest and subsequent apoptosis in tumors. Dosing is 300 mg IV every 21 days in heavily pre-treated patients. Dose reductions are at 50 mg steps. Side effects are mainly hematologic.

○ Cabozantinib (Cabometyx): a small molecule inhibitor of VEGFR-2 and c-Met among other tyrosine kinases. Dosing is 60 mg PO daily.

- mTOR inhibitors

○ Temsirolimus (Torisel): this is an ester analog of rapamycin. Temsirolimus binds to and inhibits the mammalian target of rapamycin (mTOR), resulting in decreased expression of mRNAs necessary for cell cycle progression and arresting cells in the G1 phase of the cell cycle. mTOR is a serine/threonine kinase that plays a role in the phosphoinositide-3 kinase (PI3K)/AKT pathway that is upregulated in some tumors. Dosing: 25 mg IV weekly.

○ Everolimus (Afinitor): it is an mTOR serine–threonine kinase inhibitor, and binds to intracellular FKBP-12 resulting in inhibition of formation with mTOR complex 1 thus inhibiting translation of 4EBP-1 and S6K1 that regulate proteins in the cell cycle, angiogenesis, and glycolysis. Dosing: 10 mg PO daily.

○ Ridaforolimus (AP23573): it is an MTOR kinase inhibitor. Dosing: 40 mg PO daily for 5 days/week or 12.5 mg IV daily for 5 days every 2 weeks.

○ Sirolimus (Rapamune): it is an mTOR kinase inhibitor. Dosing is 5 mg PO daily if patient weight is greater than 40 kg, or 1 mg/m²/day if patient weight is less than 40 kg after a loading dose of 3 mg/m^2 if weight is less than 40 kg or 15 mg if weight is greater than 40 kg.

- Notch inhibitors: the Notch signaling pathway plays an important role in cell-fate determination, cell survival, and cell proliferation.
  - MK0752: this is a synthetic small gamma secretase inhibitor that inhibits the Notch signaling pathway, which results in growth arrest and apoptosis of tumor cells in which the Notch signaling pathway is overactivated. Dosing: 1,200 mg PO weekly
  - Demcizumab: a humanized monoclonal antibody directed against the N-terminal epitope of Notch ligand delta-like 4 (DLL4) with potential antineoplastic activity. Demcizumab binds to the membrane-binding portion of DLL4 and prevents its interaction with Notch-1 and Notch-4 receptors, inhibiting Notch-mediated signaling and gene transcription, which impedes tumor angiogenesis. Activation of Notch receptors by DLL4 stimulates proteolytic cleavage of the Notch intracellular domain (NICD); after cleavage, NICD is translocated into the nucleus and mediates the transcriptional regulation of a variety of genes involved in vascular development. The expression of DLL4 is highly restricted to the vascular endothelium. Dosing: 3.5 to 5 mg/kg IV weekly days 1, 8, 15 of a 28-day cycle.
  - REGN421 (Enoticumab): an anti-DLL4 monoclonal antibody. This is a human monoclonal antibody directed against DLL4 preventing its binding to Notch receptors and inhibiting Notch signaling, which may result in defective tumor vascularization and the inhibition of tumor cell growth. DLL4 is the only Notch ligand selectively expressed on endothelial cells. Dosing: 3 mg/kg IV every 2 weeks
- EGFR inhibitors: EGFR is overexpressed on the cell surfaces of various solid tumors.
  - Cetuximab (Erbitux): this is a recombinant, chimeric monoclonal antibody directed against EGFR. Cetuximab binds to the extracellular domain of EGFR, preventing the activation and subsequent dimerization of the receptor; the decrease in receptor activation and dimerization results in an inhibition in signal transduction and antiproliferative effects. This agent may inhibit EGFR-dependent primary tumor growth and metastasis. Dosing: 400 mg/m^2 1 week before starting cytotoxic chemotherapy, then 250 mg/m^2 weekly.
  - Trastuzumab (Herceptin): is a recombinant humanized monoclonal antibody directed against the human epidermal growth factor receptor 2 (HER2). After binding to HER2 on the tumor cell surface, trastuzumab induces an antibody-dependent cell-mediated cytotoxicity against tumor cells that overexpress HER2. Elimination is renal and toxicities are a rash or CHF (1% to 29%). Dosing: 4 mg/kg IV loading dose with maintenance dosing at 2 mg/kg IV once weekly for 12 to 18 weeks. Maintenance dosing continues at 6 mg/kg IV every 3 weeks starting 1 week after completion of combination cytotoxic therapy.
  - Pertuzumab: it is a humanized monoclonal antibody inhibiting HER-2 binding with HER family members HER1, HER3, and HER4 preventing downstream signal transduction to PI3K. Elimination is renal and toxicities

are rash or CHF. Dosing: 840 mg loading dose IV day 1, then 420 mg IV every 21 days subsequently in combination with other chemotherapies. Low HER3 mRNA expression has been shown to be a positive predictive factor for response.

- Tyrosine kinase inhibitors (TKIs):
  - Sunitinib (Sutent): this is a selective tyrosine kinase inhibitor that blocks the tyrosine kinase activities of VEGFR-2, PDGFRb, and c-kit, thereby inhibiting angiogenesis and cell proliferation. This agent also inhibits the phosphorylation of fms-related tyrosine kinase 3 (FLT3), another RTK expressed by some leukemic cells. Dosing: 50 mg PO daily for 4 weeks, then 2 weeks off
  - Crizotinib (Xalkori): this is an orally available aminopyridine-based inhibitor of the receptor tyrosine kinase anaplastic lymphoma kinase (ALK). Crizotinib also binds to c-MET/hepatocyte growth factor receptor (HGFR), disrupting c-MET signaling. It binds in an ATP-competitive manner, and inhibits ALK kinase and ALK fusion proteins. It has activity in ALK positive patients and vaginal sarcoma ALK mutation positive patients. Dosing: 250 mg BID
  - Lenvatinib: is an oral multitargeted tyrosine kinase inhibitor of VEGFR 1 to 3, FGFR 1 to 4, PDGFR beta, RET, and KIT, and antagonizes neovascularization via downregulating angiopoietin signaling by binding to ligands ANG 1-2. Dosing: 24 mg PO daily
- Serine/threonine kinase inhibitors:
  - XL418: this is a selective, orally active small molecule, targeting protein kinase B (PKB or AKT) and ribosomal protein S6 Kinase (p70S6K), with antineoplastic activity. XL418 inhibits the activities of PKB and p70S6K, both acting downstream of PI3K. Inhibition of PKB induces apoptosis, while inhibition of p70S6K results in the inhibition of translation within tumor cells. Dosing: 6.4 mg/kg PO daily
- Multikinase inhibitors: PI3K/mTOR inhibitors:
  - SF1126: 1,110 mg/m^2 twice weekly for 4 weeks of a 28-week cycle.
  - BEZ235: 300 mg PO BID for 8 days every 4 weeks.
  - Gedatolisib (PF-05212384): is an inhibitor of PI3K and mTOR (TORC1/2) kinase activity. It is given once weekly IV with an MTD of 154 mg. Side effects are mucosal inflammation, nausea, hyperglycemia. It has shown to be effective in recurrent uterine cancer.
- Dual mTOR/AKT:
  - MKC1: is an oral cell cycle inhibitor that binds to and inhibits the importin-beta proteins and, tubulin preventing mitotic spindle formation. Dosing: 150 mg PO daily for a 28-day cycle
- WEE1 inhibitors: inhibition of WEE1 activity prevents the phosphorylation of CDC2 and impairs the G2 DNA damage checkpoint. Unlike normal cells, most p53 deficient or mutated human cancers lack the G1 checkpoint as p53 is the key regulator of the G1 checkpoint and these cells rely on the G2 checkpoint for DNA repair to damaged cells. Termination of the G2 checkpoint may therefore sensitize p53 deficient tumor cells to genotoxic/antineoplastic agents through deregulation of the G2/M checkpoint and enhancing their cytotoxic effects.
  - AZD1775: a WEE1 inhibitor. This selectively targets and inhibits WEE1, a tyrosine kinase that phosphorylates cyclin-dependent kinase 1 (CDK1,

CDC2) at the G2 checkpoint to inactivate the CDC2/cyclin B complex. Dosing: 225 mg daily to BID 5 days/week for 14 days of a 21-day cycle. Activity may be enhanced in *BRCA* mutated patients.

- Tol receptor-death ligand (TolR) agonists:
  - Entolimod (toll-like receptor 5 [TLR5] agonist CBLB502): a polypeptide derived from the *Salmonella* filament protein flagellin with potential radioprotective and anticancer activities. As a TLR5 agonist, entolimod binds to and activates TLR5, stimulating TNF production and activating nuclear factor kappa B (NF-kB). This induces NF-kB-mediated signaling pathways and inhibits the induction of apoptosis. This may prevent apoptosis in normal, healthy cells during XRT and may allow for increased doses of ionizing XRT. In addition, entolimod may inhibit XRT independent proliferation in TLR5-expressing tumor cells. Dosing: 30 mcg/day days 1, 4, 8, and 11; IV every 2 weeks
  - Motolimod (VTX2337): a small molecule agonist of toll-like receptor 8. This molecule is supposed to mobilize the immune system by directly activating myeloid dendritic cells (DCs), monocytes, and natural killer (NK) cells, resulting in production of mediators that integrate both the innate and adaptive antitumor responses to cancer. Dosing in phase II studies for some tumor sites is: 2.5 mg/m^2 SC weekly days 1, 8, and 15 of a 28 day regimen with cetuximab.
  - ANA773 tosylate (Toll-like receptor 7 agonist [TLR7]). The tosylate salt form of ANA773, a TLR7 agonist pro-drug with potential immunostimulating activity. Upon administration, ANA773 is metabolized into its active form that binds to and activates TLR7, stimulating DCs and enhancing NK cell cytotoxicity. This activation results in the production of proinflammatory cytokines, including interferon alpha, and enhanced antibody-dependent cellular cytotoxicity (ADCC). TLR7 is a member of the TLR family, which plays a fundamental role in pathogen recognition and activation of innate immunity. Dosing: 400 to 800 mg PO QOD for 14 days of a 28-day cycle.
- AKT inhibitors:
  - Perifosine: a loading dose of 100 mg PO q6h on day 1 followed by daily dosing at 50, 100, or 150 mg for 20 days.
  - MK2206, GSK2141795, GSK112021, and ARQ092.
- PI3K Inhibitors:
  - Pilaralisib: 400 to 600 mg PO daily
  - BKM120, BYL719, BEZ235, and XL147
- Folate receptor inhibitors
  - Farletuzumab: monoclonal antibody that binds to folate receptor alpha. The therapeutic index is present as folate receptor alpha is overexpressed in some tumor cells but absent in normal tissue. Dosing: 2.5 mg/kg IV weekly
- Imatinib Mesylate (Gleevec): inhibits the protein tyrosine kinase Bcr-Abl. Primary toxicities are nausea, vomiting, muscle cramps, skin rash, diarrhea, and heartburn with a secondary toxicity of fluid retention. It is eliminated via the hepatobiliary system. Dosing: 400 mg/day PO for chronic myeloid leukemia (CML), and 600 mg/day for blast crisis CML or gastrointestinal stromal tumor (GIST)

- Poly ADP ribose polymerase (PARP) inhibitors: selectively bind to and inhibit PARP, inhibiting PARP-mediated repair of single strand DNA breaks. PARP catalyzes posttranslational ADP-ribosylation of nuclear proteins and can be activated by single-stranded DNA breaks. The PARP family of proteins detect and repair single strand DNA breaks by the base-excision repair pathway. PARP inhibition enhances the cytotoxicity of DNA-damaging agents and reverses tumor cell chemoresistance and radioresistance.
  - ○ Olaparib (AZD2281): a small molecule inhibitor of PARP 1 and 2 with potential chemosensitizing, radiosensitizing, and antineoplastic activities. Dosing: 400 mg PO BID
  - ○ Veliparib (ABT-888) A PARP-1 and -2 inhibitor with chemosensitizing and antitumor activities. Veliparib inhibits PARPs, thereby inhibiting DNA repair and potentiating the cytotoxicity of DNA-damaging agents. Dosing: 400 mg PO BID
  - ○ Rucaparib (CO338, AGO14699, and PF01367338): a tricyclic indole PARP1 inhibitor with chemosensitizing, radiosensitizing, and antineoplastic activities. Rucaparib selectively binds to PARP1 and inhibits PARP1-mediated DNA repair. Dosing: 600 mg PO BID
  - ○ Niraparib (MK-4827): an inhibitor of PARP 1 and 2, enhancing the accumulation of DNA strand breaks and promoting genomic instability and apoptosis. The specific PARP family member target for MK4827 is unknown. Dosing: 300 mg PO daily
- CDK 4/6 inhibitors:
  - ○ Palbociclib (Ibrance): is an inhibitor of CDK 4/6 and works intranuclearly. Indication for treatment is for ER+/HER2- cancers. Dosing: 125 mg PO daily. It is usually given in combination with an aromatase inhibitor for a 28-day cycle for which palbociclib is taken for 21 days and the aromatase inhibitor (AI) for the full 28 days. Side effects are neutropenia and VTE.
- Epithelial cell adhesion molecules:
  - ○ Catumaxomab (Removab): a rat–mouse hybrid monoclonal antibody binding to antigens CD3 and EpCAM. It is used to treat malignant ascites and is administered IP. Dosing: 10, 20, 50, and 100 mcg given as a 6-hour IP infusion on days 0, 3, 7, and 10

Immunotherapies

Immunotherapy uses antibodies to block cytotoxic T-lymphocyte-associated antigen 4 (CTLA-4) and programmed cell death protein 1 pathways (PD-1/PD-L1)—they are checkpoint inhibitors. Normally, CTLA-r is upregulated on the plasma membrane where it functions to downregulate T-cell function and induce T-cell arrest. Mice deficient in CTLA-4 die from fatal lymphoproliferation. PD-1 is a negative regulator of T-cell activity that limits T cell activity when it interacts with PD-L1 and PD-L2. PD-1 inhibits effector T-cell activity in the effector phase within tissue and tumors. Antibodies that disrupt the PD-1 axis include those that target PD-1 and those that target PD-L1 (6).

- **FANG vaccine:** this is a vaccine consisting of autologous tumor cells transfected with a plasmid expressing recombinant human granulocyte macrophage-colony stimulating factor (rhGM–CSF) and bifunctional short hairpin RNA (bi-shRNA) against furin, with potential immunostimulatory and antineoplastic activities. Upon intradermal vaccination of bi-shRNA-furin/GM–CSF-expressing autologous tumor cell vaccine, expressed GM–CSF protein, a potent stimulator of the immune system, recruits immune effectors to the site of injection and promotes antigen presentation. The furin bifunctional shRNA blocks furin protein production. Decreased levels of furin lead to a reduction in the conversion of transforming growth factor (TGF) beta into TGF beta1 and beta2 protein isoforms. In turn, as part of the negative feedback mechanism, reduced furin protein levels inhibit TGF-beta1 and TGFbeta2 gene expression, thereby further decreasing TGF levels. As TGFs are potent immunosuppressive cytokines, reducing their levels may activate the immune system locally and this may eventually cause a CTL response against the tumor cells.

- **Tremelimumab:** a human IgG2 monoclonal antibody directed against the human T-cell receptor protein CTLA-4, with potential immune checkpoint inhibitory and antineoplastic activities. Tremelimumab binds to CTLA-4 on activated T-lymphocytes and blocks the binding of the antigen-presenting cell ligands B7-1 (CD80) and B7-2 (CD86) to CTLA-4, resulting in inhibition of CTLA-4-mediated downregulation of T-cell activation. This promotes the interaction of B7-1 and B7-2 with another T-cell surface receptor protein CD28, and results in a B7-CD28-mediated T-cell activation that is unopposed by CTLA-4-mediated inhibition. This leads to a CTL-mediated immune response against cancer cells. CTLA-4, an inhibitory receptor and member of the Ig superfamily, plays a key role in the downregulation of the immune system. Dosing: 15 mg/kg IV every 90 days

- **Avelumab:** This is a human IgG1 monoclonal antibody directed against the human immunosuppressive ligand PD-L1 protein, with potential immune checkpoint inhibitory and antineoplastic activities. Upon administration, avelumab binds to PD-L1 and prevents the interaction of PD-L1 with its receptor PD-1. This inhibits the activation of PD-1 and its downstream signaling pathways. This may restore immune function through the activation of CTLs targeted to PD-L1-overexpressing tumor cells. In addition, avelumab induces an ADCC response against PD-L1-expressing tumor cells. PD-1, a cell surface receptor belonging to the Ig superfamily expressed on T-cells, negatively regulates T-cell activation and effector function when activated by its ligand, and plays an important role in tumor evasion from host immunity. PD-L1, a transmembrane protein, is overexpressed on a variety of tumor cell types and is associated with poor prognosis. Dosing: 10 mg/kg IV every 2 to 3 weeks

- **Pembrolizumab (Keytruda):** this is a humanized monoclonal IgG4 antibody directed against human cell surface receptor PD-1 with potential immune checkpoint inhibitory and antineoplastic activities. On administration, pembrolizumab binds to PD-1, an inhibitory signaling receptor expressed on the surface of activated T cells, and blocks the binding to and activation of PD-1 by its ligands, which results in the activation of T-cell-mediated immune responses against tumor cells. The ligands for PD-1 include PD-L1, overexpressed on certain cancer cells, and PD-L2, which is primarily expressed on APCs. Treatment has been approved for patients with unresectable or metastatic melanoma, whose tumors express PD-L1 and who have disease progression on or after platinum-containing chemotherapy, or patients with EGFR or ALK genomic tumor aberrations. Dosing: 2 mg/kg IV every 3 weeks

- **Nivolumab (Opdivo):** a fully humanized IgG4 monoclonal antibody directed against the negative immunoregulatory human cell surface receptor PD-1 with immune checkpoint inhibitory and antineoplastic activities. Nivolumab binds to and blocks the activation of PD-1, by its ligands PD-L1, and PD-L2. This results in the activation of T-cells and cell-mediated immune responses against tumor cells or pathogens. Nivolumab resulted in a 32% overall response rate (ORR) in a phase III melanoma study compared to 11% for chemotherapy that included DTIC or carboplatin/paclitaxel. Dosing: regimens may differ but is recommended at 3 mg/kg IV every 2 weeks

- **Ipilimumab (Yervoy):** a CTLA-4 inhibitor. It is a recombinant human IgG1 monoclonal antibody directed against the human T-cell receptor CTLA-4, with immune checkpoint inhibitory and antineoplastic activities. Ipilimumab binds to CTLA-4 expressed on T-cells and inhibits the CTLA-4-mediated downregulation of T-cell activation. This leads to a CTL-mediated immune response against cancer cells. Ipilimumab was significant in melanoma patients for improving overall survival (OS; 18% vs. 5% 2Y OS). Dosing: regimens may differ but a common therapy is 3 mg/kg IV every 3 weeks (7)

- **Pidilizumab:** this is a humanized, IgG1 monoclonal antibody directed against human inhibitory receptor PD-1, with potential immune checkpoint inhibitory and antineoplastic activities. Pidilizumab binds to PD-1 and blocks the interaction between PD-1 and its ligands, PD-L1 and PD-L2. This prevents the activation of PD-1 and its downstream signaling pathways. This may restore immune function through the activation of NK cells and CTLs against tumor cells. Dosing varies but one regimen was 1.5 mg/kg every 42 days.

- **Adoptive T-cell therapy (ACT):** this involves infusion of autologous tumor-reactive T cells. This has been used in the treatment of some B-cell malignancies, cervical cancer, and metastatic melanoma. T-cell cultures were generated from HPV-positive cancers and selected for HPV oncoprotein-reactive cultures for administration to patients. Treatment included lymphocyte-depleting conditioning chemotherapy regimen (cyclophosphamide 60 mg/kg IV daily for 2 days, fludarabine 25 mg/m² daily for 5 days, followed by HPV-TIL infusion IV as a single dose, and aldesleukin 720,000 IU/kg/dose IV boluses every 8 hours to a tolerance of a maximum of 15 doses. T cell cultures were initiated from fragments of metastatic tumor and expanded using IL-2 containing culture media. Cultures with lymphocyte outgrowth were tested for reactivity against HPV-16 or HPV-18 E6 and E7. There was a 30% ORR. The magnitude of HPV reactivity the infusion produced, measured by IFN-gamma production, ELISPOT, or CD137 upregulation, was associated with clinical response.

- **Oregovamab:** a CA-125 specific murine monoclonal antibody. Administered 2 mg IV over 20 minutes at weeks 0, 4, 8, and then every 12 weeks until recurrence up to 5 years. A phase III trial failed to show prolongation of time to recurrence as maintenance monoimmunotherapy (10.3 months vs. 12.9 months for placebo with $p = 0.29$ log rank test) (8).

- **Abagovomab:** this is a murine monoclonal antibody used as a surrogate antigen, and when administered, enables the immune system to identify and attack tumor cells displaying the CA-125 protein. It is given 2 mg IV once every 2 weeks for 6 weeks then once every 4 weeks for maintenance up to 21 months or until recurrence. A phase III study noted a measurable immune response but did not prolong recurrence-free survival (RFS) or OS (9).

TREATMENT OF EXTRAVASATION INJURY

- **Cisplatin:** thiosulfate should be injected into the skin site at 1/3 to 1/6 molar solution. For every 100 mg extravasated, 2 mL should be injected.
- **Doxorubicin:** cold compresses should be applied immediately to the site for 60 minutes with consideration of an injection of 150 U hyaluronidase into the site. Cold topical DMSO can also be applied. This agent can cause extensive ulceration and treatment is debridement of the primary and recurrent ulcers.
- **Etoposide:** consider an injection of 150 U of hyaluronidase into the site.
- **Mitomycin C:** topical DMSO should be applied every 6 hours × 14 days.
- **Vinblastine:** warm compresses should be applied immediately to the site for 60 minutes with consideration of an injection of 150 U of hyaluronidase into the site. Corticosteroids can also help if injected into the site.
- **Vincristine:** warm compresses should be applied immediately to the site for 60 minutes with consideration of an injection of 150 U of hyaluronidase into the site.

VACCINATIONS IN CANCER PATIENTS

- Influenza inactivated virus: recommended for all patients greater than 6 months old except those receiving induction or consolidation chemotherapy for acute leukemia and those receiving anti-B-cell antibodies and 4 to 6 months after completion of chemotherapy.
- Pneumococcal conjugate 13 valent vaccine: recommended for children and adults based on immune status assessment on a case by case basis starting 6 to 12 months after completion of therapy. Pneumococcal polysaccharide vaccine 23 should then be administered to adults and children greater than 2 years old and at least 8 weeks after the indicated dose(s) of pneumococcal conjugate 13 vaccine at minimum 12 months after completion of chemotherapy.
- Inactivated vaccines (DTaP, Hib, Hep A, and Hep B) may be give together at the same time but can be delayed in patients receiving greater than 20 mg of prednisone daily.
- Zoster vaccine: is recommended 24 months after completion of chemotherapy only if no ongoing immunosuppression and patient is seronegative for varicella.
- Vaccines administered during cancer chemotherapy should not be considered valid doses unless documentation of a protected antibody level.

- Live viral vaccines (measles, mumps, rubella [MMR]) should not be administered during chemotherapy. They can be administered starting 24 months after completion of chemotherapy and if the patient has no ongoing immunosuppression and is seronegative for MMR. Can give Zoster and MMR together.
- If patients are receiving anti-B-cell antibodies, vaccinations should be delayed at least 6 months (Table 5.1).

Table 5.1 Vaccine Recommendations During Chemotherapy

Inactivated vaccine	Recommended timing after chemotherapy (months)	Number of doses
Influenza	4–6	1 annually
TDaP	6–12	3
Hep A	6–12	2
Hep B	6–12	2
Pneumococcal		
Conjugated 13-valent	6–12	3
Upon completion of Prevnar series, then pneumococcal polysaccharide vaccine 23	>12	1
Haemophilus influenza type B (Hib)	6–12	3
Meningococcal conjugate	6–12	1
Live vaccines		
Zoster	>24	1
MMR	>24	1–2

MMR, measles, mumps, and rubella.

REFERENCES

1. Vay A, Kumar S, Seward S. Therapy-related myeloid leukemia after treatment for epithelial ovarian carcinoma: an epidemiological analysis. *Gynecol Oncol.* 2011;123(3):456-460.
2. Hobohm U. Fever and cancer in perspective. *Cancer Immunol Immunother.* October 2001;50(8):391-396.
3. Monk BJ, Poveda A, Vergote I, et al. Anti-angiopoietin therapy with trebananib for recurrent ovarian cancer (TRINOVA-1): a randomised, multicentre, double-blind, placebo-controlled phase 3 trial. *Lancet Oncol.* 2014;15:799-808.
4. Matei D, Sill MW, Lankes HA, et al. Activity of sorafenib in recurrent ovarian cancer and primary peritoneal carcinomatosis: a gynecologic oncology group trial. *J Clin Oncol.* 2011;29:69-75.

5. Coleman RL, Moon J, Sood AK, et al. Randomised phase II study of docetaxel plus vandetanib versus docetaxel followed by vandetanib in patients with persistent or recurrent epithelial ovarian, fallopian tube or primary peritoneal carcinoma: SWOG S0904. *Eur J Cancer.* 2014;50:1638-1648.

6. Stevanović S, Draper LM, Langhan MM, et al. Complete regression of metastatic cervical cancer after treatment with human papillomavirus-targeted tumor-infiltrating T cells. *J Clin Oncol.* May 10, 2015;33(14):1543-1550.

7. Postow MA, Callahan MK, Wolchok JD, et al. Immune checkpoint blockade in cancer therapy. *J Clin Oncol.* June 10, 2015;33(17):1974-1982.

8. Berek J, Taylor P, McGuire W, et al. Oregovomab maintenance monoimmunotherapy does not improve outcomes in advanced ovarian cancer. *J Clin Oncol.* January 20, 2009;27(3):418-425.

9. Sabbatini P, Harter P, Scambia G, et al. Abagovomab as maintenance therapy in patients with epithelial ovarian cancer: a phase II trial of the AGO OVAR, COGI, GINECO, and CIECO—The MIMOSA study. *J Clin Oncol.* April 20, 2013:12:1554-1561.

RADIATION TYPES

There are different types of radiation currently used in medicine.

- X-rays are extranuclear radiation. They occur from the bombardment of an atom/target by another source—usually high-speed electrons.
- The alpha particle demonstrates cluster decay where a parent atom ejects a defined daughter collection of nucleons. These have a typical kinetic energy of 5 MeV. Because of their relatively large mass, their +2 electric charge, and relatively low velocity, alpha particles are very likely to interact with other atoms and lose their energy. Their forward motion is effectively stopped within a few centimeters of air or paper. This particle is the same as a helium-4 particle (two protons and two neutrons).
- Beta particles are high-energy, high-speed electrons emitted by certain types of radioactive nuclei. Beta particles are ionizing radiations. They are stopped by millimeters of tissue. The production of beta particles is termed beta decay.
- Gamma particles are a form of ionizing radiation that originates from the decay of the nucleus of a radioactive isotope. Energies range from 10,000 (10^4) to 10,000,000 (10^7) electron volts.
- An isotope is one of two or more atoms having the same number of protons but a different number of neutrons. This makes the nucleus unstable. The atom then spontaneously decomposes/decays and excess energy is given off by emission of a nuclear electron or helium nucleus and radiation, to achieve a stable nuclear composition. Some of these isotopes include radium-226, cesium-137, iridium-192, cobalt-60, and gold-198.
- Electron energy comes from outside the nucleus. Electrons are used to treat tumors en face—close to the skin.

DEFINITIONS

- Roentgen is the amount of photon radiation that causes 0.001293 g of air to produce one electrostatic unit of positive or negative charge. It can also be defined as: the amount of photon energy required to produce 1.61×10^{12} ion pairs in 1 cm^3 of dry air at 0 degree C. It is a unit of exposure, not an amount of energy that ionizing radiation imparts to matter.
- Kinetic energy related to mass (KERMA) is the transfer of energy from photons to particles. Particles transfer this energy to tissue and this is defined as absorbed dose.
- Radiation Absorbed Dose (Rad): is the amount of energy that radiation imparts to a given mass. A rad is a dose of 100 ergs of energy per gram of given material.

The SI unit for rad is the gray (Gy) which is defined as a dose of one joule per kilogram. One joule equals 10^7 ergs, and one kilogram equals 1,000 grams, thus 1 Gy equals 100 rads

- Relative biologic effectiveness (RBE) is the ratio of the dose required for a given radiation to produce the same biologic effect induced by 250 kV of x-rays.
- Isodose is the line that connects structures, which receive equal radiation dose.
- Source to skin distance (SSD) is usually defined at 80 to 100 cm from the machine to the patient. Radiation is dosed at a fixed point from the patient and thus there needs to be standardization of distance for treatment.
- Isocenter is a fixed point in the patient around which treatment is rotated.
- Dmax is the point where the maximum amount of dose from one beam is deposited. The dose at Dmax is defined at 100%. The depths of Dmax for some common energies are 4 MV, 1.2 cm; 6 MV, 1.5 cm; 10 MV, 2.5 cm; and 18 MV, 3.2 cm.
- Percent depth dose is the change in dose with depth within the patient.
- Gross tumor volume (GTV): direct tumor volume by measurement. The GTV requires a high dose of radiation to treat the primary or bulky tumor. This dose is usually 80 to 90 Gy.
- Clinical target volume (CTV): this includes any region that has a high likelihood of harboring malignancy but appears clinically normal. The CTV requires a lower dose than GTV. This dose is usually around 45 to 54 Gy and is adequate to treat occult or microscopic disease.
- Planning target volume (PTV) is a margin added to account for organ motion and daily setup error.

RADIATION EFFECTS

There are two basic types of energy transfer that may occur when x-rays interact with matter:

- Ionization, in which the incoming radiation causes the removal of an electron from an atom or molecule leaving the material with a net positive charge.
- Excitation, in which some of the x-ray's energy is transferred to the target material leaving it in an excited (or more energetic) state.

There are three important processes that can occur when x-rays interact with matter. These processes are the photoelectric (PE) effect, the Compton effect, and pair production

- The PE effect produces energy in the eV to keV range. This type of radiation occurs when atoms absorb energy from light and emit electrons. This form of radiation is used for diagnostic x-rays and to simulate radiation treatment beams. The PE effect occurs when photons interact with matter with resulting ejection of electrons from the matter. PE absorption of x-rays occurs when the x-ray photon is absorbed resulting in the ejection of electrons from the atom. This leaves the atom in an ionized state. The ionized atom then returns to the neutral state with the emission of an x-ray characteristic of the atom. Photoelectron absorption is the dominant process for x-ray absorption up to energies of about 500 keV.
- Pair production occurs when the x-ray photon energy is greater than 1.02 MeV. An electron and positron are created with the annihilation of the x-ray photon. Positrons are very short lived and disappear (positron annihilation) with the

formation of two photons of 0.51 MeV energy. Pair production is of particular importance when high-energy photons pass through materials with high atomic numbers. This type of energy is not used clinically.

- The Compton effect is when an incident photon interacts with an outer electron. The energy that results is shared between the ejected electron and the scattered photon. Compton scattering is important for low atomic number specimens. At energies of 100 keV to 10 MeV, the absorption of radiation is mainly due to the Compton effect. This type of energy is used for the radiation treatment of cancers. Photons are harvested from the decay of a source. First, the source has intrinsic decay. The electrons from this decay are used to bombard tungsten causing the Compton effect. The resultant photon is the radiation we use in linear accelerator machines.

ENERGY EQUIVALENCES

1 Gray (Gy) is equal to 1 J/kg of tissue.
1 Gy is equal to 100 cGy.
100 radiation absorbed doses (Rads) are equal to 1 Gy.
1 Rad is equal to 1 cGy.

RADIATION DELIVERY

- External beam radiation is delivered using a linear accelerator machine. These machines deliver 4 to 24 MeV. Total radiation dose is administered via a daily divided dose called a fraction. Common daily doses/fractions are 1.8 to 2 Gy. A total dose of 90 Gy is needed to sterilize most tumors. Noncancerous tissues cannot tolerate this total dose from external beam radiation, so brachytherapy is needed to locally deliver radiation directly to the tumor.
- Brachytherapy is the local, and often internalized, delivery of radiation. For gynecologic cancers, radiation is often delivered using tandem and ovoids, vaginal cylinders, or interstitial needles. Brachytherapy is delivered at a low-dose rate (LDR) or a high-dose rate (HDR).
  - LDR is defined as 0.4 to 2 Gy/hr; HDR is defined as a dose greater than 12 Gy/hr or greater than 20 to 250 cGy/min (12–15 Gy/hr). The dose conversion from LDR to HDR is 0.6.
  - HDR is more common now because of a number of patient-based reasons: treatment time is shorter, treatment is delivered on an outpatient basis, there is no need for bed rest, there is better ability to retract the rectum for shorter periods of time, and therefore better patient acceptance and comfort. Clinically, there is better implant reproducibility and a greater degree of certainty that the sources will remain stable during treatment. The HDR applicators are less bulky, so patients with narrow vaginas do not necessarily have to be treated with interstitial implants. The smaller source size also allows for finer increments in source location and weighting and a better ability to shape the dose distribution.
  - Isotopes: Iridium-192 is the most commonly used isotope. The half-life of iridium is 74 days. Cesium-137 is no longer available but its half-life is 30 years. Cobalt-60 is also no longer used but its half-life is 5.26 years. Radium-226 has a half-life of 1,626 years and has little use in modern radiation oncology.

TUMORICIDAL BASICS

- Radiation dose is proportional to the time the patient is exposed to the dose. The dose is also proportional to the distance from the source (the inverse square law): $1/r^2$. Dosing used to be mg/hr based. It is now dosimetry based.
- In the log cell kill model, each dose—called a fraction—kills a fixed amount of cells. Radiation works by causing breaks in the DNA backbone via one of two types of energy, a photon or a charged particle (an electron). This damage is either direct or indirect with ionization of the atoms that make up the DNA chain. Indirect ionization is the result of the ionization of water, forming free radicals, notably hydroxyl radicals, which then damage the DNA. Direct ionization is the result of electrons causing single-stranded DNA breaks. These single-stranded breaks need to be on opposing strands of DNA in close proximity to each other in order to create a double-stranded break. Oxygen free radicals modify radiation damage making it irreparable. Oxygen is transported to tumors via the blood system, so adequate hemoglobin (Hg) levels are needed. Without oxygen, the cell survival curve shifts to the right.
- There are two cell survival/dose-response curves, the linear and the linear-quadratic. The linear "curve" is a straight line and this is represented by LDR. LDR is delivered over a protracted period of time and cell kill is by a single electron. The linear quadratic curve demonstrates cell kill caused by two breaks in the DNA from either by the same electron or by two different electrons. This cell survival curve is straight initially and then curves, representing HDR-type delivery.
- The linear quadratic equation: $-\ln S = alphaD + betaD^2$. The alpha component is the nonreparable damage, whereas the beta component represents reparable damage. S is the surviving fraction of cells. The dose at which the cell kill is due to equal linear and quadratic components is called the alpha beta ratio.
- The biologically equivalent dose (BED) is used as a guide to determine optimal dosing. The BED = $D[1 + d/(alpha/beta)]$, where D is the total dose and d is the dose per fraction. Early side effects demonstrate an alpha/beta ratio of 10 whereas late side effects and tumor control assume an alpha/beta of 3.
- The cell can respond to radiation differently depending on its phase in the cell cycle. Late S phase is the most radioresistant phase and M phase is most radiosensitive. There are two possible outcomes after exposure to radiation: survival or death. If the cell survives there is cell cycle arrest and DNA repair.
- There are three types of cell death. The first is apoptotic, which is ordered programmed cell death. A lot of tumors have mutations in apoptotic pathways and thus do not respond to apoptotic signals easily. The second type of cell death is mitotic. Mitotic death may take days. The third is senescence. Senescence is when cell proliferation is irreversibly arrested and death eventually ensues.

THE FOUR R'S OF RADIATION

- Repair: radiation in fractionated doses is not as lethal as if it were delivered in one high dose. Sublethal repair occurs when a certain percentage of cells are killed, and those that survive can repair their damage and continue to divide.
- Reassortment: radiation kills cells best when they are in the late G_2 and M phases, which are the most radiosensitive cycles. Other cycles are relatively radioresistant. After a dose of fractional radiation, the cells that were in the

more radioresistant phases (and survived) reassort themselves into their next cell cycle. They then become more radiosensitive and when the next dose of radiation is delivered, they have a higher likelihood of death.

- Repopulation is when the surviving population of cells that are not lethally damaged divide and replace those that were killed.
- Reoxygenation is when the tumor generates new blood vessels to bring in a higher oxygen tension via Hg. Oxygen must be present during radiation to generate the free radical that yields DNA damage. Low oxygen tension makes cells more radioresistant.

DISEASE SITE RADIATION TREATMENT

Cervical Cancer

All stages of cervical cancer can be treated with definitive radiation therapy (XRT).

- Anatomical dosing is based on the paracervical triangle—the lateral vaginal fornices and the apex of the anteverted uterus. Dosing is directed at two common points. Point A is 2 cm superior and 2 cm lateral to the external cervical os. This correlates anatomically to where the ureter and the uterine artery cross. Point B is 2 cm superior and 5 cm lateral to the external cervical os. This point corresponds to the obturator lymph node (LN) basins. Point T is inside point A. It is 1 cm superior to the external cervical os and 1 cm lateral to the tandem; it receives a dose 2 to 3× the dose to point A. Point P is located along the bony pelvic sidewall at its most lateral point and represents the minimal dose to the external iliac LNs. Point C is 1 cm lateral to point B and is approximate to the pelvic sidewall. Point H is an HDR point: it originates from a line that connects the mid-dwell position of the ovoids and intersects with the tandem. Then move superiorly the radius of the ovoids (to top of ovoids) + 2 cm, and then 2 cm perpendicularly. The vaginal surface is where the lateral radius of the ovoid and ring applicator falls. This receives a dose 1.4 to 2.0 times the point A dose.
- CT-based planning and conformal blocking is the current standard of care. External beam radiation therapy (EBXRT) volumes should cover gross disease, parametria, uterosacral ligaments, at least 3 cm of vaginal margin, presacral nodes, and other nodal basins at risk. If negative LN are determined via surgical staging or imaging, the radiation volume should include all of the internal and external iliac, and the obturator LN basins. If bulky or residual tumor is present or there were positive pelvic LN found at surgical staging, the radiation volume should cover the common iliacs as well. If common iliac or PA LN involvement is identified, extended field pelvic and para-aortic radiation therapy (PA-XRT), up to the renal vessels is advised.
- Intensity-modulated radiation therapy (IMXRT) is a highly conformal dosing method, which can minimize the dose to vital pelvic organs (bowel, bladder) while maximizing dose at risk of involved sites.
- Current definitive dosing for cervical cancer prescribes a total dose to point A of 85 to 90 Gy with 60 Gy dosed to point B.
  - External beam radiation provides 45 to 50.4 Gy to point A via whole pelvic radiation therapy (WP-XRT) with a 15-Gy boost when appropriate. The dose to point A is brought up from 50.4 Gy using external beam radiation to the total desired dose of 80 Gy in small volume, and 85 to 90 Gy for large volume tumors, with brachytherapy.

○ If LDR is used, the brachytherapy dose is 50 to 60 cGy/hr with 40 Gy total given. If HDR is used, the dose is 30 Gy. The brachytherapy dose per HDR fraction to point A is 3 to 10.5 Gy. The total number of fractions is 2 to 13. The number of fractions per week is 1 to 3. The morbidity is lower for fractions less than 7 Gy. Gynecologic Oncology Group (GOG) protocols use 6 Gy × 5 fractions to point A. Radiation Therapy Oncology Group (RTOG) protocols allow more variation depending on the external beam radiation dose with brachytherapy fraction sizes of 5.3 to 7.4 Gy using 4 to 7 fractions. Platinum-based chemotherapy should be used in the definitive management of cervical cancer.

○ Microscopic nodal disease demands an EBXRT dose of 45 to 50.4 Gy in 1.8 to 2 Gy daily fractions. 10- to 15-Gy boosts can be given to residual disease, bulky adenopathy, or the parametria.

○ Sequencing of brachytherapy with external beam radiation is based on tumor size, patient anatomy, and practitioner discretion. For nonbulky disease, HDR is often integrated after 20 Gy of external beam therapy around the second week of treatment. Alternatively, some deliver WP-XRT to 50.4 Gy followed by five HDR insertions.

○ Brachytherapy most commonly uses the tandem and ovoid system. There are 48 dwell positions in the tandem. The radiation sources are usually spaced 2.5 to 5 mm apart. The dwell position is where the source is driven to stop. The longest tandem possible should be used. The tandem should be loaded so the sources reach the uterine fundus. This enables adequate distribution to the lower uterine segment, the paracervical tissues, and obturator LNs. The tandems have three curvatures (15°, 30°, and 45°); the greatest curvature is used in cavities measuring greater than 6 cm. A flange is added to the tandem after insertion into the uterine cavity and approximates the exocervix. The keel is then added and prevents rotation of the tandem after packing.

○ Vaginal ovoids come in four different sizes. The largest sized ovoid that the patient can tolerate is placed as far laterally and cephalad as possible. This gives the highest tumor dose possible. The mini-sized ovoid is 1.6 cm in diameter, the small is 2 cm in diameter, the medium is 2.5 cm in diameter, and the large is 3 cm in diameter. The mini does not have any shielding to protect the bladder. A wide separation of the ovoids is desired as this increases the dose to the pelvic sidewall. A 10-mg protruding source is recommended if the vaginal ovoids are separated by more than 5 cm. Optimal positioning is: on the AP view, the tandem is midline and unrotated, the tandem is midway between the colpostats, the keel is in close proximity to the gold seed markers fiducials placed in the cervical stroma, and the colpostats are placed high in the vaginal fornices; on the lateral view, the tandem bisects the colpostat, there is sufficient anterior and posterior packing, and the tandem is equidistant from the sacral promontory and the pubis.

○ The anterior bladder point is determined by placement of a Foley catheter with 7 mL of radiopaque material placed into the balloon. The balloon is then pulled down against the urethra creating this point.

○ The posterior rectal point is determined by packing the vagina with radiopaque packing and moving 5 mm posterior to that line.

○ The vaginal surface dose should be kept below 140 Gy.

• In the postoperative posthysterectomy setting, patients can be broken into two risk categories: (a) those with intermediate-risk factors (LVSI, DOI, and tumor size), per GOG 92 and (b) those with high-risk factors (2+ positive LNs, lesion size >2 cm, margins ≤5 mm, positive margins, or parametrial involvement proven histologically) per GOG 109. WP EBXRT should be considered for those with intermediate-risk factors, and concurrent platinum-based chemotherapy in addition to WP EBXRT for those with high-risk factors. Some centers treat both groups with combination therapy. The adjuvant dose is 45 to 50.4 Gy EBXRT. The fields include the upper 4 cm of vaginal cuff, the parametria, and the internal and external iliac LN basins. If LN metastasis is documented, the upper border of the field should be increased to the next nodal basin or 7 cm higher than the involved LN and bulky LN should be boosted with an additional 10 to 15 Gy.

- Types of applicators:
  - Fletcher-Suit and Henschke tandem and ovoids are commonly used. The Delclos applicator uses the mini ovoids. The Henschke applicator uses hemispheroidal ovoids, and the tandem and ovoids are fixed together. This creates an easier applicator for shallow vaginal fornices.
  - The Fletcher-Suit and Delclos cylinders are used for narrow vaginas, when ovoids are contraindicated. They are also used to treat varying lengths of the vagina mandated by vaginal spread of disease. Cylinders vary in size from 2 to 4 cm in diameter.
  - Ring applicators are an adaption of the Stockholm technique. There are three sizes: the small is 36 mm, the medium is 40 mm, and the large is 44 mm diameter. It is important to not activate all positions in the ring, as this will increase the dosing to the bladder and rectum. Often, four dwell positions are activated on each side of the smallest ring, five dwell positions on each side of the medium ring, and six dwell positions on each side of the largest ring. Tandems are available in lengths of 2 to 8 cm and the tandem angles are available with 30°, 45°, 60°, and 90°.
  - Interstitial applicators are used if there is a narrow or obliterated vagina, obliterated vaginal fornices, bulky or barrel-shaped cervical tumors, parametrial disease, vaginal disease, or if there is recurrent unresectable disease. This method of radiation delivery uses iridium-loaded stainless steel or plastic needles. There are a few different applicators. One is the Martinez universal perineal interstitial template (MUPIT). Another is the Syed–Neblett template, which has three different templates consisting of 36, 44, or 53 needles. If LDR is used, the dosing is 60 to 80 cGy/hr with a total dose of 23 to 40 Gy over 2 to 4 days. If HDR is used, the dosing is 60% of the total LDR dose given in 1 to 2 fractions per day over 2 to 5 days. External beam radiation usually precedes implantation.

Uterine Cancer

- Brachytherapy for uterine cancer is commonly used in the adjuvant setting. Fletcher colpostats, or a variety of vaginal cylinders, are used. The upper one half to one third of the vagina is treated after a hysterectomy.
- When using Delclos or Burnett vaginal cylinders, treatment is to the upper 4 to 5 cm of the vagina. The dose distribution conforms to the shape of the cylinder. The dose is specified either at the mucosal surface or to 0.5 cm deep. Studies have shown that 95% of the vaginal lymphatics are located within

3 mm of the vaginal surface. The LDR dose is 80 to 100 cGy/hr to the surface and 50 to 70 cGy/hr if treated to 0.5 cm deep. Treatment to the vagina in the adjuvant setting is usually limited to a total HDR dose of 21 Gy in three doses of 7 Gy to the surface, or 5 Gy in six doses to 0.5 cm deep.

- Bulky stage II or IIIB uterine cancer should be preoperatively treated with XRT. Radiation is dosed at 85 to 90 Gy with 45 to 50.4 delivered by EBXRT and 21 to 30 Gy by brachytherapy.

- Medically inoperable uterine cancer is a rare occurrence. Radiation treatment is with the placement of double or triple intrauterine tandems, or Heyman–Simons capsules in combination with external beam radiation. Total dosing follows that for the primary treatment of cervical cancer.

- Residual postoperative vaginal disease less than 0.5 cm may be treated with brachytherapy cylinders or ovoids to 45 or 50.4 Gy. If there is thicker residual vaginal disease, external beam or interstitial radiation therapy is needed.

- Recurrent vaginal disease should be treated with EBXRT followed by brachytherapy. Doses over 80 Gy are usually needed. Recurrent pelvic disease can be treated with EBXRT.

- Indications for treatment in the adjuvant setting are based on stage and patient risk factors.
  - For high-intermediate risk disease, patients are stratified by age and pathological risk factors to include G2/3, LVSI, or outer 1/2 to 1/3 myometrial involvement.
  - If there is cervical stromal involvement (stage II), a combination of EBXRT and brachytherapy is recommended.
  - For stage IIIA with adnexal metastasis, EBXRT alone can give an 85% 5Y survival (YS). For stage IIIB parametrial or pelvic peritoneal disease, EBXRT with brachytherapy with/without chemotherapy can be considered. For stage IIIC, a combination of EBXRT and chemotherapy should be considered. Evidence supports the use of combined modality therapies as adjuvant therapies for patients with extrauterine disease (1).
  - For early stage patients with aggressive histology (serous or clear cell), XRT in combination with platinum-based chemotherapy has been used. For those with stage I disease and any residual tumor, brachytherapy and chemotherapy have been used. For those staged II or higher, external beam radiation has been used with chemotherapy (2).

Vulvar Cancer

- Indications for treatment of the pelvic and groin LN basins are the following:
  - International Federation of Gynecology and Obstetrics (FIGO) stage IIIB and greater lesions.
  - In the neoadjuvant setting in combination with platinum-based chemotherapy for select T2 and advanced T3/T4 lesions. If the patient has clinically negative or resectable groin LNs, pre-treatment groin LN dissection can be considered. If all groin LNs are negative, patients can receive radiation therapy to only the primary tumor.
  - Adjuvant primary tumor bed radiation can be considered if positive margin(s) are present after resection, although this has not been shown to

increase OS. Patients with close margins of 0.8 mm or less can also be counseled on adjuvant perineal radiation.
- Treatment: radiation is prescribed to a total dose of 50.4 Gy in 1.8 Gy fractions 5 days/week in the adjuvant setting. For unresectable T3/4 disease, 57.6 Gy with radiosensitizing chemotherapy should be administered. In select cases, doses can be boosted to 60 to 70 Gy. Brachytherapy can occasionally be prescribed as a boost. A 20-Gy boost to each groin can be applied. Gross tumor probably requires a dose of at least 70 Gy. Patients should be simulated supine in the frog-leg position with a full bladder.

Vaginal Cancer
- Treatment is indicated for all FIGO stages and definitively for stage II and higher. Treatment is usually a combination of EBXRT dosed at 45 to 50.4 Gy in 180 cGy fractions daily for 4 to 5 weeks, followed by brachytherapy or interstitial implants with an additional 21 to 30 Gy. Concurrent platinum-based chemotherapy should be considered.

Ovarian Cancer
- There are minimal uses for radiation therapy for epithelial ovarian tumors. Isolated local recurrence or residual tumor after completion of chemotherapy are debatable indications.
- For germ cell tumors, radiation has a slightly higher indication. Dysgerminomas are highly radiosensitive and treatment can be considered for primary or recurrent disease.
- Sex cord stromal tumors can also benefit from radiation therapy. This has been studied in recurrent granulosa cell tumors. There are data to support a 43% response rate (3).

Brain Metastasis
- Symptoms: facial droop, cranial nerve (CN) II-X deficits, ataxia, arm drift, and expressive aphasia.
- Evaluate and confirm with MRI, with and without contrast.
- Treatment: decadron and whole brain radiation therapy (WB-XRT) for multiple metastases, Decadron and stereotactic radiation for solitary metastasis. Inpatient management is recommended for midline shift, herniation, or hemorrhage. Outpatient management is possible if the patient is compliant with support at home and none of the above contraindications.
- Dosing:
  - WB-XRT: 30 Gy in 10 fractions is considered standard treatment per RTOG-6901 protocol in a palliative fashion.
  - Decadron: mild symptoms: 4 to 8 mg/day. Moderate to severe symptoms from edema and intracranial pressure: 16 mg/day. Taper over a 2 to 7 week period based on symptom resolution. Side effects can include: Cushing's syndrome, candidiasis, psychiatric disorders, hyperglycemia, and peripheral edema. A common dose is: 8 mg PO daily-BID (based on severity) × 4 days, 4 mg PO BID for 4 days, then 2 mg/day until completion of radiation.

DESIGN OF EXTERNAL BEAM RADIATION FIELDS

The external beam fields are designed in a four-field box as anterior-posterior/posterior-anterior (AP/PA) fields plus lateral fields. These are customarily outlined as 15×15 cm^2 for the AP/PA fields and 8 to 9 cm wide for the lateral fields. The intent of the four fields is to use narrow lateral beams to avoid some small bowel and a portion of the rectum posteriorly. CT- or MRI-based planning can accurately outline the radiation targets and simultaneously spare vital organs using mobile blocks called collimators. A collimator is a device that narrows a beam of particles and multiple collimators are used to vary the radiation fields. Radiation is dosed with a 0.7 to 1 cm expansion around the involved LN, bone, and muscle (CTV) except for the groin LN where there should be a 2-cm margin. The PTV should have an additional 1-cm margin. In general, the principle of extending node treatment volume one nodal echelon proximal to the level of clinical involvement is a prudent guideline. IMRT is now being used in a significant number of centers to decrease side effects to vital structures. IMRT uses computer-controlled x-ray accelerators to distribute precise radiation doses to malignant tumors or specific areas within the tumor. The pattern of radiation delivery is determined using highly tailored computing applications.

CERVICAL CANCER

- **Cervical cancer fields**
  - **Conventional fields:** the superior border for nonbulky stage IB/IIA disease is S1/L5. For bulky or more advanced disease the border is L4/5. There are data to suggest that in 87% of patients the bifurcation of the common iliac vessels was above the L5 prominence (4). Thus, it may be necessary to extend the upper field border to L2/3. The inferior border is the mid or lower border of the obturator foramen or 3 to 4 cm below the most distal vaginal component of disease. It is important to cover the inguinal LN if the distal vagina is involved. The lateral borders are 2 to 2.5 cm lateral to the pelvic brim. The anterior border is the pubic symphysis. It may be necessary to extend this coverage to 2 cm anterior to the pubis in order to cover the external iliac arteries. The posterior border is conventionally set posterior to S2/S3. A study found that in stages IB and II, the most common inadequate margin was the posterior border at the S2/3 interface and there was no increase in rectal complications when the entire sacrum was included in the radiation field (5). Treatment is 85 to 90 Gy using combined external beam radiation and brachytherapy. External beam radiation is dosed at 45 to 50.4 Gy and brachytherapy is dosed at 30 Gy for HDR and 40 Gy for LDR. Some studies have shown that 79% of patients treated with conventional fields had inadequate coverage. CT-based planning was then able to cover 95% of patients appropriately.
    - Midline blocks are used to increase the dose to the parametria or pelvic sidewalls while shielding the bladder, distal ureters, and rectosigmoid. Some customize the midline block at the 50% isodose line that passes through point A. Some feather the block at specific isodose intervals. Most use rectangular blocks 4 to 5 cm in width, as this is the distance between the distal ureters. A margin of 0.5 cm lateral to the lateral ovoid surface is recommended in designing the width of the midline block.

- A parametrial boost of an additional 15 Gy is recommended if there is bulky parametrial disease or pelvic sidewall disease. This is done after completion of WP radiation. Doses needed to eradicate parametrial disease are about 60 Gy.
- An LN boost is dosed at 15 Gy to enlarged or known positive LN. Data have shown that 16% of patients with biopsy-proven positive LN, treated with chemotherapy and radiation, have residual disease after 45 Gy even with a 15-Gy boost (6).
- Extended field radiation defines coverage of the para-aortic LN basins. The superior margin of this field is T12/L1 and the inferior margin is L4/5, laterally the spinous vertebral processes, and 2 cm anterior to the vertebrae. The dose is 45 Gy plus an extra 15-Gy boost for positive LN.

○ CT-based planning is considered the standard of care using EBXRT. Radiation volumes should cover the gross disease, parametria, uterosacral ligaments, a minimum 3-cm vaginal margin from the gross disease, the presacral nodes, and other nodal basins involved or at risk. If surgically or radiologically negative nodes, the radiation volume should include the external iliac, internal iliac, and obturator LN basins. For patients with larger tumors or positive nodes in the true pelvis, the radiation volume should be increased to cover the common iliacs. In patients with documented common iliac and/or para-aortic nodal involvement, extended-field pelvic and PA-XRT to the level of the renal vessels (or even more cephalad) as directed should be applied.

○ IMRT: the TIME-C trial (RTOG-1203, NCT01672892) is comparing posthysterectomy patients receiving adjuvant XRT to evaluate gastrointestinal (GI) toxicity in IMRT versus standard 3D CT XRT.

UTERINE CANCER

- Uterine cancer fields are as follows:
  ○ Conventional anatomic fields: superiorly the L4/5 interface, inferiorly the mid or lower obturator foramen, laterally 2 to 2.5 cm lateral to the pelvic brim, anteriorly the pubic symphysis, and posteriorly S2/3 of the sacrum. EBXRT covers the upper one half to two thirds of the vagina, the parametria, and the pelvic LNs. Stage II cancers are recommended to have both external beam and brachytherapy.
  ○ CT-guided fields: this is the standard of care currently. XRT should target gross residual disease if present and cover the lower common iliac vessels, the internal and external iliac vessels, the parametia, the upper vagina/paravaginal tissue, the presacral LN (especially if stage II) with extended fields to cover the para-aortic LN basins if involved. The upper border of the extended para-aortic fields should at least be to the level of the renal vessels.
  ○ Brachytherapy to the vaginal cuff alone can be given up to 50 Gy. If used in the adjuvant setting, HDR brachytherapy is usually dosed at 21 Gy: consisting of 7 Gy for 3 fractions to a vaginal depth of 0.5 cm or 6 Gy for 5 fractions— initiated as soon as the cuff is healed and no more than 12 weeks after surgery.

- External beam dosing: adjuvant treatment of microscopic extrauterine disease should be 45 to 50.4 Gy with a 15-Gy boost to involved parametria or positive LN basins. Primary radiation therapy for bulky stage II disease or definitive therapy in nonoperative candidates should total 75 to 80 Gy with combined EBXRT and brachytherapy.
- To decrease vital organ complications, the patient can be treated in the prone position with a full bladder or with use of a belly board.

VULVAR CANCER

- Vulvar cancer fields:
  - Conventional fields: the superior field is no lower than the sacroiliac (SI) joints or higher than the L4/5 junction unless pelvic LN are involved; if so, the upper border should be raised to 5 cm above the most cephalad positive LN. The superior border should extend as a horizontal line at the level of the anterior superior iliac spines (ASIS). The lateral border extends in a line connecting the femoral head and the ASIS with an additional 2 cm lateral margin. The medial border is 3 cm from the body's midline. The inferiolateral inguinal nodal border is parallel to the inguinal crease and inferior enough to encompass the inguinofemoral nodal bed to the intertrochanteric line of the femur or 1.5 to 2 cm distal to the saphenofemoral junction. The inferior vulvar border should be: inferiorly 2.5 cm below the ischial tuberosity or 2 cm below the most inferior portion of the primary vulvar tumor. A narrow posterior field is used with 15 to 18 MV and a wide anterior field is used with 6 MV and an additional 12 MeV dose is prescribed to each groin. If the patient is thin and the depth of the inguinal vessels is less than 3 cm, an electron patch may be used. There is an 11% rate of femoral neck fracture or necrosis with these doses.
  - CT-based planning:
    - Vulvar field: is any gross vulvar disease plus any visible or palpable extension to the vagina. Bolus dosing should be used to adequately cover the superficial target volume.
    - Groin field CTV: is laterally from the inguinofemoral vessels to the medial border of the sartorius and rectus femoris muscles, posteriorly to the anterior vastus medialis muscle and medially to the pectineus muscle or for 2.5 to 3 cm medial from the vessels. Anteriorly the volume should extend to the anterior border of the sartorius muscle. The caudal extent is the top of the lesser trochanter of the femur.
    - The pelvic nodal CTV: includes the bilateral external iliac, obturator, and internal iliac nodal basins with 7 mm of symmetrical expansion excluding bone and muscle. If pelvic nodes are involved, the upper border can be raised to 5 cm above the most cephalad positive node.
- Dosing: doses are commonly 50.4 Gy in 1.8 Gy fractions daily. For unresectable disease, doses can be given to 59.4 to 64.8 Gy in 1.8 Gy fractions with a boost to 70 Gy if indicated.

VAGINAL CANCER

The fields are similar to that of cervical cancer: superiorly the L5–S1 interface; inferiorly to 2 cm below the lesion, and then 2 cm lateral to the pelvic brim. For lesions that include the lower one third of the vagina the groins should be included. The lateral field margins should extend in a line connecting the femoral heads and the ASIS to include the inguinal nodes.

OVARIAN CANCER

The fields are that of site-directed radiation or whole abdominal radiotherapy (WAR).

WHOLE ABDOMINAL RADIOTHERAPY

WAR is not commonly given as adjuvant therapy. It can be given for salvage treatment. The total dose is 30 Gy in fraction sizes of 1.5 to 1.7 Gy/day. The field margins are 1 to 2 cm above the diaphragm superiorly (with heart shielding), 1 to 2 cm lateral to the peritoneal reflection, and inferiorly 2 cm below the inguinal ligament. Usually, whole pelvic radiation therapy (WP-XRT) follows with a dose of 45 to 50 Gy. The kidneys should be blocked at 15 Gy and the liver blocked at 25 Gy.

RADIATION EFFECTS

- The definition of an **early complication** is occurrence less than 3 months after completion of XRT. A **late complication** is defined as onset after 3 months. Late effects are usually due to capillary damage (endarteritis obliterans).
- **Skin toxicity** is usually delayed for 2 to 3 weeks. Most patients get moist desquamation about 2 weeks into treatment. There can also be erythema. Dry desquamation can occur after the fourth week. Toxicity is enhanced by actinomycin D and doxorubicin. Treatment is sitz baths, diarrhea control, calendula lotion, or Aquaphor cream as well as sulfa-based barrier creams. The epidermis returns in 14 days. Late effects can be depigmentation and telangiectasias.
- **Vaginal toxicity** can be manifested with a yellow-white discharge due to mucositis. This can continue for 6 months. Treatment is with hydrogen peroxide douches, antibiotics, or hyperbaric therapy. Remember to rule out radiation necrosis and possible fistula—these complications may require a flap or even exenteration. The distal vagina is less tolerant with a maximum dose of 80 to 90 Gy versus a maximum dose of 120 to 150 Gy for the proximal vagina. Narrowing and shortening of the vagina is a late effect and can occur in 80% of patients. Symptom is pain. Diagnosis is with examination. Treatment is with frequent intercourse, vaginal dilators, and estrogen cream. Neovaginal reconstruction is complicated with high rates of failure and potential fistula.
- **Urinary tract toxicity** can present with frequency, urgency, and dysuria from decreased bladder capacity. Pyridium may help.
  - Spasms can be relieved by smooth muscle relaxants such as B&O suppositories or urospas. Always rule out infection. The urinalysis (UA) can show radiation cystitis with white blood cells (WBC) and red blood cells (RBC) present, but without bacteria. Focal ulcerations, hyperemia, and edema occur at greater than 30 Gy. Above 60 Gy hematuria occurs due to telangiectasias.

- ○ Hemorrhagic cystitis occurs in 1% to 5%. Treatment is with continuous irrigation with normal saline, cautery ablation via cystoscopy, methylene blue instillation, formalin instillation, alum 2% instillation, hyperbaric oxygen, or Elmiron. Surgical diversion with a conduit is a last resort.
- ○ Ureteral stricture occurs at a rate of 2.5% at 20 years. A unilateral stricture is more common. Symptoms include pain, or an increasing blood urea nitrogen (BUN)/creatinine. Diagnosis is via laboratories, intravenous pyelography (IVP), or CT imaging. Treatment is with stenting, dilation, or surgical resection and reanastomosis.
- **Fistula formation** can occur from the GI or urinary systems. Symptoms are spontaneous stool or urinary loss from an improper orifice. Diagnosis is with a full clinical examination, examination under anesthesia (EUA) with biopsies if necessary. A fistulogram, CT, MRI, or PET scan may be helpful.
  - ○ Conservative management of bowel fistula is with: NPO status, total parenteral nutrition (TPN), somatostatin 50 to 200 mcg SC TID, H_2 blockers, Questran, and tincture of opium BID. Surgical intervention is with colostomy, repair, and excision of the fistulous tract. TPN and bowel rest is often tried but rarely efficacious.
  - ○ Treatment of urinary fistula requires diagnosis of the location of the fistula, diversion with a Foley catheter or nephrostomy tube, and resection of the fistula and tract. A neobladder can be constructed as last resort.
- **Bowel toxicity** is primarily diarrhea, which is due to shortened villi and loss of their absorptive function. The dose tolerance of the small bowel is 45 Gy, the large bowel 70 to 75 Gy, and the anus 60 to 65 Gy.
  - ○ Acute radiation enteritis is demonstrated by watery diarrhea, which starts during the second or third week of treatment at about 20 Gy. There is increased flatulence and noisy bowel sounds. Treatment is with a low-residue diet, hydration, and antimotility agents. Somatostatin and bowel rest may be indicated. Chronic diarrhea is managed with dietary changes.
  - ○ Small bowel injury can occur as stricture or stenosis. It can present as a partial small bowel obstruction (SBO) or a complete SBO. These occur in 5% of patients, with the terminal ileum and cecum being the most common site because they are anatomically fixed. Symptoms of a partial obstruction are delayed postprandial cramping, nausea, vomiting, and diarrhea. Diagnosis is with clinical examination or imaging with upper gastrointestinal (UGI) and small bowel follow through (SBFT), or a CT scan. Treatment is with bowel resection and reanastomosis.
  - ○ Malabsorption can occur from excess bile salts reaching the colon. These are cathartics, so treatment with cholestyramine may help.
  - ○ Rectosigmoid toxicity can be symptomatic with a stricture causing a partial or complete large bowel obstruction. Diverting colostomy may be a treatment of last resort.
  - ○ Rectal toxicity can present with tenesmus, mucus production, pain, worsening of hemorrhoids, and proctitis. It occurs in 2% to 3% of patients. Treatment is with antispasmodics or steroid suppositories or enemas. Telangiectasia's can cause bleeding and ulceration. Treatment of these is with cortisone rectal

suppositories, sulfasalazine enemas, mesalamine (Rowasa) suppositories BID for 6 weeks, and hyperbaric oxygen.
- ○ Gastric outlet obstruction can occur from progressive fibrosis and can even lead to perforation.
- **Ovarian failure occurs** between 2.5 and 6 Gy for the germ cell components, presenting as permanent sterility. The stromal support cells fail at 24 Gy. Attempts to prevent ovarian failure are occasionally successful. Options include midline oophoropexy (surgical placement behind the uterus), surgical transposition to the upper pelvis (with a 40%–71% rate of success), cortical stripping and cryopreservation, oocyte retrieval with cryopreservation, or in vitro fertilization and embryo cryopreservation.
- **Bone marrow toxicity** can present as follows:
  - ○ Pancytopenia. This is because 40% of the marrow is in the pelvis. Symptoms can include fatigue (anemia), increased susceptibility to infections (leukopenia), and bruising or bleeding (thrombocytopenia). Patients need weekly monitoring of the complete blood count (CBC).
  - ○ Insufficiency fractures can also occur. The tolerance for the femoral head is 45 Gy. Fractures most commonly occur in the sacrum, ileum, pubic bones, and acetabulum. Asymptomatic fractures occur at a rate of 34% to 39% and symptomatic fractures at a rate of 13%. Symptoms are the sudden onset of pain which worsens with weight bearing. MRI is the best means for diagnosis. Treatment is surgical stabilization.
  - ○ The femoral neck can develop avascular necrosis. Treatment for this is hip replacement.
- **Liver toxicity** can present as follows:
  - ○ Veno-occlusive disease. This is due to platelet coagulation causing congestion and thrombocytopenia.
  - ○ Radiation hepatitis may occur and present with an elevated alkaline phosphatase 3 to 10× normal. Small portions of the liver can receive up to 70 Gy. The whole liver should not receive more than 30 Gy.
- **Renal toxicity** usually manifests as a nephrotic syndrome. Toxicities present as hypertension (HTN), leg edema, proteinuria, or a normocytic normochromic anemia. The kidney should not receive more than 18 to 20 Gy. To avoid toxicity, preferentially load 70/30 AP/PA and block the kidneys completely after 18 to 20 Gy.
- **Fetal toxicity:** in utero exposure of the fetus invariably occurs during the diagnosis and treatment of gynecologic malignancies in pregnancy. If treatment occurs at 1 to 2 weeks of pregnancy, the effect is all or nothing with spontaneous abortion, or continuation of pregnancy without effect. At 2 to 6 weeks, congenital anomalies and death can occur, with a 2-Gy dose yielding 70% mortality. At 6 to 16 weeks, growth retardation and mental retardation occur with a risk of 40% per Gy. After 30 weeks, no gross malformations tend to occur. The risk of leukemia is increased if exposure is in the third trimester. The risk is about 6% per Gy. A dose less than 1 mGy is negligible. For the entire gestational period, no more than 0.5 cGy exposure should occur (Table 5.2).

CERVICAL CANCER AND RADIATION THERAPY DELIVERY TIME

The prolongation of overall treatment time and timing of brachytherapy can impact the outcome of radiation therapy. The pelvic recurrence rate when treatment time is per Tables 5.3 and 5.4.

Table 5.2 Radiation Tolerance of Organs	
Organ	TD_{50} (Gy)
Bone marrow	5
Ovary	10
Kidney	25
Lung	30
Liver	50
Heart	60
Intestine	62
Spinal cord	60
Brain	65
Bladder	65

Table 5.3 Cervical Cancer Recurrence Rate Stratified by Radiation Treatment Duration				
Stage	<7 wks (%)	7–9 wks (%)	>9 wks (%)	p values
IB	7	22	6	$p < 0.01$
IIA	14	27	36	$p = 0.08$
IIB	20	28	34	$p = 0.09$
III	38	44	49	$p = 0.18$
III when point A dose >80 Gy	32	40	51	$p = 0.08$

Table 5.4 10Y Cause-Specific Survival by Treatment Time				
Stage	<7 wks (%)	7–9 wks (%)	>9 wks (%)	p value
IB	86	78	55	$p = 0.01$
IIA	73	41	48	$p = 0.01$
IIB	72	60	70	$p = 0.01$
III	42	42	39	$p = 0.43$
III (patient A dose >80 Gy)	46	44	37	$p = 0.016$

REFERENCES

1. Klopp A, Smith BD, Alektiar K, et al. The role of postoperative radiation therapy for endometrial cancer: executive summary of an American society for radiation oncology evidence-based guidelines. *Pract Radiat Oncol.* 2014;4:137-144.
2. Kelly MG, O'Malley DM, Hui P, et al. Improved survival in surgical stage I patients with uterine papillary serous carcinoma (UPSC) treated with adjuvant platinum-based chemotherapy. *Gynecol Oncol.* 2005;98(3):353-359.
3. Wolf JK, Mullen J, Eifel PJ, et al. Radiation treatment of advanced or recurrent granulosa cell tumor of the ovary. *Gynecol Oncol.* 1999;73(1):35-41.
4. Greer BE, Koh WJ, Figge DC. Gynecologic radiotherapy fields defined by intraoperative measurements. *Gynecol Oncol.* 1990;38(3):421-424.
5. Greer BE. Expanded pelvic radiotherapy fields for treatment of local-regionally advanced carcinoma of the cervix: outcomes and treatment complications. *Am J Obstet Gynecol.* 1996;174(4):1141-1149.
6. Houvenaeghel G, Lelievre L, Rigouard AL. Residual pelvic lymph node involvement after concomitant chemoradiation for locally advanced cervical cancer. *Gynecol Oncol.* 2006;102(3):523-529.

REPRODUCTIVE FUNCTION AND GYNECOLOGIC CANCER

6

Sexual Function, Fertility, and Cancer

SEXUAL DYSFUNCTION

Sexual dysfunction is common in patients who undergoing diagnosis of and treatment for gynecologic malignancies. This is due to pain, discomfort, bleeding, and/or psychological stress that may make intimacy difficult. Sexual disorders are typically not screened for effectively, thus masking the problem. Even for patients in whom sexual dysfunction is identified, there is little support to manage the problem. Comprehensive screening questionnaires have been validated as effective screening tools for different sexual disorders (1). Sexual disorders can be classified into four disorders: desire disorder, arousal disorder; orgasm disorder; pain disorder.

- Pre-treatment Workup:
  - Evaluate for which category of sexual disorder.
  - Discuss concerns related to specific cancer therapies: examples—surgical pain or altered anatomy; radiation induced vaginal stenosis; menopausal symptoms related to either or from chemotherapy.
  - Consider evaluation with the Female Sexual Function Index (SFSI) or the PROMIS Sexual Function Instrument.
  - Perform a physical exam: note points of tenderness, vaginal atrophy, and anatomic changes associated with cancer surgeries or treatments. It is important to biopsy any suspicious lesions.
- Management: guide treatment based on type of sexual disorder:
  - **Desire:**
    - Chronic medical conditions such as hypertension, diabetes, anxiety, and depression can have a negative impact on desire and should be addressed.
    - Surgical disfigurement may also be a factor in desire. For women with ostomies, the four P's approach has been applied: prepare (adjust diet in preparation for intimacy to reduce gastrointestinal problems), pouch (pouch covers are available in multiple different fabrics, including lace or silk), position (avoid positions that cause pressure on ostomy to prevent compression or spillage), and pleasure (communicate with the partner that the goal is pleasurable intimacy) (2).
  - **Arousal and Orgasm**: treatment-induced menopause and altered gonadal function from XRT or chemotherapy are among factors that may contribute. In most hormonally sensitive cancers, systemic estrogen therapy has generally been contraindicated. However, for lower risk patients, topical estrogens have been found to be effective and relatively safe for the treatment of vaginal symptoms after menopause. Other nonhormonal therapies include vaginal moisturizers and lubricants. With regard to arousal, the prescription device

EROS-CVD can be used to create gentle suction over the clitoris and has been proven beneficial in women with female arousal disorders, including those who have undergone treatment for cancer.

○ **Pain:** patients can experience pain during intercourse from vaginal foreshortening either due to surgery or XRT, or dryness from use of aromatase inhibitors (AIs). Patients may benefit from:

- The use of vaginal dilators along with the use of lubricants and possibly estrogen products, in order to lengthen and dilate the vagina.
- One method to minimize dyspareunia may be positional changes.
- Lidocaine 2% topical jelly applied to the vulva or vagina may reduce vulvodynia and dyspareunia.
- Antidepressants and neuromodulators (gabapentin) can mitigate some pain symptoms, but caution should be used as they may also cause some arousal disorders.
- Consider ospemifene for dyspareunia if the primary cancer was a nonhormone sensitive cancer.

○ Encourage partner communication: consider psychotherapy or sexual/couples counseling.

- **Brief sexual symptom checklist** for women:
  ○ Are you satisfied with your sexual function?
  ○ How long have you been dissatisfied?
  ○ The problem(s) with your sexual function is:
    - Little or no interest in sex
    - Decreased genital sensation
    - Decreased vaginal lubrication
    - Difficulty obtaining orgasm
    - Pain during sex
    - Other
  ○ Which problem is the most bothersome?
  ○ Would you like to discuss it with your physician?

OVARIAN PROTECTION DURING CHEMOTHERAPY

Ovarian protection during chemotherapy has been investigated. Primary outcomes are resumption of menstruation and prevention of chemotherapy-induced ovarian failure; with pregnancy as a secondary outcome, if desired. Ovarian reserve is assessed by drawing follicle stimulating hormone (FSH) and anti-Müllerian hormone (AMH) laboratories. Gonadal suppression with gonadotropin-releasing hormone (GnRH) agonist treatment has not been shown to significantly protect ovarian function or resumption of menses after completion of chemotherapy; no protective effect was seen based on age, type of chemotherapy, type of malignancy, or GnRH analog type. There was no evidence that gonadal suppression protected any ovarian reserve parameters including FSH, antra follicle count, or AMH levels (3).

FERTILITY PRESERVATION

- It is important to discuss the risk of infertility and fertility preservation options in those patients anticipating cancer treatment. Address fertility preservation as early as possible before treatment starts. Document the discussion in the medical record (Table 6.1).

Table 6.1 Chemotherapeutic Drugs and Risk of Infertility	
Definite	Chlorambucil Cyclophosphamide L-Phenylalanine mustard Nitrogen mustard Busulfan Procarbazine
Probable	Doxorubicin Vinblastine Cytosine arabinoside Cisplatin Nitrosoureas m-AMSA Etoposide
Unlikely	Methotrexate Fluorouracil Mercaptopurine Vincristine
Unknown	Bleomycin

- Refer those patients who express an interest, or are ambivalent about fertility preservation, to reproductive specialists.
  - Present both embryo and oocyte cryopreservation.
  - Discuss ovarian transposition if whole pelvic radiation therapy (WP-XRT) is part of recommended therapy: surgical manipulation/transposition should be performed close to the initiation of XRT due to potential remigration of the ovaries to the pelvis.
  - Inform patients there are insufficient data on GnRH analogs as a fertility preservation method.
  - Inform patients of conservative surgical options:
    - Radical trachelectomy: for cervical cancer patients with 1A2 to 1B1 tumors less than 2 cm in diameter, negative frozen section endocervical curettage (ECC), non–high-risk histology, and variably with invasion less than 1 cm.
    - Ovarian cystectomy can be considered for early ovarian cancers/low malignant potential (LMP) tumors—albeit with a higher risk of recurrence.
    - Completion hysterectomy bilateral salpingo-oophorectomy (BSO) can also be considered after completion of childbearing for early staged ovarian cancers, medically treated stage I uterine cancers, and stage 1A1 cervcial cancers treated with conization.
- For children: use established methods of fertility preservation (oocyte cryopreservation) for postpubertal minor children, with patient assent, if appropriate, and parent or guardian consent.
- Ovarian tissue cryopreservation and transplantation: harvesting of oocytes can be rapidly stimulated and is cycle-day independent now. Ovarian stimulation

protocols using aromatase inhibitors may reduce the concern for stimulation of estrogen receptor–positive cancers (gynecologic and breast).

- Pregenetic screening: if patient is known positive for a mutation (e.g., *BRCA*), then embryo screening can be recommended.
- In patients of reproductive age with intact reproductive organs, birth control should be administered due to the high risk of teratogenicity from cytotoxic chemotherapeutics as well as biologics (4).
- Cervical cancer exclusive of neuroendocrine and adenoma malignum
  - Stage IA1:
    - Lymphovascular space invasion (LVSI) absent: a cold knife cone (CKC) (preferably) or loop electrosurgical excision procedure (LEEP) with 3 mm negative margins is adequate therapy. If margins on the CKC are positive, repeat CKC should be performed. Consideration of simple trachelectomy if fertility is desired is another option.
    - LVSI present: a cone biopsy with negative 3 mm margins with a pelvic lymph node dissection (P-LND) and consideration of para-aortic (PA) LND can be performed. A radical trachelectomy with P-LND can also be considered.
  - Stage IA2:
    - Radical trachelectomy with P-LND with/without PA-LND
    - Consideration of CKC/LEEP: with 3 mm of negative margins; if positive margins: repeat CKC or simple trachelectomy with P-LND with/without PA-LND or
  - Stage IB1: a radical trachelectomy with P-LND with/without PA-LND can be considered. The standard maximum tumor size is <2 cm and should not be of a high-risk pathology. Some studies have shown outcomes in patients with larger tumor sizes, but the risk of needing adjuvant therapies was 64% and subsequent infertility follows.
- Uterine cancer
  - Hormonal therapy: PO high-dose progestins (180–600 mg divided doses daily) or a high-dose intrauterine device (IUD) for 3 to 6 months has been used. Repeat endometrial sampling should occur at 3 to 6 months. If regression is demonstrated, the patient can attempt conception. If persistence or progression is demonstrated, a hysterectomy with staging as appropriate should be recommended.
  - Ovarian preservation: some literature is now documenting safety of ovarian preservation at the time of staging hysterectomy. Counseling is recommended if ovarian preservation is considered. Early age of onset of uterine cancer can signal a genetic syndrome (hereditary nonpolyposis colorectal cancer [HNPCC], which has a 10% chance of ovarian cancer) and other studies have documented a 25% rate of adnexal pathology in younger patients. Without a BSO, comprehensive surgical staging is not complete and there is always the risk of undiagnosed adnexal pathology. Consider salpingectomy if ovarian preservation is performed. Cardiovascular risk factors can be modifiable, whereas cancer cannot. Consider hyperstimulation and egg retrieval with cryopreservation and a gestational surrogate if fertility is desired.

- Ovarian cancer: consider hyperstimulation and egg retrieval with cryopreservation of the unaffected ovary.
  - Early-stage epithelial, germ cell, sex cord, or stromal tumors:
    - Ovarian cystectomy or unilateral salpingo-oophorectomy (USO) with staging to include LND, staging biopsies, omental biopsy.
    - If the patient was initially unstaged:
      - Low-risk germ cell tumor: observe and treat upon identification of recurrence.
      - For epithelial, high risk germ cell, sex cord, or stromal tumors: consider staging surgery followed by recommended adjuvant therapies.
        - Advanced stage: surgical debulking with recommended adjuvant therapies.

RADIATION THERAPY AND FERTILITY

- The ovaries are the most radiosensitive organs, with only 5 to 15 Gy of XRT causing sterility.
- Age does play a role in the risk of infertility with XRT. The older a woman is when receiving XRT to the ovaries, the higher her risk of ovarian failure.
- Operative procedures performed to protect the ovaries from XRT include midline oophoropexy (moving the ovaries behind the uterus) or transposition above the pelvic brim.
- Other efforts utilized to protect the ovaries from XRT damage are pelvic shielding.
- Cortical stripping with cryopreservation, oocyte retrieval with cryopreservation, in vitro fertilization with embryo cryopreservation, or oophorectomy with cryopreservation and subsequent reimplantation of ovarian tissue are all other strategies used for fertility preservation.

REFERENCES

1. Quirk F, Haughie S, Symonds T. The use of the sexual function questionnaire as a screening tool for women with sexual dysfunction. *J Sex Med.* 2005;2(4):469-477.
2. Perez K, Gadgil M, Dizon DS. Sexual ramifications of medical illness. *Clin Obstet Gynecol.* 2009;52(4):691-701.
3. Elgindy E, Sibai H, Abdelghani A, et al. Protecting ovaries during chemotherapy through gonad suppression: a systematic review and meta-analysis. *Obstet Gynecol.* July 2015;126(1):187-195.
4. Loren AW, Mangu PB, Beck LN, et al. Fertility preservation for patients with cancer: American Society of Clinical Oncology clinical practice guideline update. *J Clin Oncol.* July 1, 2013;31(19):2500-2510.

Cancer in Pregnancy

Cancer occurs in one woman per every 1,000 live births, with approximately 4,000 cases of concurrent pregnancy and maternal malignancy each year. The most common cancer in pregnancy is breast cancer. The most common cancer of the female reproductive system in pregnancy is cervical cancer.

- If cancer is diagnosed prior to 24 weeks gestation, the patient can decide to terminate the pregnancy.
- If a malignancy is diagnosed after fetal viability, treatment can be delayed until the late second trimester, third trimester, or after delivery, depending on the specific clinical situation.

RADIATION THERAPY IN PREGNANCY

Radiation therapy (XRT) has different effects on a fetus depending on the stage of fetal development at the time of radiation exposure.

- At preimplantation, the effects are "all or nothing" meaning that XRT will either kill the embryo or not affect it at all, although there are recent reports of increased rates of fetal malformations with XRT prior to implantation.
- Organogenesis occurs 8 weeks after fertilization. The main fetal effect of XRT during organogenesis is intrauterine growth restriction but a wide array of congenital structural deformities can occur. With doses of greater than 1 Gy, morphologic anomalies, and mental retardation, may develop.
- The main effect of XRT in the fetal stage is resultant cognitive impairment. The central nervous system (CNS) is the most sensitive until about 25 weeks. Intrauterine growth restriction can also occur with doses greater than 0.5 Gy.
- The recommended maximum dose of XRT during pregnancy is 0.5 Gy (Table 6.2).
- There are three principal sources of XRT exposure to the fetus during maternal XRT: photon leakage through the treatment head of the machine, scatter XRT emanating from the imaging equipment, and internal scatter within the mother from the treatment beams. Fetal XRT exposure can be reduced by external shielding, but internal scatter cannot be modified.

CHEMOTHERAPY IN PREGNANCY

- The background rate of fetal anomalies for all pregnancies is 2% to 3%. The risk of anomalies with chemotherapy in the first trimester is 6% using a single-agent drug regimen and 17% with combination therapy. If folate antagonists are excluded, the risk is reduced to 6%.
- Chemotherapeutic agents commonly used during pregnancy are vinca alkaloids, doxorubicin, and cisplatin. Alkylators such as cisplatin and doxorubicin

Table 6.2 Fetal Radiation Dose per Radiologic Exam Type	
Type of examination	**Fetal dose range in cGy**
Chest x-ray	0.00006
KUB	0.15–0.26
Lumbar spine	0.65
Pelvis	0.2–0.35
Hip	0.13–0.2
Intravenous pyelogram	0.47–0.82
Upper GI series	0.17–0.48
Barium enema	0.18–1.14
Mammography	0.00001
CT head	0.007
CT upper abdomen	0.04
CT pelvis	2.5
99-Tc bone scan	0.15
KUB, kidneys, ureters, bladder	

can carry a 14% risk of fetal anomalies in the first trimester and 4% in the second trimester. Vinca alkaloids are particularly useful during the first trimester and do not cross the placenta. Doxorubicin can be used in the first trimester of pregnancy. The multidrug resistance (MDR1) P-glycoprotein is found in higher amounts of the endometrium and placenta. MDR1 may provide protection for the fetus. Cisplatin can cause a 50% risk of intrauterine growth restriction, bilateral neonatal hearing loss, or leukopenia. Antimetabolites can cause cranial nasal dystocia, auditory malformations, micrognathia, and limb deformities.

- Chemotherapy administration should be avoided within 3 weeks of the expected date of delivery because of: maternal myelosuppression; nadirs of blood components; increased risk of infection; and decreased wound healing for procedures such as episiotomy and cesarean section. Breastfeeding is contraindicated for women who are on active chemotherapy regimens to avoid transmission to the baby through breast milk.

CERVICAL CANCER IN PREGNANCY

- Cervical cancer occurs in approximately 1.2 to 10.6 cases per 10,000 deliveries. Pregnant patients are 3.1 times more likely to be diagnosed with stage I disease versus nonpregnant patients. There is no difference in survival in pregnant versus nonpregnant patients. Treatment of preinvasive lesions can be delayed until after delivery as the progression of dysplasia to a higher grade postpartum is 7%.
- Cervical cancer in pregnancy is diagnosed via cervical biopsy of gross lesions or colposcopic-directed biopsy of lesions concerning for invasion. Endocervical curettage is not performed during pregnancy.

- Conization is indicated if: there is persistent severe cervical dysplasia suggestive of an invasive lesion; minimal stromal invasion found on cervical biopsy; or if invasive disease cannot be ruled out by colposcopy and biopsy alone. In the first trimester, 24% of patients undergoing cervical conization experienced fetal loss (1). In the third trimester, conization was complicated by high blood loss but no loss of pregnancy, and a 10% pregnancy loss in the second trimester (2). Another report (3) detailed a 9% risk of hemorrhage and a 4% risk of delayed bleeding. There may be an increased rate of preterm deliveries. Cold knife cervical conization (CKC) is possibly better than loop electrosurgical excision procedure (LEEP) in pregnancy because it is easier to control the size of the specimen with a CKC. Furthermore, a loop is difficult to pass through the more edematous cervix that occurs with pregnancy. A coin-shaped biopsy is preferred in pregnant patients rather than a cone-shaped biopsy. The timing of the biopsy should be between 14 and 20 weeks gestation. Placement of a McDonald cerclage at the time of a cervical excision procedure may be considered.
- Progression of cancer during pregnancy is probably rare. Treatment delay can be considered for early-stage cancers diagnosed after 20 weeks. Longer delay to let an earlier pregnancy proceed to term is controversial. Spontaneous abortion occurs at doses of 40 Gy. 27% of patients do not pass the conceptus spontaneously and require evacuation. In patients with advanced stage cancers, near term, a short delay is permissible, followed by radiotherapy within 2 to 3 weeks of delivery. The mode of delivery of pregnant patients with cervical cancer is controversial. Vaginal delivery may be possible with small volume tumors. Cesarean delivery can decrease the risk of hemorrhage and obstructed labor, especially in cases where there is a large friable tumor. Vaginal metastasis or recurrence has been reported. There have been 10 cases of episiotomy site recurrence in women who have had vaginal deliveries. Fourteen percent of patients who had a cesarean section had local metastasis following delivery compared to 59% of patients who delivered vaginally. Some studies showed decreased survival with vaginal delivery (75% vs. 55% for cesarean delivery) (4).
- If a cesarean section is performed, a classical cesarean hysterotomy should be made. This can be followed by radical hysterectomy and/or ovarian transposition. A cesarean that is planned and timed is better than an unplanned delivery because of the possibility of hemorrhage and need for emergent hysterectomy, likely eliminating the opportunity for staging.

OVARIAN NEOPLASMS IN PREGNANCY

Ovarian neoplasms are detected in approximately 2% of all pregnancies and 1 in 8,000 to 20,000 deliveries. Most ovarian neoplasms found in pregnancy are simple ovarian cysts with approximately 70% resolving by the second trimester. Surgical evaluation is indicated in the second trimester if the mass persists and is greater than 6 to 8 cm, rapidly increasing in size, or complex. Torsion can occur in 5% to 15% of pregnant patients and can often occur during the time when the uterus is rapidly growing during the first 16 weeks of pregnancy or during the time of uterine involution postpartum. 17% of these masses can cause obstruction of labor, necessitating cesarean delivery. Surgical treatment, if indicated, is usually unilateral cystectomy. If malignant, at minimum, unilateral oophorectomy with staging procedures and cytoreduction is indicated.

* Malignancy is found in 2% to 6% of adnexal masses. Most ovarian cancers in pregnancy are found at stage I, likely due to incidental early detection during fetal ultrasound.
* A tumor marker that remains unchanged during pregnancy is lactate dehydrogenase (LDH). CA-125 has limited usefulness in pregnancy because it is nonspecific and levels can fluctuate throughout pregnancy.
* Germ cell tumors are the most common ovarian neoplasms found during pregnancy and mature teratomas are the most common histologic type. The most common malignant germ cell tumor is a dysgerminoma. Dysgerminomas comprise about 30% of all ovarian malignancies found during pregnancy. They have a significant rate of bilaterality (10%–15%). Because these neoplasms can rapidly increase in size, they have a tendency to cause pain, become incarcerated in the pouch of Douglas, and can acutely torse. In a study of pregnant patients with dysgerminoma, obstructed labor occurred in 33% of patients and fetal death occurred in 24% (5). Treatment of dysgerminomas is primarily surgical. At minimum, a unilateral salpingo-oophorectomy is performed along with ipsilateral pelvic and para-aortic lymph node dissection and staging biopsies. The rate of recurrence is approximately 10% for disease confined to one ovary. Other germ cell tumors that can occur during pregnancy are immature teratomas and endodermal sinus tumors. Treatment is primarily surgical and fertility preserving surgery is usually feasible.

  In patients with advanced dysgerminoma, adjuvant chemotherapy is indicated. All patients with nondysgerminoma tumors except for stage IA grade 1 immature teratoma should receive adjuvant chemotherapy. Regimens include bleomycin, etoposide, cisplatin and vinblastine, cisplatin, bleomycin, which have had favorable outcomes during pregnancy for the mother and infant.
* Sex cord stromal tumors such as granulosa cell tumors and Sertoli–Leydig tumors are uncommon during pregnancy, but when they do occur, they are associated with rupture, hemoperitoneum, and labor dystocia. Treatment is surgical, with staging and fertility preserving surgery.
* Epithelial ovarian cancers diagnosed during pregnancy have the same prognosis as in nonpregnant patients. Surgical staging should be performed. The administration of chemotherapy during the second and third trimesters is feasible if indicated for advanced disease. Ovarian tumors of low malignant potential are usually found at stage I and clinical outcomes are favorable.

OTHER GYNECOLOGIC CANCERS IN PREGNANCY

Other gynecologic malignancies are quite rare during pregnancy:

* Vaginal cancer, if diagnosed during pregnancy, may be of clear cell histology, especially if the patient had a history of diethylstilbestrol (DES) exposure. Symptoms/signs include a vaginal mass and abnormal vaginal discharge or bleeding. Treatment is with chemotherapy and radiotherapy starting postpartum for most stages.
* Vulvar cancer may present with symptoms of vulvar irritation and pruritus, or with a visible mass. Surgical treatment should be delayed until the second

trimester, with the groin node dissection occurring after delivery in order to minimize the surgical morbidity during pregnancy. Vaginal delivery is feasible after surgical excision as long as the vulvar wound is healed and there is no potential for dystocia from introital scarring.

- Endometrial cancer associated with pregnancy is usually diagnosed postpartum. The prognosis is usually favorable as most tumors are focal and well differentiated.

REFERENCES

1. Averette HE, Nasser N, Yankow SL, Little WA. Cervical conization in pregnancy. Analysis of 180 operations. *Am J Obstet Gynecol.* 1970;106(4):543-549.
2. Hannigan EV. Cervical cancer in pregnancy. *Clin Obstet Gynecol.* 1990;33(4):837-845.
3. Robinson WR, Webb S, Tirpack J, et al. Management of cervical intraepithelial neoplasia during pregnancy with LOOP excision. *Gynecol Oncol.* 1997;64(1):153-155.
4. Jones WB, Shingleton HM, Russell A, et al. Cervical carcinoma and pregnancy. A national patterns of care study of the American College of Surgeons. *Cancer.* 1996;77(8):1479-1488.
5. Karlen JR, Akbari A, Cook WA. Dysgerminoma associated with pregnancy. *Obstet Gynecol.* 1979;53(3):330-335.

SURVIVORSHIP CARE FOR GYNECOLOGIC MALIGNANCIES

7

SURVEILLANCE GUIDELINES

- At completion of primary surgery and/or initial adjuvant treatment, patients should be counseled regarding the purpose of follow-up.
- History and physical examination should include a vaginal speculum examination, bimanual exam, and rectal examination. There is no evidence for the regular use of any imaging or laboratories; these should only be obtained guided by patient symptoms or physical exam findings. Pap smears of the vaginal cuff are not recommended in patients with a history of endometrial cancer. It is not recommended to perform colposcopy for low grade, or less, Pap tests in women with a history of cervical cancer (1).
- Screening for significant anxiety and depression symptoms should be included and psychosocial support should be offered at each visit.
- Referral for palliative care for women with advanced or relapsed gynecologic cancer is important for quality of life (QOL). Avoidance of unnecessary treatments at the end of life reduces patient and family discomfort.
- In addition to cancer-specific follow-up, all women should have a primary care provider (PCP) who provides them with routine health care assessments to include hypertension (HTN), breast cancer screening, and bone density assessment. On discharge from oncologic care, women and their primary care physician should receive specific information on which symptoms to be aware of and to seek additional assessment for.
- Cost of surveillance in ovarian cancer: an additional $26 million will be needed to identify the 5% of women with recurrence seen only on CT. 95% of patients had either elevated CA-125 or office visit findings at the time of recurrence. The surveillance cost for the U.S. ovarian cancer population for 2 years after diagnosis and surgery is $32.5 billion using National Comprehensive Cancer Network (NCCN) guidelines and $58 billion if one CT scan is obtained (2).
- **Rustin Guidelines**: the EORTC 55955 reported that there was no evidence of a survival benefit with early treatment of relapse on the basis of a raised CA-125 concentration alone, and therefore the value of routine measurement of CA-125 in the survival care of patients with ovarian cancer who attain a complete response after first-line treatment is not proven. Thus, relevant therapy, not timing, is vital (3).

UTERINE CANCER

- Low-risk disease (include: stage I, grades 1 to 2): surveillance should include a history, physical exam and pelvic exam with visual inspection of the vaginal cuff. The time interval is: every 6 months for 1–2 years, then annually. Pap smears are not recommended.

- High-risk disease surveillence includes those with stage I grade 3 disease, stage II and higher—all grades. Surveillance should include a history, physical exam and pelvic exam with visual inspection of the vaginal cuff. Time interval is: every 3 months for 2 years, every 6 months up to year 5, then annually. Pap smears are not recommended.

OVARIAN AND TUBAL CANCER

- Surveillance should include a history, physical exam and pelvic exam with visual inspection of the vaginal cuff. The time interval is: every 3 months for 2 years, every 6 months up to year 5, then annually.
- Genetic testing should be performed on all high grade serous tubo-ovarian cancer patients for *BRCA 1/2* and other identified high–risk-associated genes.
- Women with germ cell tumors should have laboratory testing to include the tumor marker that was elevated at the time of presentation.

CERVICAL CANCER, VULVAR, AND VAGINAL CANCER

- Surveillance should include a history, physical exam and pelvic exam with visual inspection of the vaginal cuff. The time interval is: every 3 months for 2 years, every 6 months up to year 5, then annually.
- Vaginal screening with cytology alone should be done no more than once a year. Atypical squamous cells of undetermined significance (ASCUS) and low grade squamous intraepithelial lesions (LSIL) are low-risk results and should not be further assessed with colposcopy.
- Well-woman care should include smoking cessation.

MELANOMA PATIENTS

Melanoma patients: the earlier recommendations do not apply and follow-up should be guided by the current literature associated with cytotoxic, biologic, and immunotherapies (4,5) (Tables 7.1 through 7.4).

Table 7.1 Endometrial Cancer Surveillance Recommendation

Variable		Months			Years	
		0–12	12–24	24–36	3–5	>5
Review of symptoms and physical examination	Low risk (stage IA grade 1 or 2)	Every 6 months	Yearly	Yearly	Yearly	Yearly
	Intermediate risk (stage IB–II)	Every 3 months	Every 6 months	Every 6 months	Every 6 months	Yearly
	High risk (stage III/IV, serous or clear cell)	Every 3 months	Every 3 months	Every 6 months	Every 6 months	Yearly
Pap test/cytologic evidence		Not indicated	Not indicated	Not indicated	Not indicate	Not indicated
CA-125		Insufficient data to support routine use	Insufficient data to support routine use	Insufficient data to support routine use	Insufficient data to support routine use	Insufficient data to support routine use
Radiographic imaging (CXR, PET/CT, MRI)		Insufficient data to support routine use	Insufficient data to support routine use	Insufficient data to support routine use	Insufficient data to support routine use	Insufficient data to support routine use
Recurrence suspected		CT and/or PET scan; CA-125	CT and/or PET scan; CA-125	CT and/or PET scan; CA-125	CT and/or PET scan; CA-125	CT and/or PET scan; CA-125

CXR, chest x-ray.

Table 7.2 Epithelial Ovarian Cancer Surveillance Recommendations

Variable	Months				Years	
	0–12	12–24	24–36	3–5	>5
Review of symptoms and physical examination	Every 3 months	Every 3 months	Every 4–6 months	Every 6 months	Yearly
Pap test/cytologic evidence	Not indicated	Not indicated	Not indicated	Not indicated	Not indicated
CA-125	Optional	Optional	Optional	Optional	Optional
Radiographic imaging (CXR, PET/CT, MRI)	Insufficient data to support routine use	Insufficient data to support routine use	Insufficient data to support routine use	Insufficient data to support routine use	Insufficient data to support routine use
Recurrence suspected	CT and/or PET scan; CA-125	CT and/or PET scan; CA-125	CT and/or PET scan; CA-125	CT and/or PET scan; CA-125	CT and/or PET scan; CA-125

Table 7.3 Nonepithelial Ovarian Cancer (Germ Cell and Sex-Cord Stromal Tumors) Surveillance Recommendations

Variable		Months			Years		
		0–12	12–24	24–36	3–5	>5
Review of symptoms and physical examination	Germ cell tumors	Every 2–4 months	Every 2–4 months	Yearly	Yearly	Yearly
	Sex-cord stromal tumors	Every 2–4 months	Every 2–4 months	Every 6 months	Every 6 months	Every 6 months
Serum tumor markers	Germ cell tumors	Every 2–4 months	Every 2–4 months	Not indicated	Not indicated	Not indicated
	Sex-cord stromal tumors	Every 2–4 months	Every 2–4 months	Every 6 months	Every 6 months	Every 6 months
Radiographic imaging (CXR, CT, MRI)	Germ cell tumors	Not indicated unless tumor marker normal at initial presentation	Not indicated unless tumor marker normal at initial presentation	Not indicated	Not indicated	Not indicated
	Sex-cord stromal tumors	Insufficient data to support routine use	Insufficient data to support routine use	Insufficient data to support routine use	Insufficient data to support routine use	Insufficient data to support routine use
Recurrence suspected		CT scan, tumor markers	CT scan, tumor markers	CT scan, tumor markers	CT scan, tumor markers	CT scan, tumor markers

CXR, chest x-ray.

Table 7.4 Cervical, Vulvar, and Vaginal Cancer Surveillance Recommendations

Variable		Months			Years	
		0–12	12–24	24–36	3–5	>5
Review of symptoms and physical examination	Low risk (early stage, treated with surgery alone, no adjuvant therapy)	Every 6 months	Every 6 months	Yearly	Yearly	Yearly
	High risk (advanced stage, treated with primary chemotherapy/ XRT or surgery plus adjuvant therapy)	Every 3 months	Every 3 months	Every 6 months	Every 6 months	Yearly
Pap test/ cytologic evidence		Yearly	Yearly	Yearly	Yearly	Yearly
Recurrence suspected		CT and/ or PET scan	CT and/ or PET scan	CT and/ or PET scan	CT and/ or PET scan	CT and/ or PET scan

XRT, radiation therapy.

SURVIVORSHIP GUIDELINES

A patient is considered a cancer survivor from the time of diagnosis, through the rest of her life.

• Care of the survivor should include the following: prevention and surveillance of new and recurrent cancers, and assessment of late psychosocial and physical effects. Intervention for consequences of cancer and treatment include late effects of treatment, medical comorbidities, psychologic distress, and financial or social concerns. Coordination of care between primary care providers and specialists is necessary to ensure that all of the survivor's health needs are met.

  ○ An annual periodic assessment is recommended to determine any needs and necessary interventions. This review is to include current disease status, performance status, medication review, medical comorbidity management, and potential reversible causes for any symptoms due to prior treatment.

  ○ Symptom review should include assessment of the following:

   ▪ Cardiac toxicity: shortness of breath (SOB), chest pain, paroxysmal nocturnal dyspnea, especially if there is a history of anthracycline administration.

   ▪ Anxiety and depression: bothered more than half the day with little interest or pleasure in doing things, days feeling down, depressed, or hopelessness, or not being able to control or stop worrying.

- Cognitive function: is there difficulty multitasking or paying attention, difficulty remembering things, or is the thought process slower?
- Fatigue: is there persistent fatigue despite a good night's sleep and does the fatigue interfere with usual activities?
- Pain: is there any pain score that should be documented?
- Sexual function: are there any concerns regarding sexual function or activity in the patient or with the partner, and are these concerns causing distress personally or within the relationship?
- Sleep: are there problems falling asleep or staying asleep? Is there excessive sleepiness? Is snoring a problem? Does the partner notice sleep apnea?
- Healthy lifestyle: is regular physical activity worked into each day? Is a healthful diet eaten each day?
- Vaccination: seasonal flu vaccine and other indicated vaccinations.
- Secondary malignancies may occur in survivors due to: genetic predisposition, environmental exposures, prior oncologic therapy (radiation therapy [XRT], alkaloid cytotoxic therapy). Screening for secondary malignancies should be shared between the PCP and the oncology providers.
- Specific toxicities:
  - Cardiac:
    - Causes: often due to anthracycline, can be induced by receptor-targeted therapies (Herceptin), chest irradiation (left-sided breast or mantle XRT), and can take up to 10 years to become evident
    - There are four stages:
      - Stage A:
        - Cardiac risk factors are present but no structural heart disease. Risk factors are: HTN, dyslipidemia, family history of cardiomyopathy, age greater than 65, smoking, obesity, alcoholism, comorbid cardiac diseases (atrial fibrillation, coronary artery disease [CAD], baseline structural heart disease, and personal history of rheumatic fever), and diabetes.
        - Pre-treatment Workup: thorough clinical screening for heart failure should occur within 1 year of completion of anthracycline therapy. A cardiac ECHO should be obtained.
        - Treatment: primary prevention with early detection is suggested. Diet, exercise, blood pressure control, cholesterol lowering medications, and consideration of cardiac remodeling/cardio protective agents.
      - Stage B:
        - Structural heart disease present but no signs or symptoms of heart failure: patients may have left ventricular hypertrophy (LVH), left ventricular diastolic dysfunction, asymptomatic valvular disease, or had a previous myocardial infarction.
        - Pre-treatment Workup: as in stage A with referral to cardiologist for further diagnosis and management.
      - Stage C:
        - Signs and symptoms of heart failure are present with underlying structural heart disease.
        - Management: refer to cardiologist for further diagnosis and management.

- □ Stage D:
  - – Signs and symptoms: advanced structural heart disease with significant symptoms of heart failure are present at rest despite maximal medical therapy and interventions.
  - – Management: refer to cardiologist for further diagnosis and management.
- ○ Pain:
  - ▪ Pre-treatment Workup: quantify, qualify, and determine the etiology and pathophysiology of the pain. It is important to discuss with the patient goals for comfort and function, and determine if it is a specific cancer pain syndrome.
  - ▪ Pain types: neuropathic from neuromas, or nerve transection. Postsurgical pains from amputation, neck dissection, mastectomy, and thoracotomy. Musculoskeletal pain: myalgias, arthralgias, bone pain, and myofascial pain. Gastrointestinal (GI) discomfort: small bowel obstruction (SBO), partial small bowel obstruction (PSBO), chronic diarrhea, or constipation. Pelvic pain or urinary pain from surgery, XRT, hydronephrosis, or infection.
  - ▪ Management is with physical therapy, pelvic floor exercise, dorsal column stimulation for chronic cystitis or pelvic pain. Neuromodulating selective serotonin reuptake inhibitors (SSRIs)/serotonin and norepinephrine reuptake inhibitors (SNRIs), or gabapentin, can be used in addition to biofeedback, and a bowel regimen to include stool softners. Massage therapy may be an additional resource. Additional means of pain modification can be use of nonsteroidal anti-inflammatory drugs (NSAIDs), narcotics, bowel regimen, a low roughage low residue diet, and hydration. Surgical options, when appropriate, are to bypass, stent, or divert bowel obstructions.
  - ▪ It is important to ensure there is no recurrent tumor with imaging and biopsy.
- ○ Lymphedema: the etiology is usually from lymph node dissection (LND) but may be from XRT, scarring, or tumor obstruction. Referral to a lymphedema specialist is indicated with assistance from compression garments, progressive resistance training, physical therapy with range of motion exercises, and manual lymphatic drainage. Temsirolimus has been shown to assist in guiding postoperative lymphatic drainage.
- ○ Anxiety and depression:
  - ▪ General anxiety disorder or adjustment disorder with anxious mood:
    - □ Symptoms are excessive anxiety that is difficult to control involving: sleep disturbances, restlessness, muscle tension, irritability, difficulty concentrating, and easy fatigue.
    - □ Management: refer for counseling for consideration of medical management.
  - ▪ Panic disorder: acute onset of ≥4 of the following:
    - □ Palpations, sweating, chills or hot flashes, trembling or shaking, sensation of SOB, chest pain or discomfort, nausea, dizziness, out of body experience/being detached from self, fear of dying, fear of losing control, and paraesthesias.

- □ Management: refer for counseling and consideration of medical management.
- Posttraumatic stress disorder:
  - □ Inclusion criteria: recurrent intrusive memory of the trauma or recurrent dreams of the event, avoidance of stimuli associated with the trauma, numbing of general responsiveness, inability to recall traumatic events, feeling of detachment from body, restricted range of emotion, sense of foreshortened future. Increased arousal can manifest as: hypervigilance, exaggerated startle, irritability, difficulty concentrating, and sleep disturbance.
  - □ Management: refer for counseling and consideration of medical management.
- Obsessive compulsive disorder:
  - □ Inclusion criteria: recurrent persistent thoughts, impulses or images that cause marked distress that the person attempts to suppress with some thought or action. This often manifests as repetitive behaviors or mental acts that a person is compelled to perform in response to the obsession to reduce stress or prevent some unrealistic dreaded event.
  - □ Management: refer for counseling and consideration of medical management.
- Major depressive disorder:
  - □ Inclusion criteria: depressed mood or a loss of interest or pleasure in daily activities for more than 2 weeks and this mood represents a change from the person's baseline. There is impaired function in social, occupational, and educational activities. Five of nine of the following specific symptoms must be present nearly every day: depressed mood or irritability present most of the day, nearly every day, as indicated by either subjective report (e.g., feels sad or empty) or observation made by others (e.g., appears tearful); decreased interest or pleasure in most activities most of each day; significant weight change (5%) or change in appetite; change in sleep with either insomnia or hypersomnia; change in activity with either psychomotor agitation or retardation; fatigue or loss of energy; feelings of worthlessness or excessive or inappropriate guilt; concentration is diminished or more indecisiveness is present; there is suicidal ideation (SI) either with SI thoughts or a suicide plan.
  - □ Management: refer for counseling and consideration of medical management versus admission if SI is present.
- ○ Nutrition and weight management: weight gain after cancer diagnosis and treatment is common. Strategies to prevent weight gain should be discussed. Weight gain can exacerbate risk or functional decline, comorbidity, and possible cancer recurrence or death, and reduce QOL. Nutritious weight gain for underweight patients should be encouraged. Weight maintenance for normal weight patients should also be encouraged.
  - Principles of weight loss: limit foods that are high in calories and low in nutrients; substitute high-calorie foods with energy-dense foods such as vegetables, fruits, soups, whole grains; portion control, smaller plates, one

serving limits; and routinely evaluate food labels. There is no evidence to support the use of weight loss supplements in cancer survivors.
- Principles of weight gain: evaluate appetite changes and eating patterns.
○ If appetite stimulants indicated:
  - Megace 40 mg daily: take care due to possible increased risk of venous thromboembolism (VTE).
  - Mirtazapine 15 mg daily (Remeron): this is also an antidepressant.
○ Assess cancer treatment effects (surgery, XRT): GI dysmotility, swallowing and dysphagia, oropharyngeal anatomic changes, and bowel dysfunction can all contribute to lower PO intake or GI absorption.
○ For ovarian cancer and post whole pelvic radiation therapy (WP-XRT) survivors: low-fiber nonbulky-vegetable diets (minimizing lettuce and cruciferous vegetables) can be encouraged. Be mindful of GI tract reconstruction/anastomoses.
○ Comorbidities that may limit exercise or modify metabolism: cardiovascular (CV) disease, arthritis, DM, renal disease, liver disease, mood disorders, thyroid disease, GI disease, medication use, dental health.

REFERENCES

1. Salani R, Backes FJ, Fung MF. Posttreatment surveillance and diagnosis of recurrence in women with gynecologic malignancies: Society of Gynecologic Oncologists recommendations. *Am J Obstet Gynecol.* 2011;204(6):466-478.
2. Armstrong A, Otvos B, Singh S, Debernardo R. Evaluation of the cost of CA-125 measurement, physical exam, and imaging in the diagnosis of recurrent ovarian cancer. *Gynecol Oncol.* December 2013;131(3):503-507.
3. Rustin GJ, van der Burg ME, Griffin CL, et al. Early versus delayed treatment of relapsed ovarian cancer (MRC OV05/EORTC 55955): a randomised trial. *Lancet.* October 2, 2010;376(9747):1155-1163.
4. Elit L, Reade CJ. Recommendations for follow-up care for gynecologic cancer survivors. *Obstet Gynecol.* December 2015;126(6):1207-1214.
5. Rimel BJ, Burke WM, Higgins RV, et al. Improving quality and decreasing cost in gynecologic oncology care. Society of gynecologic oncology recommendations for clinical practice. *Gynecol Oncol.* May 2015;137(2):280-284.

PALLIATIVE CARE

8

PALLIATIVE CARE

Palliative care is an area of health care that specifically focuses on relieving and preventing the suffering of patients from diagnosis onward. It facilitates effective communication between the patient and practitioner, and it supports the goals of cure, life prolongation, quality of life (QOL), or acceptance of death. These efforts are not initially end-of-life care but can facilitate discussion. It is also helpful in determining code status and signing of a physician orders for life sustaining treatment (POLST) form. Discussion can provide effective management of expectations, treatment-associated toxicities, and channels for supportive care within the medical field and/or community.

- The ultimate goal is to provide the best possible QOL for people facing the pain, symptoms, and stress of serious illness. It is appropriate throughout all stages of an illness. It can be provided along with treatments that are meant to cure.
- Palliative therapies not only improve a patient's QOL, but also have been shown to extend life. In a study of patients with metastatic non–small cell lung cancer, patients were randomized to receive either early palliative care integrated with standard oncologic care or standard oncologic care alone. Despite the fact that fewer patients in the early palliative care group than in the standard care group received aggressive end-of-life care (33% vs. 54%, $p = 0.05$), median survival was longer among patients receiving early palliative care (11.6 vs. 8.9 months, $p = 0.02$) (1).
- Palliative surgical or medical intervention can relieve symptoms and lead to less pain for the patient. In these instances, correction of the terminal disease is not anticipated or achieved. Approximately 10% of procedures are performed for palliative intent, not cure.

HOSPICE

Hospice care is palliative care that typically occurs when a patient is considered to be terminal, or within 6 months of death.

END-OF-LIFE DISCUSSION

It can be quite difficult discussing the implications of a life-threatening illness with a patient and the family. There are a few things to keep in mind when discussing terminal disease and end-of-life care:
- Hope is important, but not a plan.
- Emotions run high: negative emotions such as fear, anxiety, frustration, and depression are common and are manifested in a variety of ways by patients and their caregivers.
- Respect is important. Health care providers should listen to and honor the perspectives and choices of patients and their families.

MULTIDISCIPLINARY APPROACH

A multidisciplinary approach is important.

- Effective palliative care involves a team approach. This involves the patient and her physician and may also include palliative care physicians; specialists; general practitioners; nurses; nursing assistants or home health aides; social workers; chaplains; and physical, occupational, and speech therapists.

COMMUNICATION

Communication is the most important factor in terminal care.

- Timing of discussion: soon after the diagnosis of advanced or recurrent cancer. Options for palliative care should be discussed.
- Ensure that legal documents are drawn up: these include a living will, power of attorney, advance directive.
- Specific issues to address with the patient: the need for ventilatory support, total parenteral nutrition (TPN), the need for emergent surgery, interventional procedures for relief of acute symptoms, invasive procedure endpoints and indications, do not resuscitate (DNR) consent, timing for discontinuation of supportive measures, location for death (hospital vs. home).

DELIVERING BAD NEWS

SPIKES METHOD

This is a six-step protocol.

- Step 1: Set up the interview: arrange for privacy, involve significant others and family, sit down, connect with the patient and family, minimize interruptions (phone/pager on vibrate).
- Step 2: assess the patient's Perception: what is your understanding of your situation?
- Step 3: obtain the patients Invitation: how would you like for me to give you information about your test results?
- Step 4: Knowledge and information giving to the patient: provide a warning: "I'm afraid I have bad news." Ensure the appropriate level of comprehension and vocabulary of the patient. Avoid excessive bluntness. Give the information in small bites and assess the patient's understanding at each step.
- Step 5: address the patient's Emotions with empathetic response: observe and identify the patient's emotion; let the patient know you have identified the emotion.
- Step 6: Strategy and summary: establish a plan to address the patient's goals of care and QOL as well as fears. Frankly discuss expectations and goals for both patient and loved ones.

MANAGEMENT OF SPECIFIC SYMPTOMS

- Dyspnea: causes and treatment options
  - Pneumonia: antibiotics and pulmonary toilet.
  - Lymphangitic tumor: diuretics, glucocorticoids.
  - Pneumonitis, radiation therapy (XRT) or chemotherapy induced: glucocorticoids.
  - Pulmonary embolus (PE): anticoagulation, inferior vena cava (IVC) filter.

- o Pleural effusion: indwelling catheter, thoracentesis, video-assisted thoracic surgery (VATS), pleurodesis (bleomycin, talc, tetracycline).
- o Airway obstruction by tumor or adenopathy: XRT, glucocorticoids, stent.
- o Bronchoconstriction: chronic obstructive pulmonary disease (COPD)/ asthma: bronchodilators, glucocorticoids.
- o Retained or excess secretions: anticholinergic drugs.
- o Massive ascites causing SOB: paracentesis with or without indwelling catheter.
- o Anxiety manifested as hyperventilation: anxiolytics, behavioral therapy.
- o Additional measures: facial cooling with fan, chest physical therapy.
- o Consider supplemental oxygen but this does not always correlate with symptomatic resolution.
- o Systemic opioids.
- Anorexia: reversible causes: constipation, pain, medications, hypercalcemia, mucositis, and bowel obstruction. Treatments: gastrokinetic agents such as metoclopramide, low-dose corticosteroids, progestone agents (Megace), antidepressants (Remeron), cannabinoids such as dronabinol, palliative surgery with bowel diversion.
- Nausea: sixty percent of patients have nausea and vomiting. Causes: usually from various receptors in the gastrointestinal (GI) tract. It is important to rule out cerebral metastasis. Other causes are uremia, electrolyte imbalances, and hypercalcemia. Treatment: use of antiemetics at optimal dosing and route of administration, use scheduled around-the-clock dosing, and add second agent when monotherapy fails rather then switch agents
  - o Dopamine antagonist: chlorpromazine 6.25 mg PO/IM/IV q8 hours; prochlorperazine PO/PR/IM/IV 10 to 50 mg q4 to 8 hours; Metoclopramide 5 to 20 mg PO/IV q2 to 8 hours; haloperidol 0.5 to 1 mg q8 hours PO/IV.
  - o Anticholinergic: clopalamine transdermal 1.5 mg q3 days; hydroxyzine 6.25 to 25 mg qHS.
  - o H1 antihistamine: diphenhydramine POIV/IM 12.5 to 50 mg q6 hours; promethazine PO/IM 12.5 to 25 mg q8 hours.
  - o 5HT3 antagonist: ondansetron P/IV/SL 4 to 20 mg q4 to 8 hours; dolasetron 100 mg PO q24 hours; granisetron 2 mg PO q24 hours; palonosetron 0.01 mg/ kg IV q24 hours, transdermal 3.1 mg q24 hours, IV 0.25 mg q24 hours.
  - o Steroids: dexamethasone PO/IV 4 to 24 mg daily.
  - o Cannabinoids: dronabinol 7.5 to 15 mg PO q3 to 4 hours.
  - o Benzodiazepines: lorazepam IV/PO 0.5 to 2 mg q4 hours.
- Malignant ascites: treatment: paracentesis, indwelling (pleurX) drains, diuretics may relieve ascites associated with portal hypertension from hepatic metastasis. Vascular endothelial growth factor (VEGF) targeting agents reduce ascites well.
- Malignant bowel obstruction:
  - o Types: mechanical: from tumor obstruction. Compressive: from external ascites compression. Functional: from carcinomatosis coating the surface of the bowel obstructing peristalsis.
  - o Treatment:
    - Conservative management: nasogastric tube (NGT), intravenous fluid (IVF), bowel rest NPO, pain, and nausea control. Steroids may reduce bowel edema (decadron 4 mg q6 hours), and octreotide may reduce secretions.

- Surgical: release of adhesions bowel surgery—resection with reanastomosis, bypass or diversion and ostomy, bowel stent, G/J-tube, or hospice. The addition of TPN is expensive and can add an average of 4 to 6 weeks of life.
- Constipation: this can be disease related, or a side effect of antiemetics, or opioids. Treatment: stool softeners, osmotic agents, stimulants, lubricants, and enemas. Bulking agents are not as helpful.
- Terminal hemorrhage: this is defined as rapid blood loss that is internal or external with volume depletion. It occurs in 3% to 14% of patients.
  - It can be classified by cause:
    - Anatomic from tumor invasion or erosion into blood vessels or organs
    - Generalized due to coagulopathy or thrombocytopenia
    - Mixed
  - Common sites are GI, genitourinary (GU), and respiratory.
  - Treatment: volume resuscitation, correction of the underlying coagulopathy, consider interventional radiology (IR) embolization of proximal vessel(s). Specific site indications:
    - Vaginal bleeding: attempts at control can be—with vaginal packing with or without Monsels solution, XRT, IR arterial embolization, endoscopic cautery, surgical ligation of large vessels, excision of bleeding tissue.
    - Hemorrhagic cystitis: treatment can be with continuous bladder irrigation (CBI), cystoscopic coagulation, instillation of 1% alum or methylene blue, or, formalin instillation, which is 80% effective but should be used as a last resort.
    - Palliative measures: apply pressure, use dark towels and suction, consider sedatives. Midazolam is rapid acting and is given IV or SC 2.5 to 5 mg q10 to 15 minutes.
- Bone metastasis: treatment with nonsteroidal anti-inflammatory drugs (NSAIDs), directed XRT, absorptive XRT with strontium, bisphosphonates, or Denosumab is a human monoclonal antibody that binds to and neutralizes the receptor activity of NKB ligand, protecting bone from demineralization. If pathologic fracture is identified, bone stabilizing surgery may be indicated.
- Hypercalcemia: diagnosis is a serum calcium above 10.2 adjusted for albumin. Treatment: IVF, bisphosphonates, calcitonin 2 to 8 IU/kg SQ or IM q12 hours; consider administration of furosemide.
- Brain metastasis: headache is present in 40% to 50% of patients. Seizures occur in 10% to 20% of persons with brain metastasis. Nausea, vomiting, visual changes, and gait disturbance (cerebellar) are other symptoms. First-line therapy is steroids, 4 to 8 mg/day of dexamethasone, followed by XRT 48 hours after onset of steroids. For patients with one to three lesions and good control of systemic disease, targeted XRT or stereotactic radiosurgery can be considered. If stable systemic disease with good treatment options, consultation with neurosurgery for possible resection can also be considered. For patients with one to three lesions and poor control of systemic disease, whole brain radiation therapy (WB-XRT) is recommended. If 4+ lesions are present or there is unresectable disease, WB-XRT is recommended. WB-XRT is delivered in 10 fractions of 3 Gy for a total of 30 Gy, or 15 fractions of 2.5 Gy to a maximum of 37.5 Gy.
- Delirium: common causes are medications, infection, electrolyte abnormalities, hypoxia, uremia, liver failure, urinary retention, and uremia.

- ○ Subtypes
  - Hypoactive subtype: lethargy, sedation, psychomotor retardation, hypoxia, metabolic disturbances, hepatic encephalopathy
  - Hyperactive subtype: agitation, restlessness, hyperactivity, hallucinations, delusions. These symptoms should be correlated with alcohol or drug withdrawal, or potential adverse effects of medication
  - Mixed subtype
- ○ Treatment
  - Nonpharmacologic means is with orientation to the familiar, family presence, no restraints, and use of eye glasses and hearing aids.
  - Medications include haloperidol, chlorpromazine. Olanzapine and risperidone are alternatives to haloperidol. If irreversible hyperactive delirium: lorazepam 1 mg every 3 minute as needed is an option.
- Fatigue: occurs in 60% to 90% of patients, especially those undergoing chemotherapy. Commonly associated symptoms are pain, depression, and insomnia. Most pharmacologic agents have not been found to be statistically beneficial including antidepressants, coQ10, L-carnitine, or central nervous system (CNS) stimulating agents. Yoga has been the only identified exercise regimen to show improvements in fatigue.
- Insomnia: occurs in 30% to 50% of patients. Treatment can be pharmacologic as well as behavioral:
  - ○ Pharmacologic
    - Benzodiazepines (lorazepam, temazepam) and nonbenzodiazepine hypnotics (zolpidem, zaleplon, eszopiclone). These can be associated with lower QOL indices and increased severity of symptoms. Therefore, they should be used in combination with nonpharmacologic measures and for the shortest time possible.
    - Hormonal and herbal products include melatonin, ramelteon.
    - Antidepressants including trazodone, mirtazapine, and paroxetine have been tried. There was no improvement in insomnia but some improvement in depression scores.
  - ○ Cognitive behavioral therapy including stimulus control, sleep restriction, relaxation training, sleep hygiene education, and cognitive therapy can be recommended as first-line therapy. Yoga in a randomized trial demonstrated greater improvements in sleep quality.
- Chemotherapy-induced neuropathy: different prescription and over-the-counter (OTC) medications have been tried, all without much success to include: alpha lipoic acid; neurontin; carnitine.
- Agonal breathing and sounds: treatment can be with glycopyrolate 0.1 to 0.2 mg IV or SQ q4 hours; atropine 0.4 mg SQ q15 minutes, scopolamine 1.5 mg patch.
- Pain: assess and manage per the World Health Organization (WHO) pain ladder. Additional potential interventions: anticonvulsants, antidepressants, muscle relaxants, and corticosteroids.
  - ○ Acute pain syndromes are partially reversible: chemotherapy can induce some of these symptoms as can recent surgery or XRT.
    - Oxaloplatin.
      - □ Symptoms: cold-induced paresthesias and muscle cramping.

□ Prevention: with IV calcium and magnesium supplementation; glutathione may also be beneficial.

- Paclitaxel
  □ Symptoms: include diffuse aching in joints within 3 days of administration and resolve at 7 days.
  □ Prevention: consider alpha-lipoic acid (ALA) and acetyl-l-carnitine (ALC).
    ALA dosing: 600 mg IV once weekly for 3 to 5 weeks then 1,800 mg PO daily.
    ALC dosing: 1 gm PO TID for 8 weeks.
- Treatment for these and other acute pain syndromes: pregabalin titrated to target dose of 150 mg PO TID; venlafaxine 50 mg 1 hour before oxaliplatin infusion and venlafaxine ER 37.5 mg PO BID days 2 to 11: Duloxetine titrated to target dose of 60 mg PO daily for 12 weeks; acupuncture.

○ Chronic pain: 33% of patients have chronic pain after curative-intent treatment.
  - Arthralgias are common in women taking aromatase inhibitors.
  - Surgical pain: phantom pain, neuroma or scar pain, nerve injury pain or postreconstruction pain.
  - XRT pain: to include plexopathies, peripheral nerve entrapment, myelopathy, pelvic pain, osteoradionecrosis, myofascial fibrosis, restricted range of motion, dermatitis, enteritis, cystitis, proctitis, pelvic fractures, secondary malignancies, fistula.
  - Treatment: antidepressants to include tricyclic antidepressants (TCA) and serotonin-norepinephrine reuptake inhibitors (SNRIs); pregabalin and gabapentin; topical lidocaine; NSAIDS; opioids; interventional nerve blocks, intrathecal therapy, joint injection, implantable devices, and vertebroplasty are options; exercise and physical therapy/occupational therapy should be incorporated into treatment. Psychological interventions and massage can be included (2).

ACTIVE DYING (I.E., TRANSITIONING)

Patients will have increased somnolence, increased oral secretions from the inability to swallow, a decreased appetite, potential delusions and/or hallucinations, body temperature fluctuation, decreased urinary output, apnea, agonal breathing, and skin mottling (3).

ETHICAL ISSUES

When the wishes of a patient contradict the physician's management desires and compromise cannot be attained, transfer of care to another physician may be appropriate.

The involvement of a hospital ethical committee may be appropriate at times.

Ethical guidelines:
- Nonmaleficence
- Beneficence
- Autonomy
- Justice

Medical futility: after having an open discussion with the patient about the terminal disease and realistic expectations, the physician needs to determine when it is advisable to move from an aggressive therapeutic approach to supportive care. The pathway for withdrawal of care, once a decision has been made, is as follows:

- Obtain informed consent
- Plan for the procedure and potential side effects
- Address the patient's distress
- Move the patient to an appropriate setting
- Use adequate sedation
- Document the procedure
- Review the outcomes

REFERENCES

1. Temel JS, Greer JA, Muzikansky A. Early palliative care for patients with metastatic non-small cell lung cancer. *N Engl J Med.* 2010;363(8):733-742.
2. Pachman DR, Barton DL, Swetz KM, Loprinzi CL. Troublesome symptoms in cancer survivors: fatigue, insomnia, neuropathy, and pain. *J Clin Oncol.* October 20, 2012;30(30):3687-3696.
3. Landrum LM, Blank S, Chen LM, et al. Comprehensive care in gynecologic oncology: the importance of palliative care. *Gynecol Oncol.* May 2015;137(2):193-202.

STATISTICS AND REFERENCE MATERIAL

9

DEFINITIONS

- **General definitions**
  - Variable—anything manipulated in an experiment.
  - Independent variable—one varied by and under the control of the experimenter.
  - Dependent variable—one that responds to manipulation.
  - Nominal variable—a named category, for example: sex, diagnosis.
  - Ordinal variable—a set of ordered categories, for example: stages of cancer are ordered but the significance between each step is not known.
  - Interval variable—measurement in which the step between is meaningful for example: temperature, age.
  - Ratio—ratio of the numbers has some meaning.
  - Parametric—data that follow a normal distribution.
  - Nonparametric—data that do not follow a normal distribution (nominal and ordinal).
  - Incidence—current number of new events/population at risk in same time interval.
  - Prevalence—total number of events/population at risk. Prevalence should be more than the incidence.
- **Measures of central tendency**
  - Mode—value most often reported.
  - Median—value with half the responses below and half above (nonparametric).
  - Mean—average of all values.
- **Measures of dispersion**
  - Standard deviation (SD) of the mean is the square root of the variance. The smaller the SD, the less each score varies from the mean: 1 SD = 68%, 2 SD = 95.5%, 5 SD = 99%.
  - Variance—the average of the squared differences from the mean (value of point − mean)^2/total number of data points.
  - Range—the difference between the highest value and the lowest value.
  - Percentile—where the result lands out of 100.

METHODS TO ANALYZE DATA

There are two methods to analyze data. Descriptive statistics communicate results, but does not generalize beyond the sample. Inferential statistics communicate the likelihood of these differences occurring by a chance combination of unforeseen variables.

- **Null hypothesis:** by statistical convention, it is assumed that the speculated hypothesis is always wrong and that the observed phenomena simply occur by chance. It is this hypothesis that is to be either nullified or not nullified by the test. When the null hypothesis is nullified, it is possible to conclude that data support the alternative hypothesis.
- **Significance level:** the extent to which the test in question shows that the "**speculated hypothesis**" has or has not been nullified is called its significance level; the higher the significance level, the less likely it is that the phenomena in question could have been produced by chance alone.
- **Statistics for inference** (hypothesis) testing
  - ○ **Confidence intervals (CIs)**—used to indicate the reliability of an estimate. The CI is calculated by 1-alpha.
  - ○ **Standard error (SE)**—this is used to help determine if the result is true or occurs more by chance. SE = SD/square root of sample size. The SE can either be systemic, where the wrong measure is taken each time or random, where the answer is different each time the experiment is run.
  - ○ **Margin of error**—the amount the results are expected to change from one experiment to another.
  - ○ **Central limit theory (CLT)**—if the sample size is sufficiently large ($n > 10$), the mean will normally distribute regardless of the original distribution. This theory allows the parametric assessment of nonparametric data.
  - ○ **Z test**—compares the sample mean with the known population mean.
- **Sensitivity:** sensitivity relates to the test's ability to identify positive results. The sensitivity of a test is the proportion of people who have the disease who test positive for it. For example, a sensitivity of 100% means that the test recognizes all actual positives—that is, all sick people are recognized as being ill. Thus, in contrast to a high-specificity test, a negative result in a high-sensitivity test is used to rule out the disease.

  This can be written as follows:

  Sensitivity = Number of true positives/Number of true positives + Number of false negatives or

  True positives/All positive with disease

  If a test has high sensitivity, then a negative result would suggest the absence of disease.

- **Specificity:** specificity relates to the ability of the test to identify negative results. The specificity of a test is defined as the proportion of patients who do not have the disease who will test negative for it. This can also be written as follows:

  Specificity = Number of true negatives/Number of true negatives + Number of false positives or

  True negatives/All negative with disease.

  The specificity states the ability of a test to determine if the patient tests negative that the patient does not have the disease.

- **Positive predictive value (PPV):** this test reflects the probability that a positive test reflects the underlying condition being tested for.
- **Negative predictive value (NPV):** this test reflects the proportion of subjects with a negative test result who are correctly diagnosed. A high NPV means that

Table 9.1 Sensitivity, Specificity, PPV, and NPV

	Disease positive	Disease negative
Positive exp/screen	A	B
Negative exp/screen	C	D
Sensitivity—True positives/All with disease		A/(A + C)
Specificity—True negatives/All without disease		D/(B + D)
PPV		A/(A + B)
NPV		D/(C + D)
NPV, negative predictive value; PPV, positive predictive value.		

when the test yields a negative result, it is most likely correct in its assessment (Table 9.1).

- **Type I error:** this occurs when one rejects the null hypothesis ($H0$) when it is true. A type I error may be compared to a false positive. The rate of the type I error is called the size of the test and denoted by the Greek letter α (alpha). It usually equals the significance level of a test. In the case of a simple null hypothesis, α is the probability of a type I error. If the null hypothesis is composite, α is the maximum of the possible probabilities of a type I error. The rate of a type I error is related to the CI ($1 - \alpha = $ CI).
- **Type II error:** this occurs when one fails to reject a false null hypothesis. A type II error may be compared to a false negative. The rate of the type II error is denoted by the Greek letter β (beta) and is related to the power of a test ($1 - \beta = $ power) (Table 9.2).
    False positive rate (α) = Type I error = 1 – Specificity = FP/(FP 1 TN)
    False negative rate (β) = Type II error = 1 – Sensitivity = FN/(TP 1 FN)
    Power = Chance of detecting a difference that is really there = $1 - \beta$
    CI = The chance that a true value lies within the specified interval (1–alpha)
    Confidence level = The chance that, with repeated sampling, the range of values actually contains the actual parameter
    Likelihood ratio positive = Sensitivity/(1 – Specificity)
    Likelihood ratio negative = (1 – Sensitivity)/Specificity
- **Alpha** is the cutoff for the ρ value.

Table 9.2 Relations Between Truth/Falseness of the Null Hypothesis and Test Outcomes

	Null hypothesis ($H0$) is true	Null hypothesis ($H0$) is false
Reject null hypothesis	Type I error FP	Correct outcome TP
Fail to reject null hypothesis	Correct outcome TN	Type II error FN
FN, false negative; FP, false positive; TN, true negative; TP, true positive.		

- ρ **value:** a measure of the strength of the evidence against the null hypothesis.

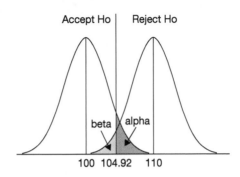

- **One- and two-tailed tests:** if the distribution from which the samples are derived is considered to be normal, Gaussian, or bell shaped, then the test is referred to as a one- or two-tailed T test.
  - A **one-tailed test** evaluates samples that fall within the curve and are excluded if they fall into one of the tails of the curve. For an SD of 95%, the full 5% falls into the single tail of the curve.
  - A **two-tailed test** evaluates samples that fall within the curve and are only excluded if they fall into either one of the tails of the curve. For an SD of 95%, 2.5% falls into each tail. It is recommended that most statistical analysis should be two tailed.
  - A test is called two tailed if the null hypothesis is rejected for values of the test statistic that fall into either tail of its sampling distribution, and it is called one sided if the null hypothesis is rejected only for values of the test statistic falling into one specified tail of its sampling distribution.

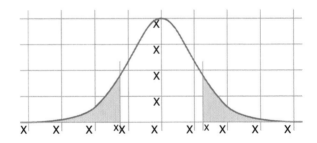

  - If the test is performed using the actual population mean and variance, rather than an estimate from a sample, it would be called a one- or two-tailed **Z test**.
- **Power** is affected by the significance criterion, the magnitude of effect, and the sample size. The beta level is usually set at 0.2. Thus, the power by convention is usually 0.8. There are two ways to perform a power analysis: a priori and posthoc. A priori (before) is the means to estimate for a sufficient sample size. Posthoc analysis is usually not recommended.

○ To decrease the amount of type I error, the alpha level can be reduced (e.g., from 0.05 to 0.01).
○ To decrease the amount of type II error, the sample size can be increased, the effect size can be changed, or the significance criterion can be changed.
- **Attributable risk**—risk of disease or death in a population exposed to some factor of interest minus the risk of those not exposed.

RECEIVER OPERATING CHARACTERISTIC

The receiver operating characteristic (ROC) is the graphical plot of the sensitivity (on the y-axis), or the true positive rate, versus $1 -$ specificity (on the x-axis), or the false positive, for a binary classifier system as its discrimination threshold is varied. The ROC can also be represented equivalently by plotting the fraction of true positives out of all positives (TPR = true positive rate) versus the fraction of false positives out of the negatives (FPR = false positive rate). It reflects the accuracy of the test. The area under the ROC curve is closely related to the Mann–Whitney U test, which tests whether the positives are ranked higher than the negatives. For an optimal test, all points should fall into the upper left quadrant.

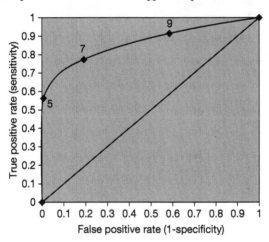

ENDPOINTS OF A STUDY

Endpoints of a study are important for evaluation of progression-free survival (PFS), overall survival (OS), and clinical response. It is necessary to choose good primary endpoints to reflect the effectiveness of the experimental therapy. Surrogate endpoints are often chosen instead because of proposed study length, study cost, and known etiologic associations with the primary endpoint.

PHASES OF TRIALS

The following are the four phases of trials:
- A **phase I trial** is a dose limiting trial. Doses of drugs are tested until a maximum tolerated dose. When 50% to 75% of patients have an adverse event (dose-limiting toxicity [DLT]), the dose one level prior to the DLT dose is

chosen as the maximum tolerated dose (MTD). The MTD is chosen as the dose to proceed with to the next phase trial.

- A **phase II trial** assesses the activity and toxicities of the drug chosen at the MTD in relation to the disease of interest.
- A **phase III trial** assesses efficacy. There are two types of phase III trials; the noninferiority trial and the equivalency trial.
  - The noninferiority trial evaluates two drugs to ensure their outcomes are similar (e.g., cisplatin vs. carboplatin with paclitaxel in ovarian cancer).
  - The equivalency trial evaluates an augmentation in care (adding platinum to radiation therapy [XRT] for cervical cancer vs. XRT alone).
  - The randomized controlled trial is the most expensive type of study. It takes a large amount of time to complete, needs a large number of subjects (150 in each arm to reduce the type II error), is prospective, provides the best level of evidence, and is the only type of trial to prove causality. Two factors can be chosen for study design: either hypothesis based (efficacy/noninferiority/equal) or outcome of interest based (efficacy or application in everyday practice).
- A **phase IV trial** is the postmarketing surveillance trial that ensures the drug is working appropriately with stated benefits.

RANDOMIZATION TECHNIQUES

There are a number of randomization techniques that can be applied: simple/coin toss, sequential digits, permuted blocks, stratified blocks, dynamic randomization, systemic nth; cluster, census, matching, restriction, quota, volunteer, cross over, split body, and factorial.

ELIGIBILITY CRITERIA

Eligibility criteria are the criteria to determine which patients to enroll in a study. These criteria serve four functions: scientific benefit, safety, logistic considerations, and regulatory considerations.

BIAS AND CONFOUNDING

To avoid bias or confounding, patients and/or investigators can be blinded, masked, adjusted for specific factors, randomized, the sample size can be increased, a placebo can be used, factors can be restricted or matched.

TRIAL SAFETY, REVIEW, AND ETHICS

- The **Data Safety Monitoring Board (DSMB)** is present for quality control, administrative capacities, and endpoint monitoring. The knowledge of any benefit or harm tends to accumulate over time and the DSMB can monitor the safety and efficacy of the trial impartially. It can also perform an interim analysis for safety and outcomes.
- The **Institutional Review Board (IRB)** was mandated in 1974 to be established locally for all government-funded research.
- Human subject rights have been established in two main doctrines. The **Belmont Report** (1979) outlines: respect for persons, justice, and beneficence. The **Nuremberg Code** (1949) outlines human subject rights to include: partici-

pation in the study be voluntary; the study be worthwhile; the study be unavailable by other means; the current state of knowledge is obtained from animals and cannot be obtained further from animal studies; there will be avoidance of unnecessary suffering; no deaths are to be expected; the risk is consistent with study benefits; appropriate precautions are taken for the study; the study is planned and reported by qualified persons; consent is ongoing; assessment of risks and benefits are ongoing; and the study is to be terminated if the risk of injury is imminent.

TYPES OF TRIALS

Trials can be broken up into the following types:

- **Prospective and retrospective** types. The prospective trials include the randomized controlled trials and the cohort trials. The retrospective trials include the case control and cross-sectional trials.
- Another way to look at trials is **randomized** trials versus **observational** trials. The observational trials are the cohort trials, the case control trials, the ecologic trials, case series, and the case report.
- **Umbrella trials:** umbrella studies are designed to test the impact of different drugs on different mutations in a single cancer type. The trial design can help to facilitate patient screening and accrual, and is quite suitable for trials examining low-prevalence diseases. The primary features of umbrella trials are as follows:
  - ○ The inclusion of multiple treatments and multiple biomarkers within the same protocol.
  - ○ A design that allows for randomized comparisons
  - ○ A design that can have flexible biomarker cohorts, and a design that can add/drop biomarker subgroups.
- **Basket trials:** basket studies are designed to test the effect of a single drug on a single mutation in a variety of cancer types. They provide a unique way of merging the traditional clinical trial design with rapidly evolving genomic data that facilitate the molecular classification of tumors. Basket trials can also screen multiple drugs across many cancer types. A basket design provides evidence for pairing a drug with a validated biomarker in a specific tumor.

TRIAL EVALUATION

- **Validity** is described in two fashions. External validity means the study results apply to the entire population. Internal validity means the study results apply specifically to those individuals studied.
- **Symmetry** means that all things between groups are similar.
- **Confounding** is the distortion of the effect of one risk factor by the presence of another
- **Bias** is any process or effect that produces results that differ systematically from the truth.
  - ○ Nondifferential bias means that the biases are the same in all study groups.
  - ○ Differential bias means that the biases are different between groups.
  - ○ There are a number of types of bias. Confounding bias is the systematic error where there is failure to account for the effect of one variable on others.

Ecological bias is the systematic error where the group average is applied to individuals. Measurement bias is when the measurement methods consistently differ between groups. Screening bias is when the disease is picked up earlier in the latent period by screening, but this screening does not affect the course of the disease. Reader bias is error of interpretation by reader inference. Sampling bias occurs when study design or execution produces errors in sampling. Zero time bias is when unintended differences exist from the beginning of the study, at enrollment.

SURVIVAL ANALYSIS

Survival analysis: there are two main types of survival analysis.
- The **time series analysis** is the parametric analysis.
- The **Kaplan–Meier** (KM) analysis is nonparametric and allows right censoring. KM analysis is used because all patients cannot start the study at the same time, there is withdrawal or loss to follow-up, patients die, and the study must end.
- The **log-rank test** compares the survival curves of two or more groups. It is a nonparametric test.
- The **Cox regression** proportional hazards test allows analysis of several risk factors affecting survival. It is a nonparametric test as well.
- The **Wilcoxon rank sum test** can be used when no censoring occurs.

CAUSALITY

Causality: there are a number of criteria for judging causality. There must be: validity of the study, strength in the study, plausibility (there is current biological support), consistency (the study can be replicated), a temporal relationship, a dose response, and alternative explanations have been ruled out.

WORLD HEALTH ORGANIZATION SCREENING GUIDELINES

World Health Organization (WHO) screening guidelines are in place to provide support for optimization of screening tests. These include: the disease history is understood; the disease is an important health problem; there is a latent stage to the disease; there is a test for the disease and it is sensitive; there is treatment for the condition; facilities are available for diagnosis and treatment; the cost to diagnosis is low and acceptable to the patient; there is an agreed policy on who to treat; and the screening is a continuous process.

PARAMETRIC VERSUS NONPARAMETRIC TESTING

- **Parametric** test means that there was random sampling, there is a normal distribution, the two populations are independent, there are quantitative variables (interval or ratio), and the variances of the normal distributions are equal. Parametric tests include the Z test (which tests the means of the populations), the one-sided t test, the t test, the paired t test, and the unpaired t test. Also included are the analysis of variance (ANOVA) (which measures differences between two or more groups), the analysis of covariance (ANCOVA) (which measures the difference between two or more groups and combines regression), the FANCOVA (which is the factorial ANOVA and allows comparison between two or more groups with each variable having at least two levels).

- **Nonparametric** tests are qualitative and measure associations. These tests include the binomial test, the sign test, the Wilcoxon test, the Mann–Whitney U test, the Fishers test, the chi-square test, the Kruskal–Wallis test, and the Friedman test.

TO QUANTIFY ASSOCIATIONS

To quantify associations, three types of tests are commonly used. The Pearson's test is for parametric data. The Spearman's rank correlation is for nonparametric data. Kendall's correlation is often used to document concordance.

MEANS OF MAGNITUDE

Means of magnitude tests refers to three ratios.
- The **odds ratio** (OR) is used in case control and logistic regression. It can be calculated as: ad/bc. It is the risk of an event happening. It can be reversed and 1/OR is the event free survival.
- The **relative risk** (RR) is used in cohort and randomized controlled trials. It can be calculated as: exposed/unexposed, or a/a + b/c/c + d. The RR is cumulative over the entire study period, or the patients' or samples' life span.
- The **hazard ratio** (HR) is the instantaneous risk. It is the time to an event.

UNIVARIATE VERSUS MULTIVARIATE TESTING

- The univariate test evaluates data on a single variable. It facilitates more advanced analysis and is the first step in looking at data analysis.
- The multivariate test looks at greater than one variable at a time. This test can reduce a large number of variables to a smaller number of factors for data modeling. It can select a subset of variables based on which original variables have the highest correlation with the principle of interest. It validates a scale by demonstrating that items load on the same factor.

Table 9.3 compares parametric tests to nonparametric tests for specific indications.

Table 9.3 Parametric Versus Nonparametric Tests				
Goal	Measurement (from Gaussian population)	Rank, score, or measurement (from non-Gaussian population)	Binomial (two possible outcomes)	Survival time
Describe one group	Mean, SD	Median, interquartile range	Proportion	Kaplan–Meier survival curve
Compare one group to a hypothetical value	One sample t test	Wilcoxon test	Chi-square or binomial test	

(continued)

Table 9.3 Parametric Versus Nonparametric Tests (*continued*)

Goal	Measurement (from Gaussian population)	Rank, score, or measurement (from non-Gaussian population)	Binomial (two possible outcomes)	Survival time
Compare two unpaired groups	Unpaired *t* test	Mann–Whitney test	Fisher's test (chi-square for large samples)	Log-rank test or Mantel–Haenszel
Compare two paired groups	Paired *t* test	Wilcoxon test	McNemar's test	Conditional proportional hazards regression
Compare three or more unmatched groups	One-way ANOVA	Kruskal–Wallis test	Chi-square test	Cox proportional hazard regression
Compare three or more matched groups	Repeated-measures ANOVA	Friedman test	Cochrane Q	Conditional proportional hazards regression
Quantify association between two variables	Pearson correlation	Spearman correlation	Contingency coefficients	
Predict value from another measured variable	Simple linear regression or nonlinear regression	Nonparametric regression	Simple logistic regression	Cox proportional hazard regression
Predict value from several measured or binomial variables	Multiple linear regression or multiple nonlinear regression		Multiple logistic regression	Cox proportional hazard regression

SURROGATE ENDPOINTS

Surrogate endpoints in tubo-ovarian cancer are now accepted outcomes. OS as a mandated primary endpoint has many problems including size, length, expense, and clinical relevance. OS remains the most objective clinical trial endpoint, but as survival increases and new cytotoxic, targeted, and immunologic therapies are emerging, OS may become less clinically relevant. A composite endpoint is integration of multiple endpoints into a single metric (OS, RR, toxicity, etc.). For trial endpoints: ineffective therapy is an RR less than 10%. Effective therapy has an RR of 25%. Safety/toxicity, duration of response, number of CR, should also be evaluated (1).

INCREMENTAL COST-EFFECTIVENESS RATIO

The incremental cost-effectiveness ratio (ICER) is a statistic used in cost-effectiveness analysis to summarize the cost-effectiveness of a health care intervention. It is defined by the difference in cost between two possible interventions, divided by the difference in their effect. It represents the average incremental cost associated with one additional unit of the measure of effect. The ICER can be estimated as: $ICER = (C_1 - C_0)/(E_1 - E_0)$ where C_1 and E_1 are the cost and effect in the intervention group and where C_0 and E_0 are the cost and effect in the control group. Costs are usually described in monetary units, while effects can be measured in terms of health status or another outcome of interest. A common application of the ICER is in cost-utility analysis, in which case the ICER is synonymous with the cost per quality-adjusted life year (QALY) gained.

REFERENCE

1. Herzog TJ, Alvarez RD, Secord A, et al. SGO guidance document for clinical trial designs in ovarian cancer: a changing paradigm. *Gynecol Oncol.* 2014;135:3-7.

SURVEILLANCE VISIT CHECKLIST: CHECKLIST FOR SURVEILLANCE OF GYNECOLOGIC MALIGNANCIES

Patient name _____

Visit date _____

Disease site and stage _____

Date of diagnosis/surgery _____

Date treatment completed _____

- Symptoms review and treatment side effects
- Pain (abdominal or pelvic, hip or back)
- Abdominal bloating
- Vaginal bleeding (also rectum, bladder)
- Weight loss
- Nausea and/or vomiting
- Cough or shortness of breath
- Lethargy/fatigue
- Swelling of abdomen or leg(s)
- Sexual dysfunction
- Neuropathy
- Fatigue

Physical examination
- General physical examination
- Lymph node assessment (axillary, supraclavicular, and inguinal)
- Pelvic examination (vulvar, vaginal speculum, bimanual, and rectovaginal exam)

Tumor markers _____

Disease status
- No evidence of disease
- Suspect recurrence
- Radiographic imaging _____
- Biopsy _____
- Refer to gynecologic oncologist _____

Routine health maintenance

Breast cancer screening
- Yearly clinical breast examination _____
- Mammogram _____
- Every 1 to 2 years starting with ages 40 to 49 years, then yearly
- Colon cancer screening

- Colonoscopy or flexible sigmoidoscopy _____
- Every 5 to 10 years beginning at the age of 50 years

Genetic screening
- Not indicated
- Recommended/completed _____

Menopausal assessment

Osteoporosis prevention

Calcium (1,200–1,500 mg) and vitamin D (800 IU)

Bone mineral density testing: begin at the age of 65 years or sooner if on gluco-corticoid therapy (World Health Organization [WHO] criteria can be used for reference)

Smoking cessation

Weight maintenance (exercise, diet)

GYNECOLOGIC ONCOLOGY REFERRAL PARAMETERS

ENDOMETRIAL CANCER

- Biopsy confirmed endometrial cancer of any grade

PELVIC MASS

- Presence of, or concern for, advanced disease
  - Omental caking (imaging-guided biopsy can be helpful).
  - Pleural effusion (cytology from thoracentesis can be helpful).
  - Ascites (cytology from paracentesis can be helpful).
  - Elevated tumor marker(s): American Congress of Obstetricians and Gynecologists (ACOG) recommends referral for a premenopausal CA-125 greater than 200 and postmenopausal CA-125 greater than 35.
- A clinically suspicious pelvic mass:
  - Simple and larger than 8 to 10 cm.
  - Larger than 4 cm and:

    Fixed

    Nodular

    Bilateral

    Excrescences

    Solid components
- Premenarchal girls with a pelvic mass
- Postmenopausal women with a suspicious mass or elevated tumor markers. Suspicious findings include a solid mass, a simple mass greater than 8 to 10 cm, or a complex mass. ACOG recommends referral for a CA-125 above 35
- Perimenopausal women with an ovarian mass, particularly when associated with an elevated CA-125
- Young patients who have a pelvic mass and elevated tumor markers (CA-125, alpha fetoprotein [AFP], human chorionic gonadotropin [hCG], lactate dehydrogenase [LDH])
- A suspicious pelvic mass found in a woman with a significant family or personal history of ovarian, breast, or other cancers (one or more first-degree relatives)

CERVICAL CANCER

- A biopsy (conization or directed) confirming invasive carcinoma.
- Women with suspicious cervical lesions should be biopsied before referral

VAGINAL CANCER

- Biopsy confirmed invasive vaginal cancer.
- Women with suspicious vaginal lesions should be biopsied before referral. Suspicious lesions include the following:
  - Nonhealing ulcers.
  - Bartholin's gland: persistent cysts in women over 40.
  - Exophytic lesions.

VULVAR CANCER

- Biopsy confirmed invasive vulvar cancer.
- Women with suspicious vulvar lesions should be biopsied before referral. These suspicious lesions include the following:
  - Nonhealing ulcers.
  - Areas of chronic pain or pruritus.
  - Areas of pigment change.
  - Grossly enlarged lesion.
- Depending on practitioner's comfort level:
  - Women with multifocal, complex, and/or recurrent vulvar intraepithelial neoplasia (VIN) 3.
  - Women with Paget's disease of the vulva.

GESTATIONAL TROPHOBLASTIC DISEASE

- Referral should occur after evacuation of the molar pregnancy if there is evidence of persistent trophoblastic disease/gestational trophoblastic disease (GTD):
  - GTD (low or high risk).
  - Choriocarcinoma.
  - Placental site trophoblastic tumor.
  - Epithelioid trophoblastic tumor.

If there is evidence of metastatic disease at initial diagnosis, referral should occur immediately.

PERFORMANCE STATUS SCALES

GYNECOLOGIC ONCOLOGY GROUP (GOG)/EASTERN COOPERATIVE ONCOLOGY GROUP (ECOG)/WHO/ZUBROD (1)

0: asymptomatic (fully active, able to carry on all pre-disease activities without restriction)

1: symptomatic but completely ambulatory (restricted in physically strenuous activity but ambulatory and able to carry out light or sedentary work)

2: symptomatic, less than 50% in bed during the day (ambulatory, capable of all self-care, unable to carry out any work activities. Up and about more than 50% of waking hours)

3: symptomatic, greater than 50% in bed, but not bedbound (capable of limited self-care, confined to bed or chair 50% or more of waking hours)

4: bedbound (completely disabled. Cannot perform any self-care. Totally confined to bed or chair)

5: dead

KARNOFSKY PERFORMANCE STATUS SCALE RATING CRITERIA (%)

100: normal; no complaints; no evidence of disease.

90: able to carry on normal activity; minor signs or symptoms of disease.

80: normal activity with effort; some signs or symptoms of disease.

70: cares for self; unable to carry on normal activity or do active work.

60: requires occasional assistance, but is able to care for most personal needs.

50: requires considerable assistance and frequent medical care. Unable to care for self; requires equivalent of institutional or hospital care; disease may be progressing rapidly.

40: disabled; requires special care and assistance.

30: severely disabled; hospital admission is indicated although death not imminent.

20: very sick; hospital admission necessary; active supportive treatment necessary.

10: moribund; fatal processes progressing rapidly.

0: dead.

ADVERSE EVENT GRADING

Common Terminology Criteria for Adverse Events (CTCAE): ctep.cancer.gov/reporting/ctc.html

RESPONSE EVALUATION CRITERIA IN SOLID TUMORS—INCLUDING IMMUNOLOGIC RECIST

Tumor response is measured via Response Evaluation Criteria in Solid Tumors (RECIST) guidelines version 1.1, 2009 (2). These are WHO criteria for measuring tumor response.

DEFINITION OF DISEASE

- Measurable disease—the presence of at least one measurable lesion. If the measurable disease is restricted to a solitary lesion, its neoplastic nature should be confirmed by cytology/histology.
- Measurable lesions—lesions that can be accurately measured in at least one dimension with longest diameter (LD) ≥20 mm using conventional techniques or ≥10 mm by spiral CT scan.
- Nonmeasurable lesions—all other lesions, including small lesions (LD <20 mm with conventional techniques or <10 mm with spiral CT scan), that is, bone lesions, leptomeningeal disease, ascites, pleural/pericardial effusion, inflammatory breast disease, lymphangitis cutis/pulmonis, cystic lesions, and also abdominal masses that are not confirmed and followed by imaging techniques.

- All measurements should be taken and recorded in metric notation, using a ruler or calipers. All baseline evaluations should be performed as closely as possible to the beginning of treatment and never more than 4 weeks before the beginning of treatment.
- The same method of assessment and the same technique should be used to characterize each identified and reported lesion at baseline and during follow-up.
- Clinical lesions are considered measurable only when they are superficial (e.g., skin nodules and palpable lymph nodes). For the case of skin lesions, documentation by color photography, including a ruler to estimate the size of the lesion, is recommended.

METHOD OF MEASUREMENT

- CT and MRI are currently the best available and reproducible methods to measure selected target lesions. Conventional CT and MRI should be performed with cuts of 10 mm or less in slice thickness. Spiral CT should be performed using a 5-mm contiguous reconstruction algorithm.
- Lesions on CXR are acceptable as measurable lesions when they are clearly defined and surrounded by aerated lung. However, CT is preferable.
- When the primary endpoint of the study is objective response evaluation, ultrasound (US) should not be used to measure tumor lesions.
- The utilization of endoscopy and laparoscopy for objective tumor evaluation is not widely accepted.
- Tumor markers alone cannot be used to assess response. If markers are initially above the upper normal limit, they must normalize for a patient to be considered in complete clinical response when all lesions have disappeared.

BASELINE DOCUMENTATION OF "TARGET" AND "NONTARGET" LESIONS

- All measurable lesions up to a maximum of two lesions per organ and five lesions in total, representative of all involved organs should be identified as target lesions and recorded and measured at baseline.
- Target lesions should be selected on the basis of their size (lesions with the LD) and their suitability for accurate repeated measurements (either by imaging techniques or clinically).
- A sum of the LD for all target lesions will be calculated and reported as the baseline sum LD. The baseline sum LD will be used as reference by which to characterize the objective tumor response.
- All other lesions (or sites of disease) should be identified as nontarget lesions and should also be recorded at baseline. Measurements of these lesions are not required, but the presence or absence of each should be noted throughout follow-up.

RESPONSE CRITERIA

- Target lesions
  - Complete response (CR) = Disappearance of all target lesions.
  - Partial response (PR) = 30% decrease in the sum of the LD of target lesions, taking as reference the baseline sum LD.

○ Progressive disease (PD) = 20% increase in the sum of the LD of target lesions, taking as reference the smallest sum LD recorded since the treatment started or the appearance of one or more new lesions.

○ Stable disease (SD) = Small changes that do not meet the preceding criteria.

- Nontarget lesions
  ○ CR = Disappearance of all nontarget lesions and normalization of tumor marker level.
  ○ SD = Persistence of one or more nontarget lesion(s) or/and maintenance of tumor marker level above the normal limits.
  ○ PD = Appearance of one or more new lesions and/or unequivocal progression of existing nontarget lesions.
  ○ SD = Small changes that do not meet these criteria.

BEST OVERALL RESPONSE

- Evaluation of "best overall response": the best overall response is the best response recorded from the start of the treatment until PD/recurrence (taking as reference for PD the smallest measurements recorded since the treatment started).
  ○ Patients with a global deterioration of health status requiring discontinuation of treatment without objective evidence of disease progression at that time should be classified as having "symptomatic deterioration." Documentation of objective progression after discontinuation of treatment should occur.
  ○ When it is difficult to distinguish between residual disease and normal tissue and evaluation of CR depends on this determination, it is recommended that the residual lesion be fine needle aspirated/biopsied to confirm status.

CONFIRMATION OF RESPONSE

- To achieve PR or CR status, changes in tumor measurements must be confirmed by repeat assessments that should be performed at least 4 weeks after the criteria for response are first met.
- The goal of confirmation of objective response is to avoid overstating the observed response rate.
- For SD, follow-up measurements must have met SD criteria at least once after study entry with a minimal interval, usually not less than 6 to 8 weeks.

DURATION OF OVERALL RESPONSE

The duration of overall response is measured from the time criteria are met for CR or PR (whichever status is recorded first) until the first date that PD is objectively documented, taking as reference for PD the smallest measurements recorded since the treatment started.

DURATION OF STABLE DISEASE

- SD is measured from the start of the treatment until the criteria for disease progression are met, taking as reference the smallest measurements recorded since the treatment started.
- The clinical relevance of the duration of SD varies for different tumor types and grades. Therefore, it is highly recommended that the protocol specify the

minimal time interval required between two measurements for determination of SD. This time interval should take into account the expected clinical benefit that such a status may bring to the population under study.

IMMUNE RESPONSE RECIST CRITERIA

- Measurement of irRC tumor burden: tumor burden is measured by combining "index" lesions with new lesions. With irRC, new lesions are purely a change in overall tumor burden. The irRC retained the bidirectional measurement of lesions that had originally been set for the WHO/RECIST 1.1 Criteria.
- Assessment of immune-related response. In the irRC, an immune-related complete response (irCR) is the disappearance of all lesions, measured or unmeasured, and the appearance of no new lesions; an immune-related partial response (irPR) is a 50% drop in tumor burden from baseline; and immune-related progressive disease (irPD) is a 25% increase in tumor burden from the lowest level recorded. All else is considered immune-related stable disease (irSD) (Table 9.4) (3).

COMMON CHEMOTHERAPY PROTOCOLS AND DOSING

Table 9.4 Common Chemotherapy Protocols	
IV paclitaxel/ carboplatin Cycle length 21 d	Paclitaxel 175 mg/m² IV, Day 1 Carboplatin AUC 5–6 IV, Day 1 Or Paclitaxel 80 mg/m², Days 1, 8, and 15 Carboplatin AUC 5–6 IV, Day 1 Or Paclitaxel 80 mg/m² IV. Days 1, 8, and 15 Carboplatin target (AUC of 2) IV. Days 1, 8, and 15
IV paclitaxel, IP cisplatin, paclitaxel Cycle length 21 d	IV paclitaxel (135 mg/m² over 24 hr) on Day 1 IP cisplatin (100 mg/m² in a liter of normal saline) on Day 2 IP paclitaxel (60 mg/m²) on Day 8 Alternative outpatient schedule: IV paclitaxel (175 mg/m² over 3 hr) on Day 1 followed by IP cisplatin (100 mg/m² in a liter of normal saline) on Day 1 IP paclitaxel (60 mg/m²) on Day 8 Dose reduction of IP cisplatin can be to 75 mg/m²
Carboplatin desensitization	Carboplatin target (AUC of _____/dose) (= _____ mg) to be infused as four separate infusions (dilutions): Dose 1—1:1,000 dilution IVPB over 60 min. Dose 2—1:100 dilution IVPB over 60 min. Dose 3—1:10 dilution IVPB over 60 min. Dose 4—remaining carboplatin IV over 60 min.
Carboplatin, liposomal doxorubicin Cycle length 28 d	Doxorubicin, liposomal 30 mg/ m² IV Carboplatin AUC of 5 IV

(continued)

Table 9.4 Common Chemotherapy Protocols (continued)	
Carboplatin, docetaxel Cycle length 21 d	Docetaxel 100 mg/m² IV Day 1 Carboplatin AUC 5–6 IV Day 1
Carboplatin, gemcitabine Cycle length 21 d	Carboplatin AUC 5 IV, Day 1 Gemcitabine 1,000 mg/m² IV Days 1, 8
Doxorubicin, liposomal Cycle length: 28 d	Doxorubicin, liposomal 40 mg/ m² IV
Cisplatin with XRT Cycle length 7 d	Cisplatin 40 mg/ m² IV (maximum of 70 mg/dose)
Cisplatin, paclitaxel, bevacizumab Cycle length 21 d	Cisplatin 50 mg/m² IV Paclitaxel 175 mg/m² IV Bevacizumab 15 mg/Kg IV
Cisplatin, topotecan Cycle length 21 d	Topotecan 0.75 mg/m² IV. Give on Days 1, 2, and 3 of each cycle. Cisplatin 50 mg/m² IV. Give on Day 1 of each cycle.
Topotecan	Topotecan 1.25–1.5 mg/m ² IV over 30 min on Days 1–5 of each cycle Cycle length 21 d Or Topotecan 4 mg/m² IV Days 1, 8, 15 (cycle length 28 d)
Gemcitabine Cycle length 21 d	Gemcitabine 1,000 mg/m² IV Days 1, 8
Olaparib	400 mg PO BID continuously may be used as monotherapy for advanced ovarian cancer with deleterious or suspected deleterious germline *BRCA* mutations in patients who have been treated with three or more prior lines of chemotherapy
Methotrexate Cycle length 14 d	Methotrexate 0.4 mg/kg/d IV or IM Days 1–5 Or Methotrexate 1 mg/kg IM Days 1, 3, 5, and 7 plus folinic acid 15 mg PO 30 hr after each MTX dose on Days 2, 4, 6, and 8
Actinomycin D Cycle length 14 d	Actinomycin D 12 mcg/kg IV Days 1–5 Or Actinomycin D 1.25 mg/m² IV

(continued)

Table 9.4 Common Chemotherapy Protocols (continued)

EMACO Cycle length 14 d	Etoposide 100 mg/m² IV over Days 1 and 2 of each cycle Methotrexate 100 mg/m² IV push Day 1 of each cycle Methotrexate 200 mg/m² IV by continuous infusion over 12 hr. Give immediately after methotrexate injection on Day 1 of cycle Leucovorin 5 mg tabs—three tablets PO every 12 hr for 2 d, starting 24 hr after beginning of methotrexate Days 1 and 2 Actinomycin D 0.5 mg IV push Days 1 and 2 of each cycle Day 8 Vincristine 1 mg/m² (maximum of 2 mg/dose) IV Day 8 of each cycle Cyclophosphamide 600 mg/m² IV Day 8 of each cycle
BEP bleomycin, etoposide, cisplatin Cycle length: 21 d	Bleomycin: 15–20 units/m² IV (maximum 30 units), Days 1, 8, 15 Etoposide: 100 mg/m² IV, Days 1–5 Cisplatin: 20 mg/m² IV, Days 1–5
VPB vinblastine, cisplatin, bleomycin, Cycle length 21 d	Vinblastine: 0.15 mg/kg on Days 1 and 2 Bleomycin: 15 units/m²/wk × 5; then on Day 1 of course 4 Cisplatin: 100 mg/m² on Day 1
VAC vincristine, actinomycin, cyclophosphamide Cycle length 28 d	Vincristine: 1–1.5 mg/m² on Day 1 Actinomycin D: 0.5 mg/d × 5 d Cyclophosphamide: 150 mg/m²/d
POMB-ACE cisplatin, vincristine, methotrexate, bleomycin actinomycin, cyclophosphamide, etoposide	POMB Day 1: vincristine 1 mg/m² IV; methotrexate 300 mg/m² 12-hr infusion Day 2: bleomycin 15 mg IV 24-hr infusion; folinic acid rescue to start 24 hr after methotrexate 15 mg every 12 hr for 4 doses Day 3: bleomycin 15 mg IV 24-hr infusion Day 4: cisplatin 120 mg/m² IV 12-hr infusion with IVF and 3 g magnesium ACE Days 1–5: etoposide 100 mg/m²/d Day 3–5: actinomycin D 0.5 mg IV Day 5: cyclophosphamide 500 mg/m² IV

(continued)

Table 9.4 Common Chemotherapy Protocols (continued)	
OMB Vincristine, methotrexate, bleomycin * Initiate with two courses of POMB followed by ACE. POMB alternates with ACE until biochemical remission, then alternate ACE with OMB. Interval between courses 9 and 11 d.	Day 1: vincristine 1 mg/m² IV; methotrexate 300 mg/m² IV 12-hr infusion Day 2: bleomycin 12 mg IV 24-hr infusion; folinic acid rescue to start 24 hr after start of methotrexate 15 mg every 12 hr IV for four doses Day 3: bleomycin 15 mg IV 24-hr infusion

AUC, area under the curve; BID, twice a day; EMACO, etoposide, methotrexate, actinomycin D, cyclophosphamide, and vincristine; IP, intraperitoneal; MTX, methotrexate; PO, orally; POMB-ACE, cisplatin, vincristine, methotrexate, bleomycin, actinomycin D, cyclophosphamide, etoposide; XRT, radiation therapy.

USEFUL FORMULAS

- The Cockcroft–Gault equation: this equation provides an estimate of creatinine clearance (CrCl) based on age, weight, sex, and serum creatinine without the need for a 24-hour urine collection.

$$CrCl = \frac{[(140 - Age) \times Weight(kg)] \times 0.85}{[0.72 \times SerumCr(mg/dL)]}$$

- The Calvert formula calculates the carboplatin dosing using the glomerular filtration rate (GFR) from the Crockcroft–Gault equation: dose (mg) = Target area under the curve (AUC) × (GFR + 25). The AUC is usually set from 5 to 7 for untreated patients and 4 to 6 for previously treated patients.
- The Jelliffe formula is good for adult patients with normal muscle mass not on hemodialysis. This calculation is not applicable to patients less than 18 years old, serum creatinine less than 0.6 mg/dL, weight less than 35 or more than 120 kg, unstable creatinine, muscle mass less than 70% or more than 130% of normal.

$$CrCl\ (female) = 0.9\ \{[98 - 0.8 \times (A-20)]/SCr\ (mg/dL)\}$$

where A = age in years; CrCl = creatinine clearance in mL/min/1.73 m². The patient's body surface area (BSA) must be determined. The CrCl value obtained by the equation must be multiplied by (BSA/1.73) to obtain the patient's CrCl in absolute terms (i.e., mL/min). Weight is in kilogram and height is in centimeter.

- BSA: the most widely used formula is the Du Bois formula:

$$BSA\ (m^2) = 0.007184 \times W^{0.425}\,kg \times H^{0.725}\,cm$$

A commonly used and simple calculation is the Mosteller formula:

$$BSA = Square\ root\ of\ (W \times H/3,600) = 0.016667 \times W0.5 \times H0.5$$

- The fractional excretion of sodium can help determine prerenal, intrinsic, or postrenal disease:
$$FENa = (UNa \times SCr)/(SNa \times UCr) \times 100$$
Below 1% indicates prerenal disease.
A value above 2% or 3% indicates acute tubular necrosis or other kidney damage.
- Serum osmolality = $2[Na] + [K] + BUN/2.8 + Glu/18$
Normal is 280 to 295 mOsm/kg
- Fe deficit = $1,000 + (15-Hgb) \times (kg\ weight)$
Normal is 2 g
- A-a Gradient = $PAO_2 - PaO_2$. The $PAO_2 = (FiO_2 \times (760 - 47)) - (PaCO_2/0.8)$
Normal is 5–10 mmHg; or less than current (age in years/4) + 4
- Corrected serum Na: measured sodium + 0.016 × (serum glucose in mg/dL – 100)

REFERENCES

1. Oken MM, Creech RH, Tormey DC. Toxicity and response criteria of the Eastern Cooperative Oncology Group. *Am J Clin Oncol.* 1982;5(6):649-655.
2. Eisenhauer EA, Therasse P, Bogaerts J. New response evaluation criteria in solid tumours: revised RECIST guideline (version 1.1). *Eur J Cancer.* 2009;45(2):228-247.
3. Wolchok JD, Hoos A, O'Day S, et al. Guidelines for the evaluation of immune therapy activity in solid tumors: immune-related response criteria. *Clin Cancer Res.* 2009;15(23): 7412-7420.

Abbreviations

5-FU	5-fluorouracil
A/C	assist-control
AABB	American Association of Blood Banks
ABC	ATP binding cassette
ABG	arterial blood gas
ACE	angiotensin-converting enzyme
ACOG	American Congress of Obstetricians and Gynecologists
ACTION	Adjuvant Chemotherapy in Ovarian Neoplasms
ADH	antidiuretic hormone
ADLs	activities of daily living
AEs	adverse events
AFFIRM	Atrial Fibrillation Follow-up Investigation of Rhythm Management
AFP	alpha fetoprotein
AGC	atypical glandular cells
AGUS	abnormal glandular cells of unknown significance
AHM	anti-Müllerian hormone
AIS	adenocarcinoma in situ
AJCC	American Joint Committee on Cancer
ALI	acute lung injury
ALK	anaplastic lymphoma kinase
ALTS	ASCUS/LSIL Triage Study
AML	acute myeloid leukemia
ANC	absolute neutrophil count
ANCOVA	analysis of covariance
ANOVA	analysis of variance
AP/PA	anterior-posterior/posterior-anterior
APD	abdominal peritoneal disease
aPTT	activated partial thromboplastin time
ARB	angiotensin receptor blockers
ARDS	acute respiratory distress syndrome
AS	adenosarcoma
ASA score	American Society of Anesthesiologists Score
ASA	acetylsalicylic acid
ASC-H	atypical squamous cells, cannot exclude high grade
ASC-US	atypical squamous cells of undetermined significance
ASCCP	American Society of Coloscopy and Cervical Pathology
ASD	atrial septal defect

ASIS	anterior superior iliac spine
AST	aspartate transaminase
ATHENA	Addressing the Need for Advanced HPV Diagnostics
ATP	adenosine triphosphate
AUC	area under the curve
AV	atrioventricular block
BED	biologically equivalent dose
BEE	basal energy expenditure
BEP	bleomycin, etoposide, cisplatin
BER	base-excision repair
BID	twice a day
BiPAP	bilevel positive airway pressure
bi-shRNAi	bifunctional short hairpin RNAi
BMI	body mass index
BMP	basic metabolic panel
BNP	brain natriuretic peptide
BOOST	Bevacizumab Ovarian Optimal Standard Treatment
BP	blood pressure
BRRS	Bannayan-Riley-Ruvaicaba syndrome
BSA	body surface area
BSE	bovine spongiform encephalopathy
BSO	bilateral salpingo-oophorectomy; buthionine sulfoximine
BUN	blood urea nitrogen
CABG	coronary artery bypass graft
CAH	complex atypical hyperplasia
CAP	cisplatin, doxorubicin, cyclophosphamide
CBC	complete blood count
CBI	continuous bladder irrigation
CC	clear cell
CCC	clear cell carcinoma
CCI	Charlson Comorbidity Index
CCR	complete clinical response
CCRT	continuous renal replacement therapies
CCU	cardiac care unit
CD	cisplatin, doxorubicin
CDP	cisplatin, doxorubicin, paclitaxel
CEA	carcinoembryonic antigen
CHAMOCA	cyclophosphamide, hydroxyurea, actinomycin D, methotrexate, vincristine, leucovorin, doxorubicin
CHF	congestive heart failure
CI	confidence interval
CIN	cervical intraepithelial neoplasia
CIR	cumulative incidence rate
CIRS	Cumulative illness index rating scale
CIS	carcinoma in situ
CIWA	Clinical Institute Withdrawal Assessment
CK	creatine kinase

CKC	cold knife conization
CKMB	creatine kinase-MB
CLT	central limit theory
CML	chronic myeloid leukemia
CMP	comprehensive metabolic panel
CMV	continuous mandatory ventilation
CNS	central nervous system
CO	cardiac output
COPD	chronic obstructive pulmonary disease
CPAP	continuous positive airway pressure
CPH-i	Copenhagen Index
CPK	creatine phosphokinase
CPR	complete pathological response
CR	complete response
CRC	colorectal cancer
CrCl	creatinine clearance
CS	carcinosarcoma
CT	computed tomography
CTC	common toxicity criteria
CTCAE	Common Terminology Criteria for Adverse Events
CTLA-4	cytotoxic T-lymphocyte-associated antigen 4
CTV	clinical target volume
CUSA	Cavitron ultrasonic surgical aspiration
CV	cardiovascular
CVA	costovertebral angle
CVA	cerebrovascular accident
CVP	central venous pressure
CXR	chest x-ray
D&C	dilation and curettage
DBP	diastolic blood pressure
dDAVP	desmopressin
DES	diethylstilbestrol
DFS	disease-free survival
DHEA	dehydroepiandrosterone
DHEAS	dehydroepiandrosterone sulfate
DIC	disseminated intravascular coagulation
DKA	diabetic ketoacidosis
DLL4	delta-like ligand-4
DLT	dose-limiting toxicity
DM	diabetes mellitus
DMSO	dimethyl sulfoxide
DNR	do not resuscitate
DOAC	direct oral anticoagulants
DOI	depth of invasion
DP	disease progression
DS	double-stranded
DSM	Data Safety Monitoring Board

DSS	disease-specific survival
DTIC	dacarbazine
DVT	deep vein thrombosis
EBL	estimated blood loss
EBXRT	external beam radiation therapy
ECC	endocervical curettage
ECHO	echocardiogram
ECOG	European Cooperative Oncology Group
EF	ejection fraction
EFS	event free survival
EGD	esophagogastroduodenoscopy
EGFR	epidermal growth factor receptor
EIA	enzyme immunoassay
EIN	endometrial intraepithelial neoplasia
EKG	electrocardiogram
ELISA	enzyme-linked immunosorbent assay
ELISPOT	enzyme-linked immunospot assay
EMACO	etoposide, methotrexate, actinomycin D, cyclophosphamide, and vincristine
EMA-CO	etoposide, methotrexate, actinomycin D–cyclophosphamide, and vincristine
EMA-EP	etoposide, methotrexate, actinomycin D–etoposide, cisplatin
EMB	endometrial biopsy
EOC	epithelial ovarian cancer
EORTC	European Organisation for Research and Treatment of Cancer
EP	etoposide, cisplatin
ER	estrogen receptor
ERT	estrogen replacement therapy
ESRD	end-stage renal disease
ESS	endometrial stromal sarcomas
ETT	epithelioid trophoblastic tumor
EUA	examination under anesthesia
EUA	exam under anesthesia
FANCOVA	factorial analysis of variance
FDG	fludeoxyglucose
FEV	forced expiratory volume
FFP	fresh frozen plasma
FGFR	fibroblast growth factor receptor
FIGO	International Federation of Gynecology and Obstetrics
FISH	fluorescence in situ hybridization
FN	false negative
FNA	fine needle aspiration
FP	false positive
FRC	functional residual capacity
FSH	follicle-stimulating hormone
G	grade
GCSF	granulocyte colony stimulating factor

GCTs	germ cell tumors
GFR	glomerular filtration rate
GI	gastrointestinal
GIS	gastrointestinal anastomosis
GIST	gastrointestinal stromal tumor
GMC	gracilis myocutaneous flap
GMCSF	granulocyte-macrophage colony-stimulating factor
GnRH	gonadotropin-releasing hormone
GOG	Gynecologic Oncology Group
GSH	glutathione
GST	glutathione S-transferase
GTD	gestational trophoblastic disease
GTN	gestational trophoblastic neoplasia
G-tube	gastrostomy tube
GTV	gross tumor volume
GU	genitourinary
H&E	hematoxylin and eosin stain
HAART	highly active antiretroviral therapy
HBOC	hereditary breast and ovarian cancer
hCG	human chorionic gonadotropin
Hct	hematocrit
HDR	high-dose rate
HER2	human epidermal growth factor receptor 2.
HERS	HIV Epidemiology Research Study
Hg	hemoglobin
HGFR	hepatocyte growth factor receptor
HGSTOC	high grade serous tubo-ovarian cancer
HIPEC	hyperthermic intraperitoneal chemotherapy
HIR	high intermediate risk
HLA	human leukocyte antigen
HNPCC	hereditary nonpolyposis colon cancer
HPF	high-power field
HPL	human placental lactogen
HPV	human papillomavirus
HR	hazard ratio
HRT	hormone replacement therapy
HSIL	high-grade squamous intraepithelial lesion
HSV	herpes simplex virus
HTN	hypertension
HUS	hemolytic uremic syndrome
IBD	inflammatory bowel disease
ICC	invasive cervical cancer
ICE	ifosfamide, cisplatin, etoposide
ICER	incremental cost-effectiveness ratio
ICG	indocyanine green
ICON	International Collaborative Ovarian Neoplasm Trial
ICU	intensive care unit

IDS	interval debulking surgery
IHC	immunohistochemistry
IHD	ischemic heart disease
IM	intramuscular
IMA	inferior mesenteric artery
IMV	intermittent mandatory ventilation
IMRT	intensity-modulated radiation therapy
INH	isoniazid
INR	international normalized ratio
IOXRT	intraoperative radiation therapy
IP	intraperitoneal
IQR	interquartile range
IRB	Institutional Review Board
irCR	immune-related complete response
irPD	immune-related progressive disease
irPR	immune-related partial response
irRC	immune-related response criteria
irSD	immune-related stable disease
ISSVD	International Society for the Study of Vulvar Diseases
IT	immature teratomas
IUD	intrauterine device
IV	intravenous
IVC	inferior vena cava
IVF	intravenous fluid
IVP	intravenous pyelography
JGOG	Japanese Gynecologic Oncology Group
JP	Jackson-Pratt
JVD	jugular venous distension
JVP	jugular venous pressure
KERMA	kinetic energy related to mass
KUB	kidneys, ureters, bladder
LAST	lower anogenital squamous terminology
LBO	large bowel obstruction
LD	longest diameter
LDH	lactate dehydrogenase
LDR	low-dose rate
LEEP	loop electrocautery excision procedure
LFT	liver function test
LLO	*listerolysin O*
LMP	low-malignant potential
LMS	leiomyosarcoma
LMW	low molecular weight
LMWH	low-molecular weight heparin
LN	lymph node
LND	lymph node dissection
LPF	low-power field
LSIL	low-grade squamous intraepithelial lesion

LV	left ventricular
LVAD	left ventricular assist device
LVEF	left ventricular ejection fraction
LVSI	lymphovascular space invasion
MAC	methotrexate, actinomycin D, cyclophosphamide
MASCC	Multinational Association for Supportive Care in Cancer
MAP	mean arterial pressure
MBP	mechanical bowel preparation
MCT	mature cystic teratoma
MD	minimal disease
MDR	multidrug resistance
MDS	myelodysplastic syndrome
METS	metabolic equivalents
MI	morphology index
MI	myocardial infarction
MIS	minimally invasive surgery
MMMTs	mixed Müllerian mesodermal tumors
MMR	measles, mumps, rubella
MODS	multiple organ dysfunction syndrome
MPA	medroxyprogesterone acetate
MPV	mitral valve prolapse
MRI	magnetic resonance imaging
MS	multiple sclerosis
MTD	maximum tolerated dose
MTHFR	methylenetetrahydrofolate reductase
MTIC	monomethyl triazeno imidazole carboxamide
MTP	massive transfusion protocol
MTX	methotrexate
MUDPILES	Methanol, Uremia (chronic renal failure), Diabetic ketoacidosis, Propylene glycol, I (infection, iron, isoniazid, inborn errors in metabolism), Lactic acidosis, Ethylene glycol, Salicylates
MUGA	multigated acquisition
MUPIT	Martinez universal perineal interstitial template
MVP	mitral valve prolapse
NCCN	National Comprehensive Cancer Network
NCI	National Cancer Institute
NCIC	National Cancer Institute of Canada
NFT	no further treatment
NGT	nasogastric tube
NICD	notch intracellular domain
NIF	negative inspiratory force
NK	natural killer
NMBA	neuromuscular blocking agent
NNRTI	non-nucleoside reverse transcriptase inhibitor
NOS	not otherwise specified
NPO	nothing by mouth

NPV	negative predictive value
NRTI	nucleotide reverse transcriptase inhibitor
NS	not statistically significant
NSAID	nonsteroidal anti-inflammatory drug
NTG	nitroglycerin
O/E	observed-to-expected ratio
OCP	oral contraceptive pills
OR	odds ratio
OR	operating room
OR	overall response
ORR	overall response rate
OS	overall survival
OTC	over-the-counter
PA-LND	para-aortic lymph node dissection
PA	pulmonary artery
PA	para-aortic
PA-XRT	para-aortic radiation therapy
PAC	premature atrial contraction
PALN	para-aortic lymph node
PAOP	pulmonary artery occlusion pressure
PAP	Papanicolaou
PAP Diastolic	diastolic pulmonary arterial pressure
PAP mean	mean pulmonary arterial pressure
PAP Systolic	systolic pulmonary arterial pressure
PARP	poly ADP ribose polymerase
PAWP	pulmonary artery wedge pressure
PCC	prothrombin complex concentrate
PCN	percutaneous nephrostomy
PCP	*pneumocystispneumonia*
PCR	polymerase chain reaction
PCWP	pulmonary capillary wedge pressure
PD	progressive disease
PDA	patent ductus arteriosus
PDGFR	platelet-derived growth factor receptor
PDS	primary debulking surgery
PE	photoelectric
PE	pulmonary embolus
PEEP	positive end-expiratory pressure
PEF	peak expiratory flow
PEG	polyethylene glycol
PET	positron emission tomography
PFI	progression free interval
PFS	progression-free survival
PFT	pulmonary function test
PFTC	primary fallopian tube cancer
PHTS	PTEN hamartoma tumor syndrome
PI	protease inhibitor

PI3K	phosphoinositide-3 kinase
PICC	peripheral centrally inserted catheter
PJ	Peutz–Jeghers syndrome
PLAP	placental alkaline phosphatase
PLD	pegylated liposomal doxorubicin
P-LND	pelvic lymph node dissection
PLUMSEEDS	Paraldehyde, Lactate, Uremia, Methanol, Salicylates, Ethylene glycol, Ethanol, Diabetic ketoacidosis, Starvation
PMPB	postmenopausal bleeding
PO	orally
POD	postoperative day
POISE	Perioperative Ischemic Evaluation Study
POMB-ACE	cisplatin, vincristine, methotrexate, bleomycin, actinomycin D, cyclophosphamide, etoposide
PPC	primary peritoneal cancer
PPE	palmar plantar erythema
P PA-LND	pelvic and para-aortic lymphadenectomy
PPV	positive predictive value
PR	partial response
PRBC	packed red blood cells
PS	pressure supported
PSTT	placental site trophoblastic tumor
PT	prothrombin time
PTCA	percutaneous transluminal coronary angioplasty
PTSD	posttraumatic stress disorder
PTT	partial thromboplastin time
PTU	propylthiouracil
PTV	planning target volume
PVB	cisplatin, vinblastine, bleomycin
PVC	premature ventricular contractions
PVI-FU	prolonged venous infusion of 5-FU
PVR	post void residual
QALY	quality-adjusted life year
QID	four times a day
QOL	quality of life
RA	room air
RAM	rectus abdominis myocutaneous flap
RBBB	right bundle branch block
RBC	red blood cells
RBE	relative biologic effectiveness
RECIST	response evaluation criteria in solid tumors
RFS	recurrence-free survival
rhGM-CSF	recombinant human granulocyte macrophage-colony stimulating factor
RM	restricted means
RMI	risk of malignancy index
RMST	restricted mean survival time

ROCA	risk of ovarian cancer algorithm
ROMA	risk of ovarian malignancy algorithm
RR	relative risk
RR	response rate
RRBSO	risk-reducing bilateral salpingo-oophorectomy
RRSO	risk reducing salpingo-oophorectomy
RTK	receptor tyrosine kinase
RTOG	Radiation Therapy Oncology Group
SBE	subacute bacterial endocarditis
SBO	small bowel obstruction
SBP	systolic blood pressure
SC	subcutaneous
SCD	sequential compression device
SCIA	superficial circumflex iliac artery
SD	stable disease; standard deviation
SE	standard error
SEER	Surveillance Epidemiology and End Results
SEPA	superficial external pudendal artery
SG	specific gravity
SIADH	syndrome of inappropriate antidiuretic hormone secretion
SIL	squamous intraepithelial lesion
SIMV	synchronized intermittent mandatory ventilation
SIRS	systemic inflammatory response syndrome
SIS	saline infusion sonography
SCJ	squamnocolumnar junction
SL	sublingual
SLL	second-look laparotomy
SLN	sentinel lymph node
SLND	sentinel lymph node dissection
SMA	superior mesenteric artery
SOB	shortness of breath
SOCQER	Surgery in Ovarian Cancer Quality of life Evaluation Research study
SOFA	sequential organ failure assessment
SPECT	single-photon emission CT
SSD	source to skin distance
SSI	surgical site infection
STDs	sexually transmitted diseases
STEMI	ST elevation myocardial infarction
STIC	serous tubal intraepithelial carcinoma
STSG	split thickness skin grafts
SVR	systemic vascular resistance
SVT	superficial vein thrombosis
TA	thoracoabdominal
TACO	transfusion-associated circulatory overload
TAH	total abdominal hysterectomy

TAP	paclitaxel, doxorubicin, cisplatin
TB	tuberculosis
TBW	total body water
TCA	trichloroacetic acid; tricyclic antidepressant
TE	thromboembolism
TG	triglycerides
TGF	transforming growth factors
TH-BSO	total hysterectomy bilateral salpingo-oophorectomy
TIA	transient ischemic attacks
TID	three times a day
TN	true negative
TNM	tumor, node, metastasis
TP	true positive
TPN	total parenteral nutrition
TRALI	transfusion-related acute lung injury
TSH	thyroid-stimulating hormone
TVUS	transvaginal ultrasound
UA	urinalysis
UAD	upper abdominal disease
UFH	unfractionated heparin
UNC	ureteroneocystostomy
US	ultrasound
USO	unilateral salpingo-oophorectomy
UTI	urinary tract infection
UU	ureteroureterostomy
UUS	undifferentiated uterine sarcoma
V/Q	ventilation/perfusion
VAC	vincristine, doxorubicin, cyclophosphamide
VAIN	vaginal intraepithelial neoplasia
VAP	ventilator acquired pneumonia
VEGF	vascular endothelial growth factors
VIN	vulvar intraepithelial neoplasia
VIP	etoposide, ifosfamide, cisplatin
VPB	vinblastine, cisplatin, bleomycin
VSD	ventricular septal defect
VTE	venous thromboembolism
WAR	whole abdominal radiotherapy
WB-XRT	whole brain radiation therapy
WBC	white blood cell
WHO	World Health Organization
WIHS	Women's Interagency HIV Study
WP	whole pelvic
WP-XRT	whole pelvic radiation therapy
XRT	radiation therapy
Y	year
YS	year survival

Index